Statistics for Biotechnology Process Development

Statistics for Biotechnology Process Development

Edited by

Todd Coffey
Harry Yang

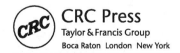

CRC Press
Taylor & Francis Group
Boca Raton London New York

CRC Press is an imprint of the
Taylor & Francis Group, an **informa** business

A CHAPMAN & HALL BOOK

Chapter 5 © David Lansky

CRC Press
Taylor & Francis Group
6000 Broken Sound Parkway NW, Suite 300
Boca Raton, FL 33487-2742

© 2018 by Taylor & Francis Group, LLC
CRC Press is an imprint of Taylor & Francis Group, an Informa business

No claim to original U.S. Government works

International Standard Book Number-13: 978-1-4987-2140-0 (Hardback)

Library of Congress Cataloging-in-Publication Data

Names: Coffey, Todd, editor.
Title: Statistics for biotechnology process development / edited by Todd Coffey, Harry Yang.
Description: Boca Raton, Florida : CRC Press, [2018] | Includes bibliographical references and index.
Identifiers: LCCN 2018002841| ISBN 9781498721400 (hardback : alk. paper) | ISBN 9781315120034 (ebook) | ISBN 9781498721417 (web pdf) | ISBN 9781351646345 (epub) | ISBN 9781351636803 (mobi/kindle)
Subjects: LCSH: Biotechnology--Data processing.
Classification: LCC TP248.25.A96 S73 2018 | DDC 660.60285--dc23
LC record available at https://lccn.loc.gov/2018002841

**Visit the Taylor & Francis Web site at
http://www.taylorandfrancis.com**

**and the CRC Press Web site at
http://www.crcpress.com**

Contents

Preface

Over the past 20 years, the need for statistical thinking in chemistry, manufacturing, and controls (CMC) for the biotechnology industry has greatly increased. With the release of the FDA's 2011 Guidance for Industry on Process Validation, recognition of the value of statistical expertise has accelerated, and further increased demand seems likely. Unfortunately, there are not enough statisticians fluent in statistical methods and scientific approaches to process and analytical development, manufacturing, formulation, and quality control. Thus, many scientists and engineers—especially those at emerging companies—are left without strategic or day-to-day guidance on important statistical issues.

Although other books on statistical methods for CMC have been written, this is the first to be geared directly toward scientists and engineers. With this book it is our intention to bring statistical thinking to you. When compared with other books, this one is lighter on formulas and heavier on case studies and examples. While statisticians will benefit from these eleven chapters, we have purposely written this book for an audience of practitioners by removing or explaining much of the statistical lingo. It is our desire that this book be referred to often when needs arise.

The themes selected for this book include the prominent considerations and methods used throughout bioprocess; formulation; and analytical development, manufacturing, and QC. We begin in Chapter 1 with a wide-range introduction to statistics that provides a foundation for the rest of the book. Statistical intervals, p-values, hypothesis testing, sample size and power, and distributions and outliers are among the topics in this chapter. Chapters 2 and 3 discuss how to design experiments using both classical and modern approaches to design of experiments (DOE), the former in the framework of process development and the latter for formulation development. Analytical and bioassay method development and validation are discussed in Chapters 4 and 5. We provide statistical guidance for developing these critical methods and then validating them. Setting specifications requires statistical input, and we consider this topic in Chapter 6. Next, in Chapter 7, we provide a comprehensive review of stability studies, with many case studies implemented using the JMP software. Chapter 8 treats a subject—continued process verification (CPV)—that is currently of great interest; in this chapter, we review the methods that enable a successful CPV program. The last three chapters include statistical methods that have been around for a long time but may be less recognized by CMC scientists and engineers. Chapter 9 describes pattern-finding techniques using multivariate analysis that are useful in understanding and troubleshooting bioprocesses. Chapter 10 reviews approaches to evaluate method robustness, and Chapter 11 closes the book with a discussion of various types of sampling. The references at the end of each chapter provide other options for gaining further knowledge.

The contributors for this book were selected for their expertise and a demonstrated track record of working closely with scientists and engineers in applying statistics. Each chapter has at least one author with more than a decade of experience in the biotechnology industry. These seasoned veterans provide not only statistical knowledge, but are also experienced in the same types of experiments, data sets, and questions that challenge you. We hope you will appreciate their accumulated wisdom.

It may be a surprise to many scientists and engineers that statisticians do not always agree on the most appropriate approach to a question that requires their expertise.

As editors, we have not sought to standardize practice but instead to allow the author of each chapter to express his or her own perspectives. Because of this choice, there are some areas in the text where different approaches are advocated. We believe the discussion of different methodologies is healthy and allows statisticians, scientists, and engineers to think critically about their specific purposes and come to a more refined approach. For example, while classical methods for Design of Experiments (Chapter 2) have been used successfully for decades, newer methods (Chapter 3) are being used more often. There are advantages and disadvantages to each technique. Practitioners may wish to try multiple approaches and decide for themselves which works best for their needs.

   We hope this book will soon be worn out from consistent use. We wish you success in applying statistics to develop the medicines of tomorrow.

Todd Coffey
Meridian, ID

Harry Yang
Gaithersburg, MD

Editors

Todd Coffey (PhD, Biostatistics) made major contributions to BLA and MAA submissions while working as a nonclinical statistician for over a decade in the biopharmaceutical industry. While continuing to advise CMC organizations of biotechnology companies from multiple continents on the development, regulatory strategy, and commercial manufacture of biological products, Todd has subsequently started a university-wide statistical consulting center and then became the chair of research and biostatistics at Idaho's first medical school.

Harry Yang, PhD, is senior director and head of statistical sciences at MedImmune, where he provides statistical support for drug discovery, preclinical and clinical study design, biomarker identfication, immunogenicity assessment, analytical method and biopharmaceutical development, manufacturing control, and regulatory submission. Dr. Yang has published 4 statistical books, 14 book chapters, and 90 peer-reviewed papers.

Contributors

Bruno Boulanger
Arlenda
Pharmalex Statistical Solution
Mont-Saint-Guibert, Belgium

Richard K. Burdick
Elion Labs
Division of KBI Biopharma, Inc.
Louisville, Colorado

Todd Coffey
Idaho College of Osteopathic Medicine
Meridian, Idaho

Katherine Giacoletti
SynoloStats, LLC
Fleming, New Jersey

David Lansky
Precision Bioassay
Burlington, Vermont

Pierre Lebrun
Arlenda
Pharmalex Statistical Solution
Mont-Saint-Guibert, Belgium

Xavier Lories
Arlenda
Pharmalex Statistical Solution
Mont-Saintt-Guibert, Belgium

Jean-François Michiels
Arlenda
Pharmalex Statistical Solution
Mont-Saint-Guibert, Belgium

Steve J. Novick
Statistical Sciences
MedImmune, LLC
Gaithersburg, Maryland

Laura D. Pack
CMC Statistics
Seattle Genetics, Inc
Bothell, WA

Lorin Roskos
Global Clinical Pharmacology and DMPK
MedImmune, LLC
Gaithersburg, Maryland

Eric Rozet
Arlenda
Pharmalex Statistical Solution
Mont-Saint-Guibert, Belgium

Tara Scherder
SynoloStats, LLC
Fleming, New Jersey

Perceval Sondag
Arlenda
Pharmalex Statistical Solution
Mont-Saint-Guibert, Belgium

Harry Yang
Statistical Sciences
MedImmune, LLC
Gaithersburg, Maryland

Binbing Yu
Statistical Sciences
MedImmune, LLC
Gaithersburg, Maryland

Lingmin Zeng
Statistical Sciences
MedImmune, Inc.
Gaithersburg, Maryland

Jianchun Zhang
Statistical Sciences
MedImmune, LLC
Gaithersburg, Maryland

1

Interpretation and Treatment of Data

Harry Yang, Steven J. Novick, and Lorin Roskos

CONTENTS

1.1 Background

The biopharmaceutical industry is strictly regulated. According to governmental regulations, before marketing approval of a new drug by regulatory agencies such as the U.S. Food and Drug Administration (FDA) and European Medicines Agency (EMA), the drug must be shown to be both safe and efficacious (Peltzman 1973). For this reason, sufficient clinical and non-clinical data are generated in support of the premarketing approval. Furthermore, regulations such as the U.S. current Good Manufacturing Practice (cGMP) also stipulate that modern standards and technologies be adopted in the design, monitoring, and control of manufacturing processes and facilities to ensure a consistent supply of high-quality drug products to the consumer or public (FDA 1995). These include use of statistics for process validation, justification of process changes post-approval, product release testing, and root cause analysis. Adherence to government regulations such as cGMP is an essential step in ensuring a consistent supply of high-quality drug products to patients, as shown in following sections.

1.2 Biopharmaceutical Development

Bioprocess development is an integral part of the overall biopharmaceutical research and development phases. For a biological drug to be tested in preclinical and clinical studies, it has to be formulated to ensure bioavailability and hence the activity of the drug. For this purpose, formulation studies are conducted to understand the effects of excipients on the properties of the formulation, such as stability and solubility. The processes by which the biologic products are manufactured are often referred to as *bioprocesses*. In general, bioprocesses can be divided into upstream and downstream processes. The former is concentrated on cell isolation, cultivation, banking, culture expansion, and harvest; the latter is primarily concerned with treatment of cell harvests from the upstream to ensure that purity and quality requirements are met (Gronemeyer et al. 2014). As the drug advances in clinical development, parallel efforts are made to optimize bioprocesses to ensure successful scale-up of the product for clinical trial purposes and ultimately commercial use. To ensure that product quality meets regulatory requirements, the testing of raw materials, bulk, and the finished product need to be performed. All of these efforts rely on reliable and accurate analytical methods. Consequently, development of these analytical methods is of critical importance. Taken together, these processes are commonly referred to as *chemistry, manufacturing, and control* (CMC).

1.3 Statistics in Bioprocess Development

For most processes there are no theoretical or mechanistic models that can be used to fully describe the process performance (Haaland 1989). As a result, successful development of robust CMC processes relies on trial-and-error through well–thought-out design of experiment (DoE). Scientific questions are addressed using the data collected from various experiments. As data are usually complex, incomplete, inherently variable, and random, parsing information and knowledge from one experiment and using it to guide the next study can be challenging. Statistics concerns itself with "learning from data" or "translating data into knowledge." It consists of a set of analytical techniques that can be used to collect, analyze, and present data in the face of measurement uncertainty. In addition, as bioprocess development is often limited by resources and tight timelines, it is essential to apply good statistical practice (GSP) to gain experimental efficiency and confidence in decision-making. Studies designed based on GSP not only help minimize impact of variations and bias, but also control the producer's and consumer's risks. Often a formal sample size calculation is needed to ensure that a proper amount of data is collected to address the issue at hand. The choice of statistical method for extracting information from data needs to reflect the design of the study.

As noted in USP <1010> (USP 2012), in addition to adherence to GSP in data collection and analysis, assurance of the quality of pharmaceuticals is achieved through combining a number of practices. Sound documentation not only makes data collection and analysis traceable and reproducible, but also helps facilitate the efforts of addressing regulatory inquiries, stemming from regulatory filings or site inspections. Data and statistical rationale used to design studies and analyze data should be documented, as should the methods of analysis and model assumptions. In fact, it is preferable to have a statistical analysis plan developed and incorporated into the study protocols before their execution because choosing methods of analysis after data collection can introduce bias. Other practices that help ensure the accuracy of data collection, analysis, and interpretation include the use of reference standards, system performance verification, and method validation. Applications of these laboratory practices also rely on use of sound statistical methods. For example, where use of a new reference standard is to be adopted for an analytical method, it needs to be shown to be comparable to the current standard, based on rigorous statistical tests. It is equally important to bring statisticians onboard in the planning stage of an experiment. There are no better words than the famous Sir Ronald Fisher quote, "To call in the statistician after the experiment is done may be no more than asking him to perform a postmortem examination; he may be able to say what the experiment died of."

1.4 Statistical Inferences

Analytical data are collected with the intent to estimate or make inferences about the true performance characteristics of a process, which are usually unknown. Because of variability in the data, neither the estimation nor inference can be made with 100% precision or certainty. However, statistical analysis makes it possible to quantify how accurate and precise an estimate is, and how likely a conclusion made about the process performance characteristic is correct. In this section, we introduce several important statistical concepts and methods that are often used to describe analytical data, assess process performance, and ensure product quality. They include random variables, distributions, statistical sampling, statistical estimation, and hypothesis testing.

1.4.1 Example

Consider a direct fluorescent focus assay (FFA) for measuring the potency of the biological product of a live virus. The FFA combines a number of antibody-binding steps, resulting in the fluorescence staining of virus-infected cells. The assay counts the fluorescent foci representing infected cells, which express a marker protein of the product virus on their surfaces. It is assumed that each focus is caused by a single infecting particle. The "infecting particle" is defined as a unit, which is indivisible on further dilution. Therefore, the assay directly estimates the number of infecting particles in a test sample. The FFA is used to determine the potency of both monovalent bulk lots and trivalent finished product, with the test result being expressed on a log–scale, commonly referred to as a $\log_{10}$ titer. Figure 1.1 consists of several plots generated from a real data set, illustrating observations from a series testing of the assay. For a monovalent lot, if one sample is tested, the test result

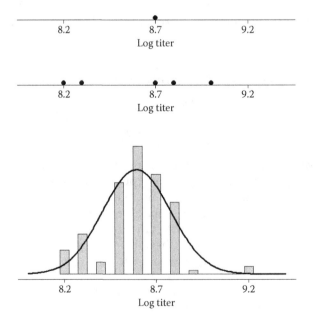

FIGURE 1.1
Log titers of FFA test of a monovalent lot. Data appear variable but form a pattern after a sufficient number of test results are plotted.

is a point on the log–titer axis as shown in the top plot. Results of four additional tests are plotted in the second plot, and they appear to vary. However, after 120 samples from the lot are tested, a pattern of the test results emerges as is shown in the last plot. Several observations can be made from the plots: (1) Potency measurements vary from sample to sample; (2) the majority of the test results center on 8.6 $\log_{10}$ titer, and are within the range of 8.2 $\log_{10}$ titer and 9.0 $\log_{10}$ titer; (3) the pattern appears to be symmetric. The reason that the titer varies from sample to sample is that there are many factors influencing the test results. Some factors, such as reagent and incubation time, are known, but many others are unknown. The spread of the pattern reflects how variable the assay is while the center of the pattern is a potential measure of the true potency value of the lot.

In statistics, the log titer is called a *random variable*, and the pattern is its distribution. It is of great interest to find out how the distribution can be used to approximate the true potency value. Note that the difference between the analytical measurement and the true value is not only due to measurement variability but also to systematic variation or bias of the analytical test. Statistical methods based on representative measurements make it possible to quantify various sources of variations in analytical measurements, thus understanding of the true process performance.

1.4.2 Random Variables

A random variable is a variable whose value varies due to chance. A random variable can be continuous or discrete. The former can take on any value within a range, whereas the latter can assume values that are either countable or finite. For example, $\log_{10}$ titer is a quantitative continuous variable. Outcome of a sterility test is discrete, as is the number of colony-forming units (CFU). Analytical measurements of a random variable are used to study the statistical properties such as spread and central tendency of the variable. Such knowledge enables one to conjecture if the process characterized by the variable meets or complies with given requirements.

1.4.3 Continuous Distributions

A probability distribution of a random variable is a theoretical structure of the variable. A continuous distribution describes the chance for a continuous random variable to be within a prespecified range. Some probability distributions are defined by parameters. For example, the normal distribution is defined by the two parameters mean and variance. By assuming that measurements of an analytical method follow a certain parametric distribution, the performance characteristics of a process can be characterized in terms of parameters of the distribution. Samples drawn from the entire population, which are all possible outcomes of the process, contain information about these parameters. Statistical methods, based on the distribution of these samples and the way by which the samples are collected, can be constructed and used to assess the performance of the process. In statistical literature, there is a broad class of statistical methods that make inferences on sample populations without distributional assumptions. These methods, often referred to as distribution-free or nonparametric analyses, are out of the scope of this chapter. We primarily concern ourselves with inference based on parametric distributions.

1.4.3.1 Gaussian Distribution

There are many statistical distributions that are used to describe behaviors of random variables. The most well-known distribution is the Gaussian distribution, also called the normal distribution. A random variable that has a normal distribution is often referred to as a normal random variable or normally distributed random variable. Mathematically, the probability for a normal random variable X to be within the range (a, b) is given by

$$P[a < X < b] = \int_a^b \frac{1}{\sqrt{2\pi\sigma^2}} e^{-\frac{(x-\mu)^2}{2\sigma^2}} \, dx \tag{1.1}$$

where μ and σ^2 are the population mean and variance, respectively. The integrand $\frac{1}{\sqrt{2\pi\sigma^2}} e^{-\frac{(x-\mu)^2}{2\sigma^2}}$ is called the density function of a normal distribution denoted as $N(\mu, \sigma^2)$.

As depicted in Figure 1.2, a normal distribution has a single peak and is symmetric and bell-shaped. Approximately 68%, 95%, and 99.7% of the observations are within one, two, and three standard deviations of the mean, respectively. Since the distribution is entirely determined by its mean μ and variance σ^2, statistical inference about the variable X can be directly made based on estimates of the two parameters.

Many analytical measurements are normally distributed. The normality of an array of measurements can be evaluated either graphically or through formal statistical tests such as Shapiro–Wilk test (see Section 1.9.2.2). For random variables that do not follow a normal distribution, an appropriate transformation of the data such as logarithm may help make the normality assumption approximately met (Box–Cox 1964). Methods that can be used to make the transformed data approximately normal are discussed in Section 1.9.3. As an example, the potency measurement of the FFA assay discussed in Section 1.4.1 is normally distributed after $\log_{10}$ transformation. In this case, the parameter μ is the true potency value and σ^2 the variance of the entire population under evaluation. Assuming that $X_1, \ldots, X_n$ are n measured potency values, a commonly used statistical estimate of the population mean μ is the sample mean given by

$$\bar{X} = \frac{X_1 + \ldots + X_n}{n}. \tag{1.2}$$

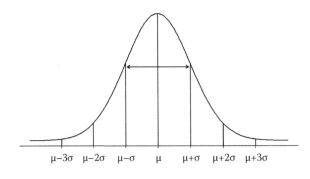

μ−3σ   μ−2σ   μ−σ   μ   μ+σ   μ+2σ   μ+3σ

FIGURE 1.2
Normal distribution. The area under the curve within an interval (A, B) represents the probability for an observation to be within the interval.

TABLE 1.1

Summary Statistics of Potency Values

N	Mean	SD	RSD
120	8.5	0.3	0.04

The sample variance below is an estimate of the population variance σ^2:

$$s^2 = \frac{\sum_{i=1}^{n}(X_i - \bar{X})^2}{n-1}. \tag{1.3}$$

Two statistical measures, sample standard deviation (SD) and relative standard deviation (RSD), are obtained as

$$s = \sqrt{\frac{\sum_{i=1}^{n}(X_i - \bar{X})^2}{n-1}} \text{ and } RSD = \frac{s}{\bar{X}}, \tag{1.4}$$

which measure variability of the potency observation and per-unit variability of the potency value, respectively. RSD, which is also referred to as coefficient of variation (CV), is particularly useful when the variability of the response is proportional to concentration. Statistical methods based on sample mean, sample SD, and sample RSD, for the interpretation of analytical data, are discussed in Sections 1.5 through 1.7. Using the summary statistics in Equations 1.2 and 1.4, data in Figure 1.1 are summarized and presented in Table 1.1.

1.4.3.2 Student's t-Distribution

Suppose a random sample $X = (X_1, \ldots, X_n)$ is taken from a normal distribution $N(\mu, \sigma^2)$. The statistic $T = \dfrac{\bar{X} - \mu}{s/\sqrt{n}}$ is a random variable, having a distribution called *Student's t-distribution* with $n - 1$ degrees of freedom. The density of this distribution is given by

$$f(x) = c\left(1 + \frac{x^2}{v}\right)^{-(v+1)/2} \tag{1.5}$$

where v is the degrees of freedom and c is a constant such that the integration of the density function over the real number is equal to 1.

Like the normal distribution, the t-distribution is also symmetric and unimodal. However, it is more spread out around its center. Figure 1.3 shows a normal distribution and t-distributions with various degrees of freedom. As seen from the plots, t-distributions have thicker tails. However, as the degree of freedom gets larger, the density function of the t-distribution gets closer to that of the normal distribution.

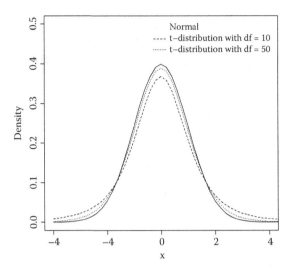

FIGURE 1.3
Density functions of standard normal and t-distributions.

As discussed in Sections 1.6.2 and 1.6.7, like the normal distribution, the t-distribution plays a very important role in statistical estimation and inference. It is often used in evaluating data for significant bias, assessing performance of an assay or process against acceptance limits, and comparing results generated from two different conditions.

1.4.3.3 Chi-Square Distribution

The chi-square distribution is another continuous distribution that has a wide range of applications in assessing process data, including construction of a confidence interval for the variance and assessment of goodness-of-fit of a statistical model to observed data. These applications rely on the fact that sample variance s^2 in Equation 1.2 has the property that $(n - 1)s^2/\sigma^2$ follows a chi-square distribution with $v = n - 1$ degrees of freedom. The distribution is characterized through the following density function:

$$f(x) = cx^{v/2-1}e^{-x^2/2} \text{ for } x \geq 0, \tag{1.6}$$

where v is the degrees of freedom and c is a normalization constant such that the area under the density function is 1.

1.4.3.4 F-Distribution

Let s_1^2 and s_2^2 be sample variances of two random samples $X = (X_1, ..., X_n)$ and $Y = (Y_1, ..., Y_m)$ from two normal distributions with the same variance. Let $F = \dfrac{(m-1)s_2^2}{(n-1)s_1^2}$. The random variable F has an F-distribution with degrees of freedom (m, n). It can be used to make inferences on the comparability of the variances of the two populations. The F statistic assumes a density function of

$$f(x) = cx^{v/2-1}e^{-x^2/2} \tag{1.7}$$

where c is a normalization constant such that the area under the density function is equal to one

1.4.4 Discrete Distributions

In process development, quality attributes can be either continuous or discrete. However, we typically use the functions of these attributes to create quantitative random variables. For example, while the result of a test may be "positive" or "negative," which are qualitative, the number of "positive" outcomes of n tests is quantitative. Two discrete distributions that are frequently used to describe counts or discrete events such as microbial excursions in a clean room are binomial and Poisson distributions.

1.4.4.1 Binomial

Suppose that $X = (X_1, ..., X_n)$ is a random sample of n independent observations from an experiment, with each of the observations assuming either one of two values such as "positive" and "negative" with probabilities p and $1 - p$, respectively. The number of "positive" results follows a binomial distribution $B(n, p)$ with the probability density function given by

$$p(x) = \binom{n}{x} p^x (1-p)^{n-x} \text{ for } x = 0, 1, ..., n. \tag{1.8}$$

When $n = 1$, the binomial distribution is known as a *Bernoulli distribution*.

1.4.4.2 Poisson

Poisson distribution is often used to describe count data. The following equation represents the density function of a Poisson distribution with λ being the mean number of counts per unit.

$$p(x) = \frac{\lambda^x e^{-\lambda}}{x!} \text{ for } x = 0, 1, ... \tag{1.9}$$

1.5 Sampling Considerations

The true value of a quality attribute, such as the potency of a batch, is usually unknown. It may be estimated by testing a sample from the batch. A sample is a subset of the population. Sample testing helps gain understanding about the population to make inferences about its characteristics. There are many ways by which a sample can be drawn. The key to proper sampling is to draw a random set of individuals that are representative of the population. For example, to assess if the potency of a lot of drugs meets the specifications or not, one could test every vial in the lot. Although perfect quality assurance can be obtained using this sampling method, it is obviously costly and impractical. A more viable alternative is to test a subset of the lot. If the sample is selected based on statistical principles, quality decisions can be made based on the test results while seeking to minimize the sample size.

1.5.1 Non-Random Sample

There are many different means to pull samples from a population. The first kind is the nonrandom convenience sample. Basically, a sample is drawn in a manner that is handy or easy for the investigator. For example, a sample consisting of the first 10 vials of a finished lot is a convenience sample. Since changes that might impact the product, such as a temperature drop, may occur during the production, such a sample is not representative of the population. Therefore, findings based on the test results from the convenience sample of 10 vials may be biased and may not be generalized to the entire lot. In general, testing of a nonrandom convenience sample often leads to biased estimates of the properties of the population and is of limited utility in making inference from sample to the population.

1.5.2 Simple Random Sampling

A more useful sampling method is called *simple random sampling*. In this method, each unit in a population is selected with an equal probability. Such a property warrants that statistical inferences based on data from the random sample are valid. For example, the sample mean and variance in Equations 1.2 and 1.3 provide consistent and unbiased estimates to the population mean and variance. Consistency means that as the sample size increases, the sample estimates get close to the true values of the population parameters.

1.5.3 Stratified Sampling

In many experimental situations, the study population consists of several subpopulations. While the subpopulation may vary, each is made up of homogeneous units. Consider a lot of drug product that is produced using three filling machines as shown in Figure 1.4. Vials

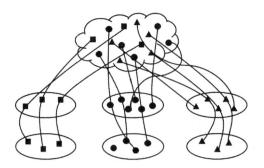

FIGURE 1.4
Stratified sampling.

of the product from each filling machine form a subpopulation or stratum. If a simple random sampling method were to be used, vials from one strata might not get selected when the overall sample size is small. In such situations, it is advantageous to take a random sample from each stratum to ensure the final combined samples are representatives of the entire lot. This method is called *stratified sampling*. It is particularly useful when there are some differences in subpopulations. It makes it possible to separate the stratum variability from measurement error, thus improving the chance of detecting differences due to changes in process conditions. Depending on what inferences are to be made, the sample sizes from each stratum must be proportional to the population size of each stratum.

1.5.4 Systematic Sampling

Systematic sampling is a method that selects a sample from a population at selected times or locations. A typical example is sampling in a clean room environment where septic product is produced. To ensure the environment is in a state of control, samples are collected at different locations in the room and at different times. Systematic sampling has several advantages. First, it is simple to carry out when compared to simple random sampling. Second, it ensures that the population is sampled evenly. This is extremely important when there are uncontrollable changes such as ambient temperature that may influence the performance of a process. Both simple random sampling and systematic sampling methods can be used in conjunction with stratified sampling to take random samples from subpopulations. It is important to point out that when analyzing data, the sampling method used to generate the data needs to be taken into account to minimize the chance of misinterpretation of data. However, systematic sampling can produce biased samples when the sampling interval or locations match or do not match a characteristic of the process. For example, one could sample every Monday and the sample would be biased if something different occurred on other days of the week.

1.6 Statistical Estimation

Because it is often either impossible or impractical to obtain all the possible observations of a population, a sample that is part of the population is used to gain understanding about the population. Figure 1.5 displays the empirical distribution or histogram of a large

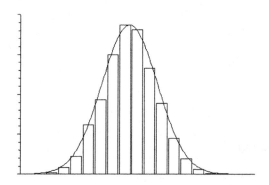

FIGURE 1.5
When sample size is large, empirical distribution closely mimics theoretical distribution.

random sample drawn from a population. The smooth curve is the theoretical distribution of the population. As seen from the plot, the empirical distribution closely approximates the theoretical distribution. Intuitively, sample mean, sample variance, and other derived statistical measures are close to the mean, variance, and other characteristics of the theoretical distribution. If the sample is a random sample, statistical theories warrant desirable properties of these estimators, which we discuss in this section.

1.6.1 Point Estimate

A point estimate is a single value estimating a population parameter of interest. It is obtained based on data from a random sample. For instance, the sample mean $\bar{X}$ and sample variance s^2 are point estimators of the mean and variance of the population, respectively. There are numerous estimators that can be constructed for a population parameter. For example, the sample median can also be used to estimate the central tendency of a distribution. To assess the qualities of these estimators, several statistical properties are suggested in the published literature. They include consistency, unbiasedness, and precision. An estimator is consistent if it tends toward the true value of the population parameter being estimated as the sample size increases. It is related to the accuracy of the estimation. An unbiased estimator is one whose expected value is equal to the population parameter. Lastly, an estimator is precise if its variance is small.

Both $\bar{X}$ and s^2 are consistent estimators of population mean and variance. It can also be shown that, for normally distributed data, the expected values of $\bar{X}$ and s^2 are equal to μ and σ^2, respectively. Furthermore, among all the unbiased estimators of μ, $\bar{X}$ exhibits the minimum variance among all the unbiased estimators of the population mean μ.

1.6.2 Interval Estimation

A point estimate is a descriptive statistical summary. Although it provides some insight about the population parameter that it intends to estimate, it does not provide a metric of uncertainty through the accuracy or precision of the point estimate. Therefore, inferences drawn from the point estimate of one sample can hardly be generated to the population. Consider a bioprocess experiment in which product yields from two experimental conditions A and B are obtained by testing 10 samples from each condition. The point estimates of the average yields of conditions A and B may suggest that condition B represents an improvement over condition A as the sample mean of the former is greater than that of the latter. However, based on the point estimates alone, one may not be able to infer with confidence that the yield from condition B is indeed greater than that from condition A. In such a situation, an interval estimate of the mean difference (B – A) may be considered. It provides a range of plausible differences between the yields produced under conditions A and B, which are consistent with the observed difference from the current sample testing. The lower and upper limits of the range represent the most conservative and liberal estimates of the difference. If the lower limit exceeds 0, this is indicative of the potential improvement of the process brought about by condition B.

1.6.2.1 Confidence Interval

A confidence interval is an interval estimate of a population parameter, say μ. It is expressed through two limits, $a(X)$ and $b(X)$, both of which are calculated from the random sample

$X = (X_1, ..., X_n)$. Given $0 < \alpha < 1$ and assuming that $(1 - \alpha)100\%$ is the desired confidence level, the $(1 - \alpha)100\%$ interval is constructed by choosing $a(X)$ and $b(X)$ such that

$$P[a(X) < \mu < b(X)] = 1 - \alpha. \qquad (1.10)$$

Since the limits $a(X)$ and $b(X)$ themselves are random variables, they vary from sample to sample. Before X is observed, there is $(1 - \alpha)100\%$ probability for the interval $[a(X), b(X)]$ to include μ. However, when X is observed with the values of X_0, the limits $a(X_0)$ and $b(X_0)$ are no longer random variables. Therefore the interval $[a(X_0), b(X_0)]$ either contains or does not contain the true value of population parameter. So the $(1 - \alpha)100\%$ confidence refers to proportion of the intervals $[a(X), b(X)]$ based on repeated sampling.

The previous concepts are illustrated in Figure 1.6. Suppose the experiments to compare the potency values of two conditions A and B is repeated many times. Each time, the observed results are used to construct a confidence interval. While each interval may with an absolute certainty cover or not cover the true mean difference between A and B, overall, the proportion of intervals containing the true difference is $(1 - \alpha)100\%$. In Figure 1.6, $(1 - \alpha)100\% = 95\%$.

1.6.2.1.1 Confidence Interval When σ^2 Is Known

Confidence intervals can be either two-sided or one-sided. The width of a confidence interval measures how reliable the point estimate is in approximating the true value of population parameter. Consider that the sample $X = (X_1, ..., X_n)$ is from a normal distribution $N(\mu, \sigma^2)$. If the variance σ^2 is known, the statistic $Z = \dfrac{\overline{X} - \mu}{\sigma/\sqrt{n}}$ follows the standard

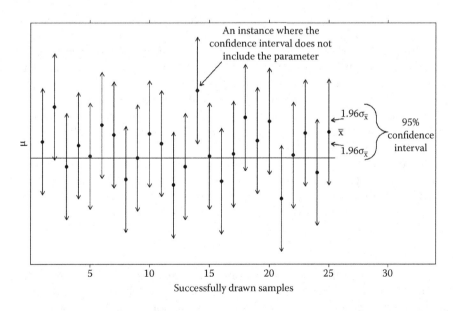

FIGURE 1.6
Ninety-five percent confidence intervals constructed using samples from repeated experiment. Each interval may or may not contain the true mean difference with 100% certainty. But the overall proportion of the intervals covering the true mean difference is 95%.

normal distribution. From Section 1.4.3.1, with $1 - \alpha$ probability Z would lie within a range given by

$$-z_{1-\alpha/2} < Z < z_{1-\alpha/2} \tag{1.11}$$

where $z_{1-\alpha/2}$ is the upper $(1 - \alpha/2)100^{th}$ percentile of the standard normal distribution. After some algebraic manipulations, Equation 1.11 can be rewritten as

$$\bar{X} - z_{1-\alpha/2}\sigma/\sqrt{n} < \mu < \bar{X} + z_{1-\alpha/2}\,\sigma/\sqrt{n}. \tag{1.12}$$

Per the definition put forth previously in this section, the following is the $(1 - \alpha)100\%$ confidence interval of μ,

$$\left(\bar{X} - z_{1-\alpha/2}\sigma/\sqrt{n}, \bar{X} + z_{1-\alpha/2}\sigma/\sqrt{n} \right). \tag{1.13}$$

1.6.2.1.2 Confidence Interval When σ^2 Is Unknown

In the case that the variance σ^2 is unknown, the statistic $T = \dfrac{\bar{X} - \mu}{s/\sqrt{n}}$ follows a t-distribution with $n - 1$ degrees of freedom. Following the same derivations as above, it can be shown that the $(1 - \alpha)100\%$ confidence interval of μ is given by

$$(\bar{X} - t_{1-\alpha/2}(n-1)s/\sqrt{n}, \bar{X} + t_{1-\alpha/2}(n-1)s/\sqrt{n}) \tag{1.14}$$

where $t_{1-\alpha/2}(n - 1)$ is the upper $(1 - \alpha/2)100^{th}$ percentile of the t-distribution with $n - 1$ degrees of freedom.

For a validated CMC process, the process variability σ^2 is usually well characterized, and so it can be assumed to be known. In this case, the confidence interval in Equation 1.13 can be used to assess the performance of the process. When the process is in its early stage of development and there is limited knowledge of the process, the interval in Equation 1.14 is preferable. The percentiles $z_{1-\alpha/2}$ and $t_{1-\alpha/2}(n - 1)$ can be easily obtained from published tables of the standard normal and t-distributions (Kenkel 1984) or statistical software packages such as SAS (SAS 2009).

As an example, we assume 10 vials are randomly selected from a batch of finished drug product to assess the potency of the batch. The test results are $(X_1, ..., X_{10}) = (94, 104, 96, 103, 103, 102, 97, 95, 107, 100)$. Using Equations 1.2 and 1.4, it can be calculated that $\bar{X} = 100.1$ and $s = 4.38$. Because of $t_{1-0.05/2}(10-1) = 2.262$, from (1.14) the 95% confidence interval of the potency of the lot is calculated to be (96.9, 103.2).

1.6.2.1.3 Central Limit Theorem

It is worth pointing out that the construction of the previous confidence interval requires the random sample independently drawn from normal distributions. In reality, there are many quality attributes such as microbial count that are not normally distributed. However, in most situations, Equations 1.13 and 1.14 can be used to obtain an approximate confidence interval. This is largely due to a probability theory called *central limit theorem* (CLT). The theory establishes that the distribution of the average of a large number of independent, identically distributed sample will be approximately normal, regardless of the underlying

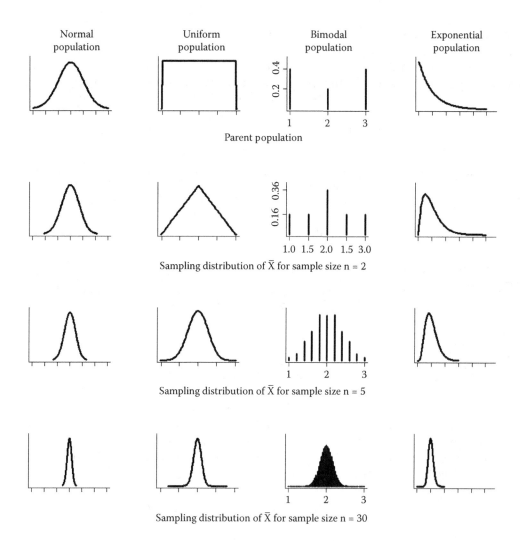

FIGURE 1.7
Effect of sample size on sampling distribution of sample mean. (Adapted from Kendel, Introductory Statistics for Management and Economics, 2nd ed., Duxbury Press, 1984.)

distribution. To demonstrate, consider four distributions, normal, uniform, bimodal, and exponential, as shown in the top row of Figure 1.7. The sampling distributions of each of the four distributions are derived and shown for sample size n = 2, 5, and 30. Regardless of the population distribution of a single observation, the sampling distribution of the sample average from the illustrated distribution appears to be normal when n = 30.

1.6.2.2 Prediction Interval

A confidence interval provides an interval estimate for the average performance of analytical method or manufacturing process. Sometimes it is of interest to predict the values of the future observations given what have been observed so far. For example, in product manufacturing, we are interested in knowing with certain probability all possible values of a lot release test given that three lots used for process validation study have passed acceptance criteria. A prediction interval is also useful for an out of specification (OOS) investigation where the behavior of a suspected outlying individual observation is of primary concern. If the OOS result is far beyond the range predicted based on data generated under normal manufacturing conditions, it is likely a real outlier. A prediction interval provides a range for the future randomly selected observations from the population to fall in with a pre-specified level of confidence. When the distribution of the population is normal with mean μ and variance σ^2, construction of the prediction interval is relatively straightforward. Let X_{n+1} be a future observation and $X = (X_1, \ldots, X_n)$ be the current data obtained by testing a random sample from the population. Because the statistic $T_{n+1} = \dfrac{X_{n+1} - \bar{X}}{s/\sqrt{1+1/n}}$ follows a t-distribution with n – 1 degrees of freedom, with probability of $1 - \alpha$ we have

$$-t_{1-\alpha/2}(n-1) < T_{n+1} < t_{1-\alpha/2}(n-1) \tag{1.15}$$

which is the same as

$$\bar{X} - t_{1-\alpha/2}(n-1)s/\sqrt{1+1/n} < X_{n+1} < \bar{X} + t_{1-\alpha/2}(n-1)s/\sqrt{1+1/n}. \tag{1.16}$$

Thus the interval

$$\left(\bar{X} - t_{1-\alpha/2}(n-1)s/\sqrt{1+1/n}, \bar{X} + t_{1-\alpha/2}(n-1)s/\sqrt{1+1/n} \right) \tag{1.17}$$

is the 100(1 – α)% prediction interval of the future observation X_{n+1}.

Now we assume that the potency specification limits are (90,110). Suppose that a test of a sample from a new batch yields a potency of 85, which is an OOS result. Is this observation an outlier? To answer the question we use the data described in the previous section to calculate the 95% prediction interval:

$$\left(100.1 - 2.262 \times 4.38/\sqrt{1+1/9}, 100.1 + 2.262 \times 4.38/\sqrt{1+1/9} \right) = (89.7, 110.5).$$

Since 85 is not within the prediction interval, it is likely that something else other than random variation has caused this outlying result.

Lastly, the previous prediction interval for a single future observation can be generalized to construct prediction intervals for all of *m* future observations or the average of *m* observations. For a detailed discussion please refer to Hahn and Meeker (1991). The generalized method is useful for comparability study after a change is made to a process, in which the acceptance criterion requires that the prediction interval of the *m* future observations be contained within the specification limits to lend confidence for the *m* batches used in the process validation study to comply with given requirements.

1.6.2.3 Tolerance Interval

Unlike a prediction interval that predicts the test outcome of a single observation, a tolerance is a numeric range which covers a proportion of a population with specified confidence. This kind of statistical interval is particularly useful when one wishes to predict long-term performances of a large proportion of samples from a population. For example, when controlling the quality of a product lot, one may wish that, with certain confidence, a large proportion of samples from the lot meet specification. Likewise, for an analytical procedure, a negative or positive sample may be used to ensure the validity of the assay. This often involves checking if the test result of a control falls within a range. The range should be set so that under the normal testing condition, a large percentage of the controls will fall within the range. For these purposes, tolerance intervals may be used.

A two-sided tolerance interval contains at least a $100p\%$ of the population with probability of $1 - \alpha$. Let $T_L(X)$ and $T_U(X)$ be the lower and upper limits of such a tolerance interval based on sample $X = (X_1, ..., X_n)$, and let X^* be a random observation from the population. Mathematically, $T_L(X)$ and $T_U(X)$ satisfy

$$P_X[P_{X^*}[T_L(X) < X^* < T_U(X)] \geq p] \geq 1 - \alpha. \tag{1.18}$$

The inside probability statement concerning the new observation $X^* P_{X^*}[T_L(X) < X^* < T_U(X)] \geq p$ implies that the interval $(T_L(X), T_U(X))$ contains at least p proportion of the future observations. The inequality in Equation 1.18 means that the probability for the above statement to be true is at least $(1 - \alpha)100\%$. As with the interpretation of confidence interval, before an experiment is carried out and data X collected, the $(T_L(X), T_U(X))$ covers $100p\%$ of the future observations with probability $1 - \alpha$. However, after the data are collected and X take on values X^*, [TL, TU] either contains or does not contain $100p\%$ of the future observation with 100% certainty. Furthermore, both quantities p and α are prespecified. Construction of a tolerance interval relies on the sampling distribution, and knowledge of the population parameters. In the case where the sampling distribution is normal with known parameters, a tolerance interval is the same as the prediction interval. For example, if $p = 0.99$ and $\alpha = 0.05$ and the sampling distribution is normal with known mean $\mu = 5$ and variance $\sigma^2 = 1$, the interval

$$(\mu - z_{0.995}\sigma, \mu + z_{0.995}\sigma) = (5 - 2.576 \times 1, 5 + 2.576 \times 1) = (2.424, 7.576)$$

is both a 99% prediction interval and a tolerance interval covering 99% proportion. This is due to the facts that

$$P_{X^*}[\mu - z_{0.995}\sigma \leq X^* \leq \mu + z_{0.995}\sigma] = 0.99$$

and

$$P_X[.P_{X^*}[\mu - z_{0.995}\sigma \leq X^* \leq \mu + z_{0.995}\sigma] \geq 0.99] = 1.$$

However, when the population parameters are unknown, construction of a tolerance interval may require advanced statistical techniques (Krishnamoorthy and Mathew 2009). For a population with a normal sampling distribution, a closed-form tolerance interval is given as follows:

$$(\bar{X} - k_{n,\alpha,p}s, \bar{X} + k_{n,\alpha,p}s) \tag{1.19}$$

where the factor $k_{n,\alpha,p}$ can be approximated by (Howe, 1969)

$$k_{n,\alpha,p} = \sqrt{\frac{v(1 + 1/n)z_{(1-p)/2}^2}{\chi_{1-\alpha,v}^2}} \tag{1.20}$$

TABLE 1.2

Values of Tolerance Factor

Sample Size (n)	Confidence Level ($1 - \alpha$)	Percent of Coverage (p)	k
22	0.95	0.9	2.264
22	0.95	0.95	1.697
30	0.95	0.9	2.14
30	0.95	0.95	2.549
50	0.95	0.9	1.996
50	0.95	0.95	2.379
75	0.95	0.9	1.917
75	0.95	0.95	2.285
100	0.95	0.9	1.874
100	0.95	0.95	2.233

with $k_{n,\alpha,p} = \chi^2_{1-\alpha,v}$ being the $(1 - \alpha)$100th percentile of the chi-square distribution with degrees of freedom v. The quantity v is the degrees of freedom of the sample variance s^2. For the sample variance SD in (1.19), $v = n - 1$. The values of $k_{n,\alpha,p}$ can be found in published tables such as Table 1.2; values of this factor are given for selected values of n, α, p.

For example, for $n = 30$, $\alpha = 0.05$, which corresponds to 95% confidence, and $p = 0.90$, the k-factor is equal to 2.140. Suppose that $\bar{X} = 100.1$ and $s = 4.38$. The tolerance interval that covers 90% of the future observations with 95% confidence is given by

$$(100.1 - 2.14 \times 4.38, 100.1 + 2.14 \times 4.38) = (90.7, 109.4).$$

1.7 Hypothesis Testing

In CMC process development, researchers may wish to test some hypothesis about performance characteristics of an analytical procedure, a formulation, or a process due to changes made to experimental conditions, components of formulations, or process parameters. Consider improvement of a cell culture system for production of monoclonal antibodies. Suppose the system has consistently produced 1 gram of the product when the incubation time is set at 35°C. Suppose that a scientist speculates that the yield will increase if the incubation time is set at 37°C. To test this hypothesis, the scientist performs an experiment at 37°C in which 20 culture units are randomly selected and their yields determined. The mean yield is calculated to be 1.1 gram, and the sample variance is 0.5. Can the scientist conclude that the increased incubation time resulted in an increase in the yield of antibody production? Or is the observed a consequence of variability in measurements? These questions can be addressed through formal statistical hypothesis testing.

Statistical hypothesis testing is a statistical procedure to evaluate two conflicting hypotheses commonly referred to as the null hypothesis H_0 and the alternative hypothesis H_1. Whereas the null hypothesis makes a claim about the true value of the population parameter, the alternative hypothesis includes all possible values of the parameter in the parameter space other than the one specified in the null hypothesis. For the above cell culture example, we formulate the following hypotheses:

$$H_0: \mu = 1 \quad \text{versus} \quad H_1: \mu \neq 1. \tag{1.21}$$

A statistical procedure to test the hypotheses in Equation 1.21 can be developed based on random samples $(X_1, \ldots, X_n)$ generated from the cell culture system when the incubation temperature is set at 37°C. It is reasonable to expect that the mean yield $\bar{X}$ is close to 1 if the null hypothesis is true. On the other hand, if the null hypothesis is not true, the observed mean value is likely to deviate from 1. However, the more variable the measured yield is, the more the sample mean $\bar{X}$ may vary. Therefore, a large difference between $\bar{X}$ and 1 can be due to the large variability in the data rather than an actual increase in yield caused by the higher temperature. Consequently, for data that are more variable, a bigger difference needs to be observed in order for one to feel comfortable to reject the null hypothesis. Alternatively, with a more powerful test, one could detect real differences that are small. A statistical test procedure is generally constructed to take into account the variability of the data to quantify and control the risk of either falsely rejecting or failing to reject the null hypothesis. Below we show the essential relationships among the probabilities of erroneous decisions, data variability, desirable difference to detect, and sample size.

1.7.1 Type I and Type II Errors

As previously mentioned, since data generated from the population contain information about the true value of the parameter, a properly devised statistical test allows us to test hypotheses with controlled risk. For a typical statistical test, there are four possible outcomes listed in Table 1.3.

Because of the variability of the data, there are uncertainties associated with the decisions made based on the statistical test. In particular, there are two types of errors that may occur. One is called Type I error, which is the error of rejecting the null hypothesis H_0 when it is true. The other is called Type II error, caused by failing to reject H_0 when H_1 is true. The former is also referred to as the consumer's risk; the latter is the producer's risk. In constructing a statistical test for hypothesis testing, one needs to bear in mind both types of risk. Specifically, to minimize both types of risk, a statistical test is often constructed such that Type I and II errors are bounded by two prespecified small positive numbers, α and β, respectively, with $0 < \alpha < 1$ and $0 < \beta < 1$. Selection of α and β depends on the research problems at hand. For example, if the experiment is a validation study to demonstrate that an analytical procedure is fit for finished product batch release testing, α may be chosen to be 5%. The smaller α value of 5% guards against the risk of passing an unreliable test for batch release. However, if the experiment is the first experiment in a series to be conducted to screen a large set of factors that potentially may have an impact on the

TABLE 1.3

Possible Outcomes of a Statistical Test

Decision	State of True Population Parameter	
	H_0 is true	H_1 is true
Do not reject H_0	Correct decision	Incorrect decision—Type II error
Reject H_0	Incorrect decision—Type I error	Correct decision

yield of a manufacturing process, a larger α or risk is acceptable. In such case, a smaller α value increases the chance of rejecting the null hypothesis of no effect claim, resulting in too many factors being carried over to the subsequent experiment. Thus a larger value, say, 10%, may be a more appropriate choice for α since there will be subsequent tests to support or contradict the initial decision.

1.7.2 Significance Test

A statistical test often consists of a test statistic based on the observed data and a decision rule. The test statistic has a distribution dependent on the population parameter whereas the decision rule, which often involves a cutoff value, decides if the null hypothesis should be rejected or not, by way of comparing the test statistic with the cutoff. For example, when the statistic exceeds the value, the null hypothesis is rejected; otherwise, the null hypothesis is not rejected. The cutoff value is chosen such that the Type I error is bounded by α, $(0 < \alpha < 1)$. Therefore, regardless of the sample size, the consumer's risk is always kept to be no more than α.

Now consider testing the null hypothesis H_0 in Equation 1.21. Suppose that the sample $X = (X_1, \ldots, X_n)$ is from a normal distribution $N(\mu, \sigma^2)$, with known variance σ^2. We use the statistic $T_0 = \dfrac{\bar{X} - 1}{\sigma/\sqrt{n}}$ to test the null hypothesis. We wish to choose a cutoff value c such that H_0 is rejected if T_0 significantly deviates from 0, in other words, $|T_0| \geq c$. To ensure that Type I error or the consumer's risk is no more than α, it is necessary for the chosen cutoff value c to satisfy

$$P[\,|T_0| \geq c \mid \text{When } H_0 \text{ is true}] = \alpha. \tag{1.22}$$

Because the statistic $T_0 = \dfrac{\bar{X} - 1}{\sigma/\sqrt{n}}$ follows the standard normal distribution when the null hypothesis is true, c is determined to be

$$c = z_{1-\alpha/2}. \tag{1.23}$$

Similarly when the variance σ^2 is unknown, we define $T = \dfrac{\bar{X} - 1}{s/\sqrt{n}}$. The statistic T follows a t-distribution with $n - 1$ degrees of freedom under the null hypothesis in Equation 1.21. Therefore a cutoff value c can be determined by solving the following equation assuming H_0 is true:

$$P\left[\left|\frac{\bar{X} - 1}{s/\sqrt{n}}\right| \geq c \mid H_0 \text{ True}\right] = \alpha. \tag{1.24}$$

It turns out

$$c = t_{\alpha/2}(n - 1). \tag{1.25}$$

Consider the example in Section 1.6.2.2 regarding assessment of potency of a batch of finished drug product based on testing 10 vials of the product from the batch. Suppose the

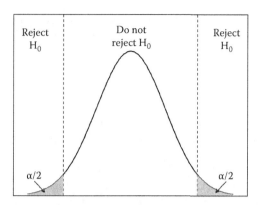

FIGURE 1.8
Acceptance and rejection regions.

disposition of the batch is based on if the hypothesis that H_0: potency = 100% is rejected or not. From the sample test results $(X_1, \ldots, X_{10})$ = (94, 104, 96, 103, 103, 102, 97, 95, 107, 100), it is calculated that $\bar{X} = 100$, $s = 4.38$, and $T = \dfrac{\bar{X} - 100}{s/\sqrt{n}} = 0$. Note that $t_{1-0.05/2}(10 - 1) = 2.262$. Thus $T < t_{1-0.05/2}(10 - 1)$ and the above null hypothesis is not rejected. The batch can be deemed to have 100% potency and good for release.

In either of the above two situations, the cutoff value $z_{1-\alpha/2}$ or $t_{\alpha/2}(n - 1)$ divides all possible values of the T_0 or T statistic into an acceptance region and a rejection region. The former contains all values of T_0 or T for which the null hypothesis is not rejected while the latter includes all possible values for which the null hypothesis is rejected. In Figure 1.8, the acceptable region is the interval $(-c, c)$, and rejection region are values which are either below $-c$ or above c.

It is worth noting that there is a fundamental difference between not rejecting the null hypothesis and accepting the null hypothesis. Failing to reject the null hypothesis does not imply that we accept that the null hypothesis is true. It may mean we do not believe it is true but there is not enough evidence to support our belief.

1.7.3 Statistical Significance

In practice, there are two ways one may carry out hypothesis testing. One is to calculate the test statistic based on the observed data. If it falls within the acceptance range, the null hypothesis is not rejected; otherwise, it is rejected. Alternatively one may calculate the probability to observe values as extreme or more extreme as the observed value of the test statistic when the null hypothesis is true. That is to calculate $P[|T| \geq T_{observed} \mid H_0 \text{ True}]$. Such probability is commonly referred to as the p-value. It is the probability for those large values of the test statistic to be caused by chance alone. This calculated p-value is compared to α. The null hypothesis is rejected if the p-value is less than α; it is not rejected if the p-value is at least α. Operationally this test is equivalent to the test that does not reject the null hypothesis if the $(1 - \alpha)100\%$ confidence interval of the difference between the mean of the sampling population and that hypothesized value conditions contains zero or not (Chow and Liu 1992).

To illustrate, we use the above example. Since the calculated T statistic is equal to 0, the associated p-value is $P[|T| \geq 0 \mid \text{mean of sampling population} = 100] = 0.5$. Since 0.5 is greater than the cutoff 0.05, the null hypothesis is not rejected. From Equation 1.14, the 95% confidence interval between the sampling population mean μ and hypothesized mean 100 is given by

$$(\bar{X} - 100 - t_{1-0.05/2}(n-1)s/\sqrt{n}, \bar{X} - 100 + t_{1-0.05/2}(n-1)s/\sqrt{n}).$$

Substituting values 100, 4.38, and 2.26 for $\bar{X}$, s, and $t_{1-0.05/2}$, respectively, in the above formula, the 95% confidence is obtained as (–3.2, 3.2). Since it contains 0, the null hypothesis is also not rejected.

The number α is also called the significance level of the test, and is usually chosen to be 5%, 1%, or 10%. However, as previously discussed, the choice should be based on the purpose of the experiment. More importantly, statistical significance does not imply practical importance. Statistically significant findings need to be interpreted within the scientific framework within which the research hypothesis is formulated.

1.7.4 Equivalence Test

1.7.4.1 Issues with Significance Test

The significance tests described in Section 1.7.3 are aimed at rejecting the null hypothesis of no difference in light of the observed data. If data are collected to demonstrate that the yield of a new process is greater than the old process, a significant test is the right statistical procedure to use as the risk of falsely claiming that the new process improves the old is bounded by α. However, in many cases, changes made to CMC processes are not intended to improve the performance characteristics of the processes in terms of accuracy, precision, yield, and so on. Instead the changes might be made due to adoption of new technologies or ease of use. For example, due to emerging technology, a manual assay may be replaced by an automated assay. Regulatory guidance requires that comparability studies be conducted to demonstrate equivalency in performance between the old and new assays. In such cases, formulating the research hypothesis as H_0: no difference between the two assays versus the alternative hypotheses H_1: there is a difference, and applying the significance test may raise several issues.

To illustrate, suppose an analytical group has developed four methods, called A, B, C, D, for measuring potency of the same product. The variability of the four methods is 10%, 10%, 5%, and 20%, respectively. Assume that ten samples were tested for each of the four methods. Using Equation 1.13, the 95% confidence interval between the mean response of each assay and the target potency value of 100 were calculated and displayed in Figure 1.9. The vertical line at zero represents the difference between old and new for each method, assuming H_0 is true. The vertical lines (± 5%) to either side of zero represent a difference considered to be practically significant. Since the confidence intervals of Methods B and D both contain zero, the new and old version of these two assays are deemed to be equivalent by the significant test. But Method D also supports the hypothesis that the difference is of practical significance since it contains the vertical line to the right of zero. Methods A and C are considered to be not equivalent as their corresponding confidence intervals do not contain zero.

There are a couple of issues associated with the above conclusions. First of all, although Method C has the least variability and lies entirely within the indifference limits (± 5%), it is deemed to be inequivalent to the old assay. By contrast, Method D is most variable, but

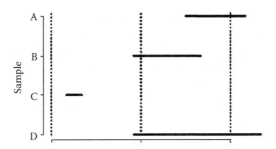

FIGURE 1.9
Confidence intervals of four analytical methods.

is considered equivalent to the old assay. Secondly, since width of the confidence intervals narrows as the sample size increases, if the sample size were to be doubled, the confidence interval of Method B would not contain zero. As a consequence, Method B would not be equivalent to the old method. The above observations suggest data collected from a small experiment or using an imprecise assay would increase the chance to declare the assay to be equivalent, which obviously does not make sense.

1.7.4.2 Alternate Test

One method known as the *equivalence test* can be used to resolve the above issues. In this test, the specification of the null and alternative hypotheses is reversed. That is,

H_0: there is a meaningful difference, versus H_1: there is no meaningful difference.

Suppose that we are interested in mean yields of a cell culture system before and after a change. The above hypotheses can be restated as

$$H_0: \mu_1 - \mu_2 \le -\delta \text{ or } \mu_1 - \mu_2 \ge \delta \quad \text{versus} \quad H_1: |\mu_1 - \mu_2| < \delta \tag{1.26}$$

where μ_1 and μ_2 are the average yields of the process before and after the changes, and δ is the change in yield which is meaningful when compared to the variability in the system. Assuming that two random samples, $X_1 = (X_{11}, \ldots X_{1n})$ and $X_2 = (X_{21}, \ldots X_{2n})$, collected from the two processes are normally distributed with means μ_1 and μ_2, and the same variance σ^2. Shuirmann (1987) suggested a two one-sided test (TOST) that reject the null hypothesis in Equation 1.26 if

$$T_L = \frac{(\bar{X}_1 - \bar{X}_2) - (\mu_1 - \mu_2) + \delta}{\sqrt{s_1^2/n + s_2^2/n}} \le -t_{1-\alpha}(2n-2)$$

or $\tag{1.27}$

$$T_U = \frac{(\bar{X}_1 - \bar{X}_2) - (\mu_1 - \mu_2) - \delta}{\sqrt{s_1^2/n + s_2^2/n}} \ge t_{1-\alpha}(2n-2)$$

where $\bar{X}_1, \bar{X}_2, s_1^2$, and s_2^2 are sample means and variances of the process before and after changes, respectively, and $t_{1-\alpha}(2n-2)$ is the $(1-\alpha)100^{th}$ percentile of a t-distribution with

2n – 2 degrees of freedom. The test has a significance level of α. As indicated previously, the TOST is equivalent to a test procedure which rejects the null hypothesis in Equation 1.26 if the $(1 - 2\alpha)100\%$ confidence interval of the mean difference $\mu_1 - \mu_2$

$$\bar{X}_1 - \bar{X}_2 \pm t_{1-\alpha}(2n-2)\sqrt{s_1^2/n + s_2^2/n} \tag{1.28}$$

is entirely enclosed in the interval $(-\delta, \delta)$.

Regardless of the sample size, the test guarantees that when there is a meaningful difference, the probability of rejecting H_0 is $100\alpha\%$. Therefore it protects the consumer's risk. Since the smaller (larger) the variability (sample sizes) of the assays is, the narrower the confidence interval in Equation 1.28 is, thus the higher the chance it would be contained within $(-\delta, \delta)$. Therefore, the equivalence test ensures that an insignificant difference claim is not the consequence of small sample sizes and large variability. However, application of this method requires that researchers provide equivalence limits, which are often determined based on scientific judgment and process variability. Applying this test to the above example, Methods B and C are equivalent as evidenced that their corresponding 90% confidence intervals are within (–5%, 5%); Methods A and D are not. However, if one were to increase the sample sizes for the evaluations of Methods A and D, they can be shown to be equivalent to the old methods as well.

1.8 Sample Size

A key question concerning design of an experiment is how large the number of observations needs to be. For estimation problems, in general, larger sample sizes result in a more precise estimate of the parameters. For testing research hypotheses, larger sample sizes increase the probability of accepting the alternative hypotheses when they are true. This probability is referred to as power of the statistical test. Sample size determination is dependent on the research objective at hand, study design, and method of analysis. It also requires researchers to make certain assumptions such as sampling distribution, effect size, variability in sample, significance level, practically meaningful difference, and so on. It is also very important to take into practical considerations in terms of cost the feasibility of running an experiment at a certain size.

1.8.1 Sample Size for Estimation

When the research objective is to estimate the average performance of a process, the sample size can be determined to ensure the mean estimate has desirable level of precision. One way to achieve this is to choose sample size such that half of the width of the $100(1 - \alpha)\%$ confidence interval (CI) is bounded by a predetermined number δ_0. Consider the case when the sample has a normal distribution with known variance σ^2. The half width of the $100(1 - \alpha)\%$ is given by $z_{1-\alpha/2}\sigma/\sqrt{n}$. Therefore, the sample size is chosen to satisfy

$$z_{1-\alpha/2}\sigma/\sqrt{n} \le \delta_0. \tag{1.29}$$

Solving the above inequality for n, we obtain the sample size

$$n \geq (z_{1-\alpha/2}\sigma/\delta_0)^2. \tag{1.30}$$

When the variance σ^2 is unknown, an estimate of σ^2 can be used in the above formula to obtain the sample size. That estimate may come from other data considered comparable.

1.8.2 Sample Size for Significance Test

To determine the sample size n for testing a hypothesis of no difference such as the null hypothesis in Equation 1.26, one needs to specify an effect size, which is the minimum difference that is deemed as practically significant. Consider the cell culture example in Section 1.7. We assume the random samples $(X_1, ..., X_n)$ follow a normal distribution with a known variance σ^2. It is further assumed that that the practically meaningful minimum difference is δ^*. As shown in Section 1.7.2, the statistical test based on statistic $T_0 = \dfrac{\bar{X}-1}{\sigma/\sqrt{n}}$ and the cutoff point $z_{1-\alpha/2}$ has significance level of α. The sample size n is chosen to ensure H_0 is rejected with a probability no less than $1 - \beta$, if the difference is δ^* or bigger. Hence

$$P\left[\left|\frac{\bar{X}-1}{\sigma/\sqrt{n}}\right| \geq z_{1-\alpha/2} \,|\, \mu = \delta^* + 1\right] = 1-\beta. \tag{1.31}$$

After some manipulations, the left-hand side of the above equation can be approximated by (Chow et al. 2008)

$$\Phi\left(\frac{\sqrt{n}\delta^*}{\sigma} - z_{1-\alpha/2}\right) = 1-\beta \tag{1.32}$$

where Φ is the cumulative probability function of the standard normal distribution.

Consequently, the sample size, providing a power of $1 - \beta$, is a solution to the equation

$$\frac{\sqrt{n}\delta^*}{\sigma} - z_{1-\alpha/2} = z_{1-\beta}. \tag{1.33}$$

Thus

$$n = \frac{(z_{1-\alpha/2} + z_{1-\beta})^2\sigma^2}{(\delta^*)^2}. \tag{1.34}$$

When the variance σ^2 is unknown, a sample size can be estimated by replacing σ^2 with an estimate. In practice, since there are practical limitations, an experiment is usually sized, taking into account both the statistical power of detecting a difference and practical considerations. Typically, a power function like the one shown in Figure 1.10 is plotted. This allows the experimenter to choose a sample size that is both practical and enables the experimenter to achieve certain study objectives. For instance, in Figure 1.10 it can be seen that with a sample size of 100, the test has 80% power to detect a difference

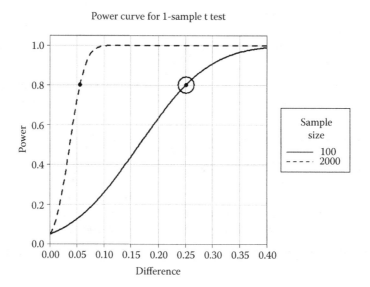

FIGURE 1.10
Power plot shows the power of a test is dependent on both sample size and size of difference.

as small as 0.25. However, to achieve the same 80% probability of detection, a test based on 100 can only detect a difference of 0.25 or larger. Alternatively, for the same difference of 0.05, tests based on 2000 and 100 observations have respective 80% and 17% powers to detect it.

The power plot is a useful tool in aiding an experimental design. It provides experimenters with a means to choose a size sample in light of experimental objectives and practical constraints.

1.8.3 Sample Size for Equivalence Test

As previously mentioned, equivalence testing is a frequently encountered problem in process development. A statistical test procedure is developed to protect both Type I (α) and Type II (β) errors. In addition, the test makes an inference about equivalence in reference to an equivalence bound δ. Similar to the sample size estimation for the significance test, the sample size for the equivalence test can be derived based on the pre-specified values of α, β, and δ, as well as assumptions about the sampling distributions. For instance, when the sampling distributions are normal and possibly have different means but are the same variance, the sample size n that warrants a significance level α and power of $1 - \beta$ for testing the hypotheses in Equation 1.26 is estimated by (Chow et al. 2008),

$$n = \frac{(z_{1-\alpha} + z_{(1-\beta)/2})^2 \sigma^2}{(\delta^*)^2}. \tag{1.35}$$

Again, the variance σ^2 can be replaced by its estimate if it is unknown.

1.9 Selection of Method for Data Analysis

Descriptive statistical summary, point and interval estimation, and hypothesis testing are all statistical techniques used to analyze data. To make sense out of data, proper statistical methods need to be selected and assumption of the methods verified. One common mistake in data analysis is that the method used does not take into account the structure of the data or the study design or sampling method by which the data were collected. This may lead to either false findings or failure to detect true statistically significant differences.

1.9.1 Example

Suppose an improvement of a potency assay is made by replacing the manual reading of the test results with an automated reader. It is expected that two assays give comparable performance in terms of accuracy and precision though the automated system is much more efficient in throughput. Before a formal validation study is carried out, an experiment is run to test the hypothesis that potency measures of the two assays are comparable. Ten samples are chosen from a reference lot and tested. Each sample is read both by the manual-reading assay and by the automated-reader assay. The results are listed in Table 1.4 along with summary statistics.

One hypothesis of interest is that there is no significant difference between the mean potencies μ_1 and μ_2 of the two assays. Mathematically we need to test the following hypotheses:

$$H_0: \mu_1 = \mu_2 \quad \text{versus} \quad H_1: \mu_1 \neq \mu_2 \tag{1.36}$$

Two statistical tests can be constructed using the test statistics

$$T_1 = \frac{(\bar{X}_1 - \bar{X}_2) - (\mu_1 - \mu_2)}{\sqrt{s_1^2/n + s_2^2/n}} \text{ and } T_2 = \frac{\bar{d} - (\mu_1 - \mu_2)}{\sqrt{s_d^2/n}} \tag{1.37}$$

where $n = 10$ is the sample size, $\bar{X}_1, \bar{X}_2, s_1^2$, and s_2^2 are sample means and variances of the two assays, and $\bar{d}, s_d^2$ are sample mean and variance based on the differences $X_{1i} - X_{2i}, i = 1,\ldots,10$.

TABLE 1.4

Potency Values of Ten Test Samples

Sample	Manual	Automated	Difference
1	103	102	1
2	104	105	−1
3	97	100	−3
4	100	102	−2
5	95	97	−2
6	93	96	−3
7	109	107	2
8	98	99	−1
9	92	96	−4
10	101	104	−3
Mean	99.2	100.8	−1.6
Variance	27.96	14.84	3.60

Under the null hypothesis of equal means, T_1 is approximately distributed according to a t-distribution with a degree of freedom of $n_0 = \dfrac{\left(s_1^2/n + s_2^2/n\right)^2}{\left[\left(s_1^2/n\right)^2 + \left(s_2^2/n\right)^2\right]/n}$ when X_{1i}, X_{2i}, $i = 1,\ldots,10$ are random samples from two normal distributions (Satterthwaite 1946) and T_2 follows a t-distribution with a degree of freedom of n − 1. Using the data in Table 1.4, it can be calculated that $T_1 = -0.773$, $n_0 \approx 16$, and $T_2 = 2.667$. From the t-table in (Kenkel 1984), $t_{1-0.05/2}(16) = 2.120$ and $t_{1-0.05/2}(9) = 2.262$. Because

$$|T_1| = 0.773 < 2.120$$

$$|T_2| = 2.667 > 2.262$$

the null hypothesis in Equation 1.36 is not rejected by the first test, but rejected by the second test.

Why do these two tests lead to two different conclusions? The answer is that the first test is a wrong test to apply. The first test is based on test is based on sampling distribution of the difference between two independent samples from two analytical procedures. However, X_{1i} and X_{2i}, ($i = 1,\ldots,10$) are not independent as they are measures of the same test sample. Even if the independence assumption is approximately true, the variability in T_1 includes variations due to both sample and analytical methods. Therefore, it is conceivably larger than the variability in T_2 which only involves analytical method precision.

By taking differences between the measures of the two assays for each sample, the paired *t* test not only creates 10 independent results but also removes sample-to-sample variability from the total error used in statistical comparison, thus increasing signal-to-noise ratio or the power of the test. Figure 1.11 shows the sampling distributions of paired and unpaired differences. The top distribution of the difference is much narrower, thereby increasing the probability of detecting a true difference greater than 0. However, the sampling distribution based on the t-statistic of the first method is wider, thereby reducing the power of the test to detect a true difference greater than 0. Therefore, it cannot conclude the difference is significantly larger or smaller than 0. Although the average difference is the same −1.6 for both sampling distributions, the variability in the unpaired distribution is much larger when compared to that of the paired distribution, resulting in a much smaller test statistic relative to its critical value.

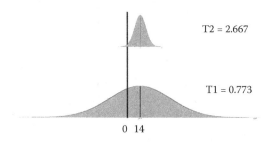

T2 = 2.667

T1 = 0.773

0 14

FIGURE 1.11
Comparison of sampling distributions of paired and unpaired differences. The top distribution shows the variability within samples while the bottom shows within-sample plus between-sample variability.

1.9.2 Test Model Assumptions

In order to make a statistical inference about a population, certain assumptions need to be made. The most common is that the samples from a population follow a normal distribution. However, before analysis is performed on data, it is necessary to evaluate whether such an assumption is correct. When comparing data from two or more groups, it is also necessary to check if the variances from the different groups remain the same. There are several methods that can serve this purpose, including Q–Q plot and nonparametric tests for normality (Chamber et al. 1983; Shapiro and Wilk 1965). Other tests are available for other assumptions (Box 1953).

1.9.2.1 Q–Q Plot

A Q–Q plot is obtained by plotting ordered observations against their corresponding quantiles of the standard normal distribution. In brief, suppose that $X = (X_1, ..., X_n)$ are the observed data. The random observation $X_1, ..., X_n$ are ordered from smallest to the largest to give rise to the ordered observations $X^{(1)} < X^{(2)} < ... < X^{(n)}$. The ith ordered observation is paired with the percentiles z_{p_i} of the standard normal distribution, where $p_i = (i - 0.5)/n$. The paired points $\left(X^{(i)}, z_{p_i} \right)$ are plotted. In statistics, if a random variable y follows a normal distribution with mean μ and variable σ^2, it can be expressed as $y = \mu + \sigma x$, where x is a random variable having the standard normal distribution. In other words, there is a linear relationship between the two variables. Consequently if the sampling distribution of the observed data is normal, the data will lie on an approximate straight line. A Q–Q plot is constructed for the potency values of a random sample from a batch of finished product in Section 1.6.2.1 and is displayed in Figure 1.12. Because the point fall close to the straight line, the data appear to be normally distributed. Thus it is reasonable to assume that the data are from a normal distribution.

This is also a significance test where H_0 is the data from a normal distribution. However, as discussed before, unless there sample size is large enough, there may not be enough power to distinguish between a normal distribution and various non-normal ones. Thus,

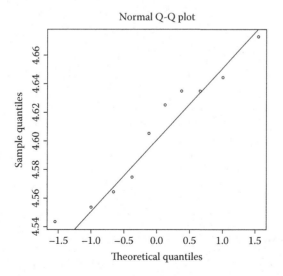

FIGURE 1.12
Q–Q plot of empirical quantiles against quantiles of the standard normal distribution.

other tests that do not rely on or tests that are robust to such assumptions can be used. Fortunately, the CLT supports the robustness of the t-tests on means.

1.9.2.2 Nonparametric Test

Whether data come from a normal distribution can also be assessed through formal statistical tests. One of these tests is called the *Shapiro–Wilk test*. It is a nonparametric test based on order statistics (Shapiro and Wilk 1965). It tests the null hypothesis to ensure the sampling distribution is normal. A *p*-value less than 0.05 is indicative of non-normality. For example, when applying the Shapiro–Wilk test, the above potency data results in a *p*-value of 0.5332. Therefore, the hypothesis that the data are normally distributed cannot be rejected.

1.9.3 Data Transformation

In most cases, continuous data generated from bioprocess development are normally distributed. When a Q–Q plot or a formal test suggests non-normality, it may be necessary to transform data so that the transformed data would have an approximately normal distribution. This improves the validity of statistical analyses that are based on the normality assumption. A necessary condition for the transformation is that it must preserve the order of the data. Such property ensures that conclusions based on the transformed data can be directly translated into conclusions concerning the original data. Commonly used transformations include natural or 10-based logarithm, square root, and reciprocal. In practice, appropriateness of a transformation can be assessed by applying the above tests for normality to the transformed data. The transformation can be more formally determined. Box–Cox (1964) suggested a method for selecting an appropriate transformation from a family of power functions as follows:

$$y^{(\lambda)} = \begin{cases} \dfrac{y^{\lambda} - 1}{\lambda \tilde{y}^{\lambda-1}} & \text{if } \lambda \neq 0 \\[2ex] \ln(y) & \text{if } \lambda = 0 \end{cases} \tag{1.38}$$

where $\tilde{y} = (y_1 \ldots y_n)^{1/n}$ is the geometric mean of the data assuming the observed values are positive.

The Box–Cox power functions include those common transformations as special cases. For example, the λ values of 1, 0.5, and 0, −0.5, and −1 correspond to no transformation, square root, nature logarithm, inverse square root, and reciprocal, respectively. Several methods for estimating the parameter λ are discussed in Haaland (1989).

1.10 Removal of Outliers

Following the 1993 Barr Decision (Longwell 2016), the OOS problem was formalized by the FDA in a draft guidance document, Investigation of OOS Test Results for Pharmaceutical Production (FDA 2006). The guidance requires that every single OOS result be investigated.

One needs to conduct laboratory investigation and look for assignable causes. If no such cause is identified, a full-scale OOS investigation should be carried out, which includes (1) Review of product; (2) additional laboratory testing; and (3) reporting testing results. Removal of outliers based on statistical analysis should be the last resort. This section discusses statistical tools that can be used in identification of outlying observations.

1.10.1 Definition

An outlier is a data point that has an abnormal distance from the others in a random sample from a population. Outliers may significantly impact conclusions. For example, in Figure 1.13, the horizontal solid line segment below the x-axis represents the specification interval. Two vertical bars correspond to reportable values excluding outliers (solid line) and including outliers (dashed line). The former is in spec but the latter is out of spec.

Outliers can be detected either graphically or through statistical analyses. Graphically, methods such as the boxplot shown in Figure 1.14 are intuitive and easy to carry out.

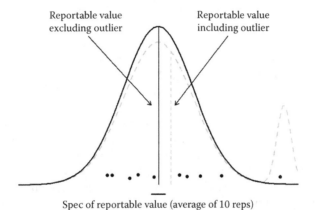

Spec of reportable value (average of 10 reps)

FIGURE 1.13
Effect of outliers.

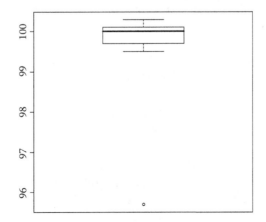

FIGURE 1.14
Use a boxplot to detect outliers.

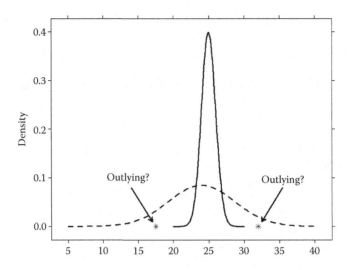

FIGURE 1.15
Outlier detection relies on reference distribution.

They can be used to identify potential outliers. The boxplot uses a specific definition of an outlier as a point more than 1.5*IQR, where IQR = interquartile range = $Q_3 - Q_1$. A histogram and normal probability plot are also useful to identify outliers and, with added lines or symbols, may also denote the mean, median, quartiles, and other percentiles.

A formal statistical analysis can assess how significant the outliers are in reference to a distribution or a well-established model. Bear in mind that a value may be an outlier in relation to one distribution but not others. For examples, the two star points in Figure 1.15 appear to be outliers for the thin distribution but not for the fat distribution.

Detection of outliers relies on the distribution of the reference sample. An outlier based on the normal assumption might not be a real outlier if the normal assumption is untrue. Therefore, it is important to evaluate if the data come from a certain distribution before an outlier test is performed. Statistical techniques described in Section 1.9.2 can be used to test the normality assumption if the data are assumed to follow a normal distribution. In the event the normality assumption does not hold, proper transformation of the data may be carried out to ensure the assumption is met. In such cases, outlier testing needs to be performed on the transformed data.

1.10.2 Outlier Tests

1.10.2.1 Grubbs' Test

Grubbs (1950) developed several outlier tests. Grubbs' tests work well with small sample sizes. Perhaps more widely used is a method based on the maximum deviation from the sample mean,

$$G = \frac{\max_{\{1 \le i \le n\}} |X_i - \bar{X}|}{s}. \tag{1.39}$$

When the data are from a normal distribution, the distribution of the statistic G can be derived, as can cutoff values for various significance levels and sample sizes. For example,

TABLE 1.5

Critical Values of Grubbs' Outlier Test

N	3	4	5	6	7	8	9	10
Critical Value	1.15	1.48	1.71	1.89	2.02	2.13	2.21	2.29

Table 1.5 lists cutoff values $G(\alpha, n)$ for a sequence of n and $\alpha = 5\%$, where n and α are the number of samples in the data set and the probability of incorrectly rejecting the suspected outlier (Grubb and Beck 1972). The suspected outlier is rejected if G is greater than the critical cutoff value.

Consider a situation in which a potency assay to release a finished trivalent influenza vaccine lot. Six samples are drawn from the lot and tested. The lot is good for release if the test result of each of the six samples and the average are within the specification (6.6, 7.5) $\log_{10}$ titer. The test results were 7.0, 7.2, 7.1, 7.4, 7.7, and 7.3 with an average of 7.3. It is suspected that 7.7 is an outlier. Grubbs' test was performed on the data, resulting in $G = 1.68$. From the above table, the critical value for G with $n = 6$ is 1.89, which is greater than 1.68. Therefore, the value 7.7 cannot be declared an outlier.

1.10.2.2 Dixon's Test

Several tests based on range calculations were suggested by Dean and Dixon (1951). Among those tests, the Dixon's Q test is more frequently utilized and effective for detecting both high and low outliers for small data sets. To perform the test, the data set $(X_1, \ldots X_n)$ are ordered such that $X_{(1)} \leq X_{(2)} \leq \ldots \leq X_{(n-1)} \leq X_{(n)}$, and statistics $\dfrac{X_{(2)} - X_{(1)}}{X_{(n)} - X_{(1)}}$ and $\dfrac{X_{(n)} - X_{(n-1)}}{X_{(n)} - X_{(1)}}$ calculated.

The larger of the two statistics is compared to the critical value in Table 1.6. The extreme value is deemed to be an outlier if the critical value is exceeded.

Using the above example, we can calculate that $r = 0.3/0.7 = 0.428$, which is below the corresponding critical value at 95% significance level. Therefore, per the Dixon's test, 7.7 is not considered as an outlier.

TABLE 1.6

Critical Values of Dixon's Q Test

N	Significance Level		
	90%	**95%**	**99%**
3	0.941	0.97	0.994
4	0.765	0.829	0.926
5	0.642	0.71	0.821
6	0.56	0.625	0.74
7	0.507	0.568	0.68
8	0.468	0.526	0.634
9	0.437	0.493	0.598
10	0.412	0.466	0.568

1.10.2.3 Other Outlier Tests

There are other outlier tests, such Hampel's tests, that may detect multiple outliers. More sophisticated outlier tests based on prediction intervals, Bayesian analysis, and multivariate methods also exist. For detail, please refer to Yang (2017).

1.10.2.4 Model-Based Method

Analysis of analytical data often involves fitting a statistical model to describe the relationship between the measured response such as potency and an independent variable such as drug concentration. Unlike the univariate case where outliers are identified in relation to the "center" of the data, detection of outliers is carried out in reference to the relationship between the response and independent variables. Therefore, outlier detection may be more challenging.

1.11 Bayesian Inference

Unlike the classical statistical methods given earlier in this chapter, which attempts to estimate a fixed, unknown population parameter value, the Bayesian method assumes that the parameters follow a statistical distribution. It is the distribution of the population parameters that the Bayesian estimates.

Bayesian inference is a branch of statistics in which Bayes' theorem is used to blend the information from current experiment results with prior knowledge of the population. Consider two events, A and B. Bayes' theorem states that the probability of the joint event of A and B occurring simultaneously can be expressed as the probability of event A, conditioned on the knowledge that event B has occurred multiplied by the probability of event B. In formulae, this is P(A and B) = P(A | B) × P(B). When using Bayesian inference, one considers the distribution of a set of parameters, conditioned on the observed data. Applying Bayes' theorem twice, this might be written as P(parameters | data) = P(data | parameters) × P(parameters) / P(data). Thus, the Bayesian theorem blends the current information, represented by P(data | parameters), with prior knowledge of the population, represented by P(parameters). The P(data) term is called the *normalizing constant* and is technically necessary to construct a proper probability distribution.

For a quick example, consider the probability p of seeing heads when tossing a coin. The classical statistician flips a coin 100 times and records the number of times that heads is observed. The classical statistician and Bayesian statistician both agree that the number of heads (out of 100) follows a binomial distribution (see Section 1.4.3.1), thus defining P(data | p). Suppose that heads is observed in 55 of the 100 coin tosses. The classical statistician will estimate p with 55/100 = 0.55, stating that this is the best estimate of the true nature of the coin. In advance of flipping the coin, the Bayesian statistician might have no idea about the true nature of the coin and assign the population parameter p a uniform chance to fall between 0 and 1, thus defining P(p). Finally, after observing 55 out of 100 coin tosses, the Bayesian statistician states that the parameter p follows a *Beta* distribution with shape parameters 56 and 46. The beta density function is given by $f(x) = cx^{a-1} (1 - x)^{b-1}$, where a and b are the shape parameters and c is a constant such that the integration of the

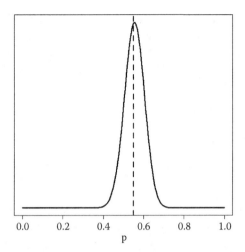

FIGURE 1.16
For the example of observing 55 heads in 100 coin tosses, the vertical dashed line shows the point estimate for
p. The solid curve shows the beta distribution with shape parameters 56 and 46.

density function over the $0 < x < 1$ is equal to 1. Figure 1.16 shows the classical statistician
point estimate of 0.55 (the vertical dashed line) for p and the Bayesian estimate of the distribution for p given the observed data. Using the Clopper and Pearson method (Clopper
and Pearson 1934), the classical statistician might calculate a 95% confidence interval for
p as (0.45, 0.65). In this example, the Bayesian statistician makes inference from the beta
distribution and will claim with 95% probability that p lies between 0.45 and 0.64, drawing
a similar conclusion.

Bayesian statistical methods are especially applicable when analyzing CMC processes.
For example, a manufacturing process may have the target to produce a compound with
potency equal to 100% of its label claim with specification limits of 80% and 120% of label
claim. Will a measured sample from a future batch fall within 80% and 120%? Given a set
of data consisting of samples from past batches, the Bayesian statistician calculates the
distribution of the parameters (say, mean μ and variance σ^2) and, from that distribution,
may directly calculate the probability that the potency value from a future batch will fall
between 80% and 120%. The classical statistician cannot easily make the same calculation,
instead relying on tools like a tolerance interval (Section 1.6.2.3).

A CMC process may be produced from multiple sources of variability, such as might
come from taking multiple samples from each batch, yielding batch-to-batch and within-
batch variability. In such a case, one might estimate a mean μ and the total variance
$\sigma^2_{Total} = \sigma^2_{Batch} + \sigma^2_{Within}$. It is difficult to calculate a tolerance interval in the presence of two
sources of variability. The Bayesian statistician, however, as before estimates the distribu-
tion of parameters (μ, σ^2_{Total}) and directly calculates the probability that the potency value
from a sample from a future batch will fall between 80% and 120%.

The Bayesian method provides simple, straight-forward solutions for calculating statistical intervals and for comparing hypotheses. So why isn't everyone using Bayesian statistics? The answer has to do with the difficulty in evaluating the expression P(data) in
calculating the distribution of P(parameters | data). Statisticians have worked out the
exact value of P(data) for only a small set of situations. For all others, special, sometimes
time-consuming computer calculations must be made to estimate P(parameters | data).

Until recent times, the necessary computer power was unavailable, but in today's modern world of parallel computing, virtually any new computer can handle the Bayesian calculations, opening the door to a different type of statistical problem solving.

1.12 Concluding Remarks

Effective development of biotechnology processes relies on good statistical practices in design of experiment, analysis, and interpretation of data. GSP not only generates information-rich and reliable data by minimizing bias and variability, but also controls consumer's and producer's risks. GSP is the foundation for making sense out of complex data and is recommended in many regulatory guidelines. Successful implementation of GSP increases the probability of success for bioprocess development. Lastly, it is important to note that this chapter discusses the basic but fundamental statistical concepts, principles, and methods for bioprocess development. There are issues that require application of more advanced statistical methods, which are discussed in Chapters 2 through 11.

References

Billingsley, P. (1995). *Probability and Measure* (3rd ed.). John Wiley & Sons.

Box, G.E.P. (1953). Non-normality and tests on variances. *Biometrika* 40 (3/4), 318–335.

Box, G.E.P. and Cox, D.R. (1964). An analysis of transformations. *Journal of the Royal Statistical Society Series B* 26, 211–252.

Chambers, J., Cleveland, W., Kleiner, B., and Tukey, P. (1983). *Graphical methods for data analysis.* Wadsworth.

Chow, S.C. and Liu, J.P. (1992). *Design and Analysis of Bioavailability and Bioequivalence Studies*. Marcel Dekker.

Chow, S.C., Shao, J., and Wang, H. (2008). *Sample Size Calculations in Clinical Research*. Chapman & Hall/CRC Press.Dean, R.B. and Dixon, W.J. (1951). Simplified statistics for small numbers of observations. *Analytical Chemistry* 23 (4), 636–638.

FDA. (1995). Current good manufacturing practice in manufacturing, processing, packing, or holding of drug: Amendment of certain requirements for finished pharmaceuticals. *Federal Registry* 60 (13), 4087–4091.

FDA. (2006). Guidance for industry: Investigating out-of-specification (OOS) test results for pharmaceutical production. From https://www.fda.gov/downloads/drugs/guidances/ucm070287 .pdf (accessed August 20, 2017).

Gronemeyer, P., Ditz, R., and Strube, J. (2014). Trends in upstream and downstream process development for antibody manufacturing. *Bioengineering* 1, 188–212.

Grubbs, F.E. (1950). Sample criteria for testing outlying observations. *Annals of Mathematical Statistics* 21(1), 27–58.

Grubbs, F.E. and Beck, G. (1972). Extension of sample sizes and percentage points for significance tests of outlying observations. *Technometrics* 14(4), 847–854.

Haaland, P. (1989). *Experimental Design in Biotechnology*. CRC Press.

Hahn, G.J. and Meeker, W.Q. (1991). *Statistical Interval: A Guide for Practitioners*. Wiley.

Howe, W.G. (1969). Two-sided tolerance limits for normal populations: Some improvements. *Journal of the American Statistical Association* 64, 610–620.

Kenkel, J. (1984). *Introductory Statitics for Management and Economics,* 2nd ed. Duxbury Press.

Krishnamoorthy, K. and Mathew, T. (2009). *Statistical Tolerance Regions: Theory, Applications, and Computation.* Wiley.

Longwell, A. (2016). *United States of American v. Barr Labs, Inc.* 812 F. Supp 458. GMP lessons from a federal judge. From http://fdclaw.com/cases/gmp/ (accessed August 20, 2017).

Peltzman, S. (1973). An evaluation of consumer protection legislation: The 1962 drug amendments. *The Journal of Political Economy* 81(5), 1051.

SAS, Inc. (2009). SAS/STAT 9.3 User's Guide.

Satterthwaite, F.W. (1946). An approximate distribution of estimates of variance component. *Biometric Bullitin* 2, 110–114.

Schuirmann, D. (1987). A comparison of the two one-sided tests procedure and the power approach for assessing the equivalence of average bioavailability. *Journal of Pharmacokinetics and Biopharmaceutics* 15(6), 657–680.

Shapiro, S.S. and Wilk, M.B. (1965). An analysis of variance test for normality (complete samples). *Biometrika* 52(3/4), 591–611.

USP. (2012). General chapter <1010> Analytical data-interpretation and treatment. USP 36-NF 31, 452–464.

Yang, H. (2017). *Emerging Non-Clinical Biostatistics for Biopharmaceutical Development and Manufacturing.* Chapman & Hall/CRC.

2

Design of Experiments (DOE) for Process Development

Todd Coffey

CONTENTS

2.1 Introduction and Overview

Since the mid-twentieth century, DOE has been the most useful statistical tool for industrial process development. Its success derives from its ability to optimize processes with many process variables using fewer resources than other approaches. It has been estimated that DOE provides a return on investment of four to eight times the cost of running one-factor-at-a-time experiments, in a fraction of the time (Branning and Torbeck, 2009). First conceived in 1926 to improve agricultural yields (Fisher, 1926), the methods were expanded and refined for industrial use over the following decades. In 1951 Box and Wilson introduced the concept of design space, and by the 1960s applications of response surface methods were appearing regularly in the literature. Although biotechnology process development was slower to adopt DOE than many other industries, it has now become an indispensable part of cell culture, purification, formulation, and analytical method development.

DOE is a systematic approach to understanding the relationship between measured response variables and the experimental factors that may affect them. From beginning to end, this process allows the experimenter to sift through a large number of variables, determine those that have the greatest effect or none at all, and pinpoint the optimal levels of each to achieve the best result for multiple responses. The designs use a mathematically derived combination of levels of input variables chosen across a comprehensive experimental grid. Ultimately, this experimentation allows the development of a statistical model that relates process variables to outcomes. The results from these models determine which factors are statistically relevant, estimate their effect, predict response values at any combination of the inputs, and discover the optimal combinations for the process or assay. Figure 2.1 illustrates the outcome of a DOE experiment: A statistical model that can predict a response as a function of multiple factors.

Entire books have been written on DOE and our purpose will be focused on outlining and illustrating with case studies the fundamental considerations for designing and analyzing experiments for bioprocess, formulation, and analytical method development. After becoming familiar with the content in this chapter, you should be able to design experiments for a variety of scenarios and analyze the resulting data. This chapter focuses

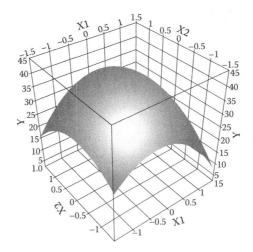

FIGURE 2.1
Statistical model relating process variables X_1 and X_2 to outcome Y.

on the designs that are traditionally thought of as DOE—fractional factorials and response surface designs for screening and process optimization. However, DOE encompasses many types of designs. In Chapter 3 we present twenty-first century designs in the context of formulation development. Other examples of DOE can be found in Chapter 10.

2.1.1 Definitions

Before we begin, it's important to define a few words that have specific meanings in DOE and that will be used frequently in this chapter.

- *Factor*: An input, also called an independent or predictor variable, that will be studied to evaluate its effect on the response.
- *Response*: An output of the experiment, also called a dependent variable or outcome.
- *Effect*: The change in the response caused by a factor. An effect can either be a main effect or an interaction.
- *Main effect*: The mean difference in the response between the high and low levels of a factor, averaged across the levels of all other factors. For example, if the response decreases by an average of 10% when factor A is increased from the lowest level to the highest level, the linear main effect would be –10%.
- *Interaction*: When the effect of one factor depends on the level of a second or even third factor. As an example, if the mean response decreases by 20% for factor A when factor B is at its low level and there is no change in the response for factor A when factor B is at its high level, we say that factor A interacts with factor B because the effect of A depends on the level of B.
- *Run*: A performance of an experimental condition using a combination of levels from each factor. The design is composed of a set of runs. Each run should be independent from all other runs.
- *Replicate*: The number of times each experimental run is performed. For example, running two replicates of the design means performing each condition twice.
- *Statistical model*: A mathematical equation that partitions the variability in the response values into that due to the factors included in the model—described by main effects, interactions, or polynomial terms—and that which cannot be explained by the model terms, called the error or residual. The error term can be further separated into replicate variation (sometimes called pure error) and lack-of-fit variation. Lack-of-fit error is the variability attributed to model terms that could be included in the model but were not.

2.1.2 General Classes of Designs

In general, DOE can be divided into three main categories of designs, each with distinct objectives: (1) Screening, (2) characterization, and (3) optimization.

The objective of screening designs is to determine which of the many potential factors have a meaningful effect on the responses of interest. These designs use a limited number of runs to determine whether there is a significant linear relationship between the high and low levels of each factor and generally only permit estimation of main effects. The main effects in these designs cannot be distinguished from two-factor interactions, which is called *aliasing*. For example, seven factors can be screened in just eight experiments but one cannot have certainty that the observed effects are due to the main effects or another interaction due to the aliasing. Figure 2.2 shows an example of the outcome of most screening designs: An estimate of the main effect of each studied factor. While many variables potentially could be important, experience has shown that for most processes and assays, only three to four factors have large effects in the studied ranges. This result is known as the *sparsity-of-effects principle* and is similar in concept to the Pareto principle or the 80/20 rule, which states that 80% of the effects are caused by 20% of the causes.

Characterization designs allow the unaliased estimation of both linear main effects and interactions. They achieve this by using sufficient runs to independently estimate the aliased terms that occur with screening designs. Typically, multiple runs of the center point are also included to make an assessment of the adequacy of the linear model. The interactions estimated from characterization designs will graphically appear as different slopes for levels of one factor plotted across a second factor, as demonstrated in Figure 2.3.

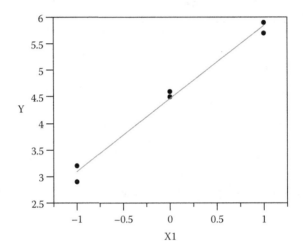

FIGURE 2.2
Estimation of a linear main effect in screening design.

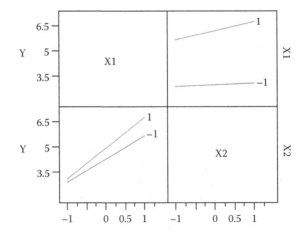

FIGURE 2.3
Estimation of two-factor interactions in characterization design.

Optimization designs are used to find the sweet spot in a process or assay and are necessary when the linear model is not adequate to describe the relationship between factors and responses. These designs include quadratic main effects and potentially quadratic terms in interactions. The need for these designs can be detected during screening or characterization when the linear model is deemed to be inadequate. Although the runs for optimization designs can be performed in a single designed experiment, it is more common to sequentially add, or augment, the screening or characterization designs. These designs are often called *response surface designs* because the quadratic nature of the statistical model reveals a multidimensional surface that can be explored to find optimal conditions. Figure 2.4 provides an example of the model that can be created from these designs. These models make predictions over every combination of variables within the design region.

The traditional way of using these designs is in the outlined sequence: Screening, characterization, and then optimization. For example, you may run a screening design to narrow down a list of ten potential factors to four. Then you conduct a characterization design to estimate the main effects and two-factor interactions. If the linear model is not adequate because the relationship between at least one factor and the response is not linear, you run an optimization design. However, the power of DOE—indeed, one reason why it's been so successful—is that these designs are often hybridized to achieve multiple objectives with greater efficiency and in a timely manner. For example, it's common to perform a design that combines screening and characterization studies or characterization and optimization designs. You can also jump directly from a screening design to optimization. Or, if you prefer, you can skip screening and go straight to either a characterization or an optimization design. Regardless of which strategy you choose, it's important to state two principles of DOE: (1) The combinations in the designs are structured—meaning not random—to achieve mathematical optimality, but (2) flexibility exists in the way the designs are constructed and performed. The methods we'll discuss allow the experimenter to build upon previous knowledge without repeating experimental runs. If you're unsure whether DOE will really save you time or money, keep reading.

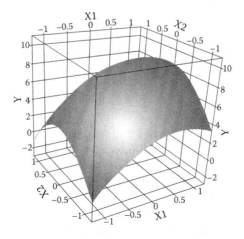

FIGURE 2.4
Response surface model from optimization design.

2.2 Before You Start: Planning for Success

You are probably ready to jump into the design for your experiment, but it's better if we first discuss some fundamentals and keys for success. Planning is crucial for any experimental program. However, it is even more vital for DOE because a carefully proposed set of experiments can result in additional savings in time and resources. This section discusses critical things to consider when planning an experiment. You should consult this section as often as needed. You can read each section consecutively or skip to those sections that are most relevant to your current work.

2.2.1 Defining the Experimental Purpose

In DOE it is critical to start with the end result in mind so you must take the time to assess what experiments are needed to address the study objective. Data generated from initial DOE studies can help choose additional combinations to study or be analyzed with experimental runs from subsequent studies. But ad hoc experimental conditions almost always don't provide useful information in the context of classical DOE, so you will want to carefully plan the full range of potential studies to come up with the best strategy. For example, the fractional factorial design (more on this in Section 2.3.3) has a valuable feature known as the *projection property*, which enables well-designed screening experiments to be projected into characterization designs. Savvy experimenters recognize this property and design their experiments to potentially save an entire set of experiments. Before beginning the study, the most important question to ask yourself is the following:

- What is my ultimate objective with these experiments?

In other words, at the end of the set of experiments, what statistical information do you want? Do you want a statistical model that will predict the optimal combination of levels for each response? Do you simply want to estimate the effect of each factor? Alternatively, do you want to know whether the range of levels for each factor produces a response that is acceptable? Perhaps you only need to eliminate factors that aren't relevant. Each of these objectives may require a different type of experiment. For example, if the ultimate goal is to predict the response at the optimal combination, a characterization or optimization experiment will be needed. If the desire is to simply estimate the effect of each factor or eliminate factors with no effect, a screening experiment may be all that is needed. And if the primary objective is to assess robustness, a screening or characterization design will likely be sufficient.

2.2.2 Selecting the Responses

There is no limit to the number of responses that can be assessed in DOE—and methods are available to analyze these responses simultaneously—but more responses mean more data and more effort to analyze, understand, and interpret. Carefully choose responses that are most meaningful for the process or assay, keeping in mind that continuous responses are optimal because they have more statistical power than responses that are binary (power is the ability to observe a specified effect in the main effect or interaction terms when the observed effect or an even greater one truly exists). Binary responses will require huge increases in sample sizes compared to continuous responses. Ordinal responses should be avoided when possible because statistical methods for analyzing them are complex.

When there is more than one response—and there almost always is—it can be helpful to prioritize the responses and assigns weights. For example, response A may be three times as important as response B and twice as important as C. We'll cover how to analyze multiple responses in Section 2.6.

2.2.3 Identifying Factors, Levels, and Ranges

The most critical step in planning—and often the most difficult—is to identify the factors and their levels that should be studied. Initially you may want to study many factors, but each additional factor increases the number of experimental runs. But you also want to find all the important factors, so you don't want to exclude factors that may prove to be important. Factors should be chosen for study that are at least somewhat likely to impact the experimental objectives. You don't have to include a factor in the study just because it may have the slight potential of showing an effect. A risk assessment should be conducted and then factors chosen that have high or medium risk. Likewise, the range of each factor to study is sometimes hard to judge, especially if DOE has not been used with the process or assay. It's important to realize that the success of DOE depends on being in the right range and that DOE itself will not necessarily find that range if it is initially missed in planning. If the range is too wide the process or assay may completely fail, while using too narrow of a range may cause no effects to be observed. The range sometimes has to be discovered by trial and error, and mistakenly selecting an improper range is the number-one cause of failure to produce the desired results. Experiments varying one factor at a time are meaningful at this initial stage to ensure that the right range is chosen. If you don't know anything about the range of the factors and jump immediately into DOE, be prepared to rerun the design when you realize you need to adjust the levels. For this reason, starting with a screening design is beneficial.

While the factors are sometimes self-evident, a handful of tools can be used to ensure all important factors have been considered. Reviewing historical data on similar processes or assays can elucidate factors that should be considered. Doing structured brainstorming from the beginning to end of the process (also called fishbone, cause-and-effect, or Ishikawa diagram) helps you to see all factors that contribute. An example of such a cause-and-effect diagram for a potential out of specification (OOS) result for an analytical method is shown in Figure 2.5. A failure modes and effects analysis (FMEA) serves a similar purpose. All of these approaches attempt to allow consideration of all the relevant factors. A winnowing of the identified factors will then have to be conducted, and often a risk assessment to rank and prioritize factors is helpful. A risk assessment can evaluate the severity, probability, or detectability of each factor. It is helpful to go through this process as a team so that all potential factors can be explored and agreement can be reached on those that are vital.

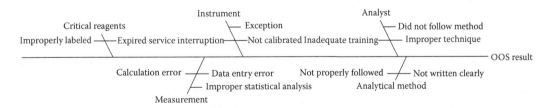

FIGURE 2.5
Ishikawa diagram for potential OOS from analytical method.

Although it seems simple, choosing the factor levels can be even more time-consuming than selecting the factors. It is common to have limited information about the effect of factors beyond the immediacy of the target conditions and the optimal ranges for some factors may be completely unknown. Although there are efficient methods to explore ranges, with today's short timelines, it's often more efficient to proceed at risk and subsequently miss the range and then be forced to redo the experiments than use alternative approaches, such as the method of steepest ascent. However, when experiments are expensive, the method of steepest ascent can be used effectively. While we won't discuss that here, other textbooks provide good explanations (see Myers, Montgomery and Anderson-Cook, 2016). The usual approach to selecting factor levels is to utilize historical data from similar processes or assays or use one factor-at-a-time experimentation to get a ballpark estimate. In experiments where much is known about the factors, it is usually undesirable to push the process or assay to failure. Instead, ranges can be chosen that would be expected to give acceptable responses based on historical data. The levels chosen are generally the high, low, and mid-point of the range. When little is known about the factor levels, an initial one-factor-at-a-time experimental approach will help avoid the failure zones.

Two other questions that you should ask yourself about factors are shown below. If you can't answer these questions at an early stage you can still use DOE effectively, but knowledge of these attributes will give you an advantage.

1. Do I expect the relationship between the factors and responses across the studied design space to be linear? If the relationship between all factors and the responses is linear, the optimization design will not be necessary because the optimal combination will be found within the selected ranges of a characterization design. This consideration could save an experimenter from jumping directly into a more costly optimization design.

2. What factors might interact with each other? If potential interactions can be identified or excluded early on, the experimental strategy can be designed to reduce the total number of runs. While it can be hard or impossible to prospectively know which interactions are likely, especially with new process development projects, a useful exercise is to consider each set of two factors, and ask the following questions: When factor 1 is at its low level, what do I expect the effect of factor 2 to be? When I change factor 1 to its high level, will the relationship between factor 2 and the response change? What will happen to that relationship when factor 1 is at its midpoint? Answers to these questions can help alias two-factor interactions that are unlikely to occur and thus make a smaller design more likely to identify meaningful interactions.

2.2.4 Fundamental Design Principles

There are three fundamental design principles that should always be considered, regardless of the chosen design.

Replication is the independent repetition of an experimental run and it is important for at least two reasons. First, it produces assurance that the response at the replicated combination can be reproduced and allows the experimenter to disregard assay variability as an explanation for unusual results. Second, having multiple measurements at a single combination provides replication variability, which has two advantages: (1) It provides a benchmark upon which to quantitatively determine which effects are greater than background noise, and (2) it permits the calculation of *p*-values for all main effects and interactions allowed by the design. Replication is most commonly implemented at the center point or target conditions.

Randomization is the process of assigning experimental units to factor combinations in a stochastic manner such that each unit has an equal chance of selection. When done properly, randomization removes or minimizes potential bias because specific factors or their combinations are not predisposed to a more or less desirable outcome. In every process or assay there are noise factors—variables that affect the response but cannot be directly measured—that impact the response. For example, the humidity or temperature at different locations in the laboratory may vary and be difficult to measure throughout the day. If temperature impacts an assay, its effects need to be minimized, eliminated, or at least balanced across the levels of each factor. If the effects cannot be measured, randomization helps prevent certain treatment combinations from being exposed to adverse temperatures that may prejudice the results. If the effects of these noise variables can be measured, other designs should be used that block or adjust for levels of the noise variables.

Blocking is the stratification of experimental runs into homogeneous units (for example, locations, instruments, time periods, environmental conditions) and can be applied on either noise variables or factors included in the design. Blocking should be applied whenever a factor is known to vary from experiment to experiment and its effect cannot be controlled. For example, if a set of older bioreactors in the lab are known to give different results than a set of reactors purchased more recently, it will be undesirable to run all conditions at the low level of one factor in the old reactors and all conditions at the high level of the factor in the new reactors because the effect of the factor will be confounded with the effect of reactor type. Conversely, when a factor is known to impact the response but is hard to vary, other experimental designs are necessary that will control the effects of this blocking factor. The split-plot design is commonly used in this situation.

2.3 Design Building Blocks

Whether your objective is screening, characterization, or optimization, classical DOE uses factorial or fractional factorial designs. It is imperative to understand the building blocks that go into these designs.

2.3.1 Design Notation

Before we discuss designs and how to choose them, it's important to introduce some notation. In DOE the most common designs and the basis for more sophisticated designs are the two-level factorial and fractional factorial. In these designs, the number of combinations is represented by 2^k for factorials and 2^{k-p} for fractional factorials. The superscript k is the number of factors being studied, and p refers to the fraction studied (1 = ½ fraction, 2 = ¼ fraction, 3 = ⅛ fraction, etc.). The use of two-level studies is common with DOE because experience has shown that most outputs have a linear relationship with the factors, as long as the factor levels are close enough together. For outputs with a quadratic or nonlinear relationship within the factor ranges under consideration, alternative designs are available, which will be discussed in Section 2.4.4.

TABLE 2.1

Factorial Design with Three Levels of A and Four
Levels of B

Level of Factor A	Level of Factor B
L1	L1
L1	L2
L1	L3
L1	L4
L2	L1
L2	L2
L2	L3
L2	L4
L3	L1
L3	L2
L3	L3
L3	L4

2.3.2 Factorial Designs

In a full factorial design, each level of each factor is combined with all other levels of all other factors. For example, if factor A has three levels and factor B has four, there are $3 \times 4 = 12$ combinations in the factorial design (see Table 2.1 as an example). Obviously, if one wishes to study many factors with many levels, the number of combinations in a factorial design will become very large. Except in situations when experimentation is inexpensive, these designs are typically only used with no more than three factors at two to three levels each.

2.3.3 2^{k-p} Fractional Factorial Designs

The basis for most designs used in biotechnology process development is the 2^{k-p} fractional factorial. As mentioned earlier, the 2 refers to the number of levels for each factor, k is the total number of factors, and p is the fraction of the two-level full factorial in the experiment. For example, if $p = 1$, it is a ½ fractional design; $p = 2$, a ¼ fractional design; $p = 3$, a ⅛ fractional design, and so forth. As the name implies, this design uses a fraction of a full factorial that is created in a systematic fashion that allows certain terms to be estimated independently of other terms. It is important to reiterate that the fraction is not chosen in a haphazard manner. This design has proven to be useful because it often identifies the key factors or their interactions without the need for the entire set of factorial combinations. Of course, taking a fraction of the factorial design means that some meaningful effects might not be identified, or what is called *aliasing*. Aliasing occurs because the formula for calculating the effect of one model term is exactly the same as that for another model term due to running too few factor combinations to separate the effects. The challenge then is to choose a design that is large enough to answer the questions of interest without aliasing meaningful effects but small enough to be feasible with the available resources. This challenge can be met using the principle of resolution.

Resolution refers to the degree of aliasing. In Resolution III designs, main effects are aliased with two-factor interactions and these designs are used for screening studies. Resolution IV designs have main effects aliased with three-factor interactions and two-factor interactions aliased with other two-factor interactions. Because the default assumption is that three-factor interactions are extremely unlikely, Resolution IV designs are often used in practice for characterization and optimization designs. If the analysis shows that additional runs are needed, the designs are augmented to include the fraction that will allow other effects to be estimated. Resolution V designs include two-level full factorial designs and fractional factorials that have main effects completely unaliased with two-factor interactions. In these designs, two-factor interactions are aliased with three-factor interactions. Fractional factorials are almost always able to identify the critical factors. While Resolution V designs are the gold standard for characterization and optimization, it is our experience that Resolution IV designs are often sufficient in CMC due to the sparsity-of-effects principle discussed previously. Table 2.2 shows the number of runs that must be performed with a given number of factors to achieve each level of resolution.

Two-level fractional and full factorial designs are usually created and analyzed using coded levels. The following formula shows how to perform the coding (denoted by z), with x as the studied level in scientific units, midpoint as the average between the high and low levels of x, and range as the difference between the high and low levels of x.

$$\text{Coded level for factor } z = \frac{x - midpoint}{range}$$

This coding puts the factorial points of each factor on a scale from −1 (low level) to +1 (high level). Using the coded levels in the analysis eliminates the potential of disparate units to distort the true effects. From a practical sense, coded factors makes it easy to determine the model terms that have the greatest effect within the studied ranges by examining their coefficients, which represent the change in the response when moving from the center of the design space to the −1 or +1 design edges.

Examples of Resolution III, IV, and V fractional factorial designs are shown in Tables 2.3, 2.4, and 2.5, respectively. Each factor is represented by a letter and factors that are aliased with other factor combinations are shown with an "=" sign, followed by the aliasing pattern. The designs in these tables are shown in what is called the standard form, that is, the way the designs were created before computers and before randomization. The astute reader will notice that each factor has an equal number of "+1" and "−1" signs and that there is a distinct pattern of alternating signs in the factors that are not aliased. Because modern software produces this design automatically we won't go into the derivation of these designs, but we will indicate that a fractional factorial is not unique. Other aliasing

TABLE 2.2

Resolution Matrix for Two-Level Fractional and Full Factorial Designs

| Runs | Number of Factors | | | | | | |
	2	3	4	5	6	7	8
4	2^2	2^{3-1} (III)					
8		2^3	2^{4-1} (IV)	2^{5-2} (III)	2^{6-3} (III)	2^{7-4} (III)	
16			2^4	2^{5-1} (V)	2^{6-2} (IV)	2^{7-3} (III)	2^{8-4} (III)
32				2^5	2^{6-1} (VI)	2^{7-2} (IV)	2^{8-3} (IV)
64					2^6	2^{7-1} (VII)	2^{8-2} (V)
128						2^7	2^{8-1} (VIII)
256							2^8

TABLE 2.3

Example of Resolution III 2^{6-3} ⅛ Fractional Factorial Design

A	B	C	D = AB	E = AC	F = BC
−1	−1	−1	+1	+1	+1
+1	−1	−1	−1	−1	+1
−1	+1	−1	−1	+1	−1
+1	+1	−1	+1	−1	−1
−1	−1	+1	+1	−1	−1
+1	−1	+1	−1	+1	−1
−1	+1	+1	−1	−1	+1
+1	+1	+1	+1	+1	+1

TABLE 2.4

Example of Resolution IV 2^{4-1} ½ Fractional Factorial Design

A	B	C	D = ABC
−1	−1	−1	−1
+1	−1	−1	+1
−1	+1	−1	+1
+1	+1	−1	−1
−1	−1	+1	+1
+1	−1	+1	−1
−1	+1	+1	−1
+1	+1	+1	+1

TABLE 2.5

Example of Resolution V 2^{5-1} ½ Fractional Factorial Design

A	B	C	D	E = ABCD
−1	−1	−1	−1	+1
+1	−1	−1	−1	−1
−1	+1	−1	−1	−1
+1	+1	−1	−1	+1
−1	−1	+1	−1	−1
+1	−1	+1	−1	+1
−1	+1	+1	−1	+1
+1	+1	+1	−1	−1
−1	−1	-1	+1	−1
+1	−1	−1	+1	+1
−1	+1	−1	+1	+1
+1	+1	−1	+1	−1
−1	−1	+1	+1	+1
+1	−1	+1	+1	−1
−1	+1	+1	+1	−1
+1	+1	+1	+1	+1

patterns could be chosen and this particular pattern was chosen based on convention. What is important to notice, however, is what happens when the columns constructed by aliasing are removed from the table. For example, in Table 2.3 this removal leaves three factors and eight runs and results in a full factorial in these three factors. Thus, if after analysis D, E, and F are determined to not be relevant, we have "projected" the Resolution III screening design into a full factorial. Notice that if A, B, and C are dropped from the table that the design is left with three factors and eight runs but that it is not a full factorial in D, E, and F. In fact, the only way to get a full factorial is by dropping the last three factors. If factors E and F can be removed, the designs projects into a Resolution IV design, which has two-factor interactions aliased with other two-factor interactions. If only factor F can be removed, the resulting design is still Resolution III but fewer interactions are aliased with main effects.

2.4 Choosing a Design

In this section we provide guidelines and insights into how to choose each type of design.

2.4.1 Screening Experiments

Strictly speaking, screening experiments are defined as Resolution III designs in which main effects are aliased with two-factor interactions. For an example, combinations are shown in Table 2.3 or displayed graphically in Figure 2.6. This aliasing means that if a main effect is shown to be important or statistically significant, it is unclear whether the interaction or main effect—or perhaps both!—are driving the observed effect. Additional experiments will be necessary to determine the real cause.

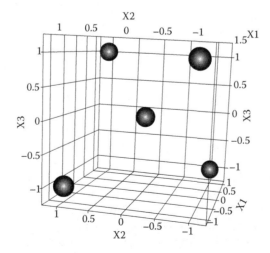

FIGURE 2.6
Graphical depiction of 2^{3-1} fractional factorial with center points. Four of eight potential factorial points were selected.

Screening designs are often fractional factorials, but other types of screening designs have been created.

The most common type of screening experiment is the Resolution III fractional factorial. These two-level designs require the number of runs to be a factor of 2^{k-p} and to be one greater than the number of factors. For example, three factors can be studied in four runs, seven factors in eight runs, fifteen in sixteen runs. While the experimental effort for completing eight runs may not be an obstacle for process or analytical method development experiments, an additional eight or sixteen runs may become prohibitive. For this reason, other types of screening designs were developed, of which the Plackett–Burman designs is the most well-known. In this design the number of runs is equal to a power of 4 (4, 8, 12, 16, 20, etc.). This additional flexibility allows experimenters to find a compromise between the 8 and 16 runs of a fractional factorial. These designs are most commonly used with the factors of 4 that do not appear with fractional factorials. The alias structure of these designs can be very messy, but the main effects are aliased with two-factor interactions as in the Resolution III fractional factorials.

Whatever design is used, we recommend adding center points to the number of runs already determined. This practice allows replication and provides a test for linearity between factors and responses. Center points are literally just what the name implies—the middle of each level of each factor is chosen such that they reside at the center of the design. Placing the point at the exact center allows the other effects to be orthogonal, or independent, of each other when the analysis is performed. When the target conditions are not at the exact center of the chosen ranges, the lack of orthogonality causes the effect estimates to change depending on which effects are in the model. Usually the bias introduced by slight modifications of the exact center point does not make the analysis overly difficult, but this feature should be recognized. We recommend running at the exact center when possible.

Up until now, we haven't differentiated between two-level designs for continuous or categorical factors because in the coded design the continuous levels are placed on a -1 to $+1$ scale so the analysis will be the same. However, for categorical factors, there is no exact center so there is a difference in how the design treats center points. In the case with only one categorical factor, the center point conditions for the remaining factors can be run at both levels of the categorical factor. This obviously doubles the number of center points needed to achieve the same level of replication—and with multiple categorical factors the number of center points greatly increases—so it may become difficult to obtain suitable replication when there is more than one categorical factor.

In addition to replication, center points add a third level to the factor ranges. Although we've chosen this third level for each factor, we run the center point condition at the third level for all the factors. Thus, the third level is not mutually independent and these designs are not considered true three-level designs. However, this shared third level is important because it allows us to test whether our assumption of a linear relationship between the high and low levels of each factor is valid. This test is called a test for curvature. Because the third level is shared, if significant, the test for linearity will not identify which factor is causing the curvature but indicates simply that the curvature is present for at least one factor. Additional optimization experiments will be necessary to understand which factors are causing the curvature. These principles are illustrated in Case Study 2.1.

CASE STUDY 2.1 SCREENING DESIGN FOR POTENCY ASSAY METHOD DEVELOPMENT

A cell-based potency assay is being developed to support lot release, product characterization, and stability testing. At a meeting with the research associates, the assay developer makes a list of six factors that the team believes may have the greatest impact on the reportable result. After an informal risk assessment, the team lists these factors in order of assumed priority: Cell density, sample incubation time, substrate concentration, substrate incubation time, biotinylation concentration, and biotinylation incubation time. After more discussion and based on some early assay development, the team agrees on the following target conditions (with low and high levels in parentheses): A cell density of 1E6 cells/ml (8.5E5–1.15E6), 30 minute sample incubation (20–40), substrate concentration of 5 mg/mL (4.5–5.5) with an incubation of 60 minutes (45–75), and a biotinylation concentration of 0.15 mg/mL (0.14–0.16) with an incubation time of 15 minutes (14–16). Their objective is to screen factors to determine which cause meaningful changes in relative potency within the studied ranges. Because they are most interested in identifying main effects, they decide to run a Resolution III 2^{6-3} fractional factorial design. They realize that due to aliasing a main effect could be indicative of an interaction but they also believe that at most three or four of the factors may be relevant. By ordering the most likely factors they hope to take advantage of the projection property of fractional factorials to unalias main effects from interactions. The factorial runs for their design were shown previously in Table 2.2. Because they can fit ten samples on a plate, they also add two center point conditions for a total of ten runs. Because they also want to estimate the precision of the assay, they decide to repeat the ten runs on two plates (one by each of two analysts) on each of three days. We typically recommended three to five replications of the center point but due to a desire to characterize the precision of the assay the team ran twelve.

2.4.2 Characterization Experiments

Characterization experiments refer to designs in which linear main effects and two-factor interactions can be determined without aliasing but for which quadratic or higher effects are not needed. If quadratic or higher effects are necessary, the optimization designs described in Section 2.4.3 are used. Characterization experiments are used for one main purpose: They allow optimization of a process or method when curvature is not present but interactions are. In some circumstances they are also used to test the robustness of process or analytical method parameters.

There are two main ways to run a characterization experiment. The simple way is to choose a Resolution V fractional factorial and add three to five center points to test for curvature as we described with screening designs. This ensures that two-factor interactions are not aliased with main effects, but this design may require more runs than is needed. The second, and perhaps more common, approach is to first run a Resolution III or IV screening design, analyze the results, and then augment the design (if necessary) to remove main effects aliased with two-factor interactions in the screening design. The advantage of this latter approach is the potential to eliminate the need for the characterization design. This elimination can occur because of the projection property of fractional factorials, as was discussed previously. This important

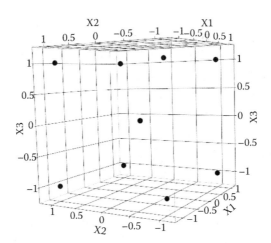

FIGURE 2.7
Graphical depiction of 2^3 factorial with center points.

property is utilized often by savvy DOE practitioners. Table 2.5 shows the combinations for a Resolution V characterization design and Figure 2.7 graphically depicts a full factorial.

Because of the potential gains used by this projection property, in practice many scientists prefer to run Resolution IV designs for screening or characterization, and with careful planning and a little luck, may be able to project that initial design into a Resolution V characterization design without aliasing. However, even if the projection property is not able to remove all aliasing, the design can still be augmented to achieve the desired design. Augmenting refers to the practice of adding runs that remove the aliasing from the two-factor interactions. We won't cover how to do this manually because modern software does it automatically. But as an intuitive explanation, the way to augment a one-half fractional Resolution IV design is to choose the other fraction that would complete the full factorial. This common approach of augmenting a fractional factorial design is called a *fold-over*. Case Study 2.2 illustrates a screening design that projects into a characterization design.

CASE STUDY 2.2   CELL CULTURE ROBUSTNESS DESIGN

A bioprocess engineer was responsible for developing a cell culture process and decided to design an experiment in bioreactors. She had already screened several factors, performed other experiments to fine-tune process parameter ranges, and determined that the titer of the process was approximately 2 grams per liter. Although not as high as she hoped, the program was moving forward and she needed to lock in the parameters of her process.

Although she had some preliminary data, some of the factor ranges had been changed from the screening experiment. She decided to run a robustness experiment on the four factors that had been shown to be most important. The purpose of this experiment was to vary the factor levels over a relatively small window to assess whether minor changes to the process could prove detrimental.

After thawing the working cell bank vial and passaging the cells through shake flasks and a seed bioreactor, cells were transferred to a 3L bioreactor for the 14-day short fill and production stages. A 2^{4-1} fractional factorial was chosen to evaluate the effect of temperature (target: 36.5°C; limits 35°C and 38°C), viable cell density (target: 1.8×10^6 cells/mL; limits 1.6 and 2.0×10^6), pH (target: 7; limits 6.8 and 7.2), and volume of feed media on day 7 (target: 6%; limits 4 and 8%). This Resolution IV design aliases two-factor interactions with other two-factor interactions but not with main effects. Screening experiments are sometimes used for robustness experiments because it is assumed that two-factor interactions are not present at the factor levels chosen. In this case the engineer and her team had enough bioreactors for the larger experiment and wanted to ensure that main effects were unaliased with two-factor interactions. The team also decided to add two replicates at the center point conditions. This had two purposes: First, it allowed the confirmation of whether the relationship between the low and high levels of each factor was linear, something that is preferable to do during the screening experiments; and second, it provides an estimate of the experimental variability. Because she had used replication in previous experiments, this replication will confirm what she had observed previously and will provide a check on the validity of the results. In total, she will study nine conditions in ten runs as shown previously in Table 2.4.

2.4.3 Optimization Experiments

In the strictest definition, optimization experiments are designs that optimize the response surface of two or more factors from a model with quadratic or higher order effects. When quadratic effects are not needed, the optimization that is performed is done with a characterization design. Optimization designs are often called *response surface designs* because the model allows the scientist to explore the curved surface of each response. The two main types of response surface methodology (RSM) designs are the central composite (CCD) and Box–Behnken. The CCD is used most commonly because it is an extension of a two-level full or fractional factorial design. The CCD can be implemented either directly or by augmenting a screening or characterization design. Examples are shown in Table 2.5 and Figure 2.8. The Box–Behnken design is a three-level design that may be preferred in rare situations of higher level interactions.

RSM designs have a variety of purposes. If an initial design has demonstrated curvature, one purpose is to understand which factors are causing the curvature.

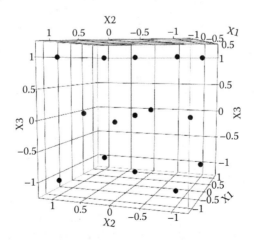

FIGURE 2.8
Graphical depiction of 2^3 face-centered central composite design.

Another purpose for these designs is to explore the entire design space and find the factor levels that produce the optimal response. Sometimes these designs are also used to find the edge of failure and gain a better understanding of the robustness of certain levels. Due to the relatively larger number of runs required to characterize curvature and explore the design space, these designs are typically only run with a few factors.

RSM designs provide, at a minimum, three independent levels. The additional levels of the CCD are called axial points and the mathematically optimal number of levels and spacing of these points is based on achieving orthogonality and rotatability (ensuring that the precision at a specified distance from the center is the same for the entire design space). Modern software will perform these calculations and typically four independent levels in addition to the shared center point are chosen. However, four or five independent levels are often more than is needed because three levels provide the ability to determine quadratic effects and most designs have factor levels spaced close enough together that cubic and higher order polynomial terms are not relevant. For these reasons, a face-centered CCD is often used in bioprocess development. This design puts the additional points on the face of a cube, as shown in Case Study 2.3.

CASE STUDY 2.3: ANTIBODY PURIFICATION OPTIMIZATION DESIGN

An antibody purification group is trying to optimize a chromatography process to maximize the yield and minimize the aggregate level of the antibody. After performing an initial screening experiment and analyzing the data, the group determined that three factors—pH, concentration of NaCl in the elution buffer, and conductivity—appeared to be scientifically relevant. After removing unimportant factors from the analysis, they are left with eight factorial runs in these three factors as well as two center points. Using the projection property of fractional factorials, the resulting design is a full factorial. However, this screening study also showed that curvature was present. To determine the factors which produce the curvature as well as map the entire response surface, the group augmented the full factorial with axial points to complete a central composite design. The group initially planned to do a face-centered CCD, but after analyzing the data from the screening experiment they wanted to reduce the ranges for some factors. Thus, they ran the axial points with narrower ranges for the elution buffer and conductivity. This strategy provides four independent levels of each of these factors in addition to the center point. The group decided to perform eight additional runs: Six axial points and two additional center points. After collecting the data, they will split the first set of experiments into one block and the second set of experiments into another block. This blocking will ensure that differences between the two sets of experiments will be accounted for in the analysis. The eighteen runs of the augmented design are shown in standard order (not randomized) in Table 2.6. Notice that the axial points consist of running two independent levels of each factor at the shared center point of the other two factors.

TABLE 2.6

Optimization Design for Case Study 2.3

Block	pH	NaCl Elution Buffer (mM)	Conductivity (mS/cm)
1	5.7	70	5
1	6.3	70	5
1	5.7	110	5
1	6.3	110	5
1	5.7	70	9
1	6.3	70	9
1	5.7	110	9
1	6.3	110	9
1	6.0	90	7
1	6.0	90	7
2	5.7	90	7
2	6.3	90	7
2	6.0	80	7
2	6.0	100	7
2	6.0	90	6
2	6.0	90	8
2	6.0	90	7
2	6.0	90	7

2.4.4 Advantages and Disadvantages of the Classical Approach

For over 50 years, the classical approach of two-level fractional factorials and response surface designs has been used to improve and optimize an innumerable number of processes in many types of industries. These designs have proven to be successful because they are easy to design and analyze, estimate interactions and curvature with a reasonable number of experiments, and are a great improvement over one-factor-at-a-time experimentation. However, these designs suffer from the disadvantage of not being flexible in the number of factorial runs. Indeed, two-level designs are typically only feasible in factors of 4, 8, 16, and 32. What if your budget or material constraints allow you to make six or ten runs but you still want the main effects to be unaliased with two-factor interactions? This situation arises frequently and is often overcome in the classical design setting by using the projection property, sparsity-of-effects principle, and scientific knowledge. Groundbreaking work done in the early 2010s provided a new approach that may become the future of industrial experimentation. This approach is called *definitive screening designs* (Jones and Nachtsheim, 2011) and in Chapter 3 we'll show how these techniques overcome inflexibility of classical DOE in the context of formulation development.

2.5 Analyzing a Single Response

2.5.1 Linear Regression Fundamentals

The statistician George Box famously wrote, "Essentially, all models are wrong, but some are useful" (Box and Draper, 1987). Also attributed to him is this quote: "All experiments are designed, most poorly." By now, we hope you have executed a well-designed experiment. In most cases, a well-designed experiment leads to a straight-forward analysis. The experiments we have designed will all be analyzed using statistical models, specifically linear regression models. These models are empirical and are intended to provide a good approximation to the observed data. Although using functional equations is sometimes possible, the empirical models we will discuss are not intended to describe a physical, chemical, or biological mechanistic phenomenon and are intended in the spirit that Box described: They are useful models to describe the observed relationship between the response and factors over the studied range. We next present the linear regression model, how it is fit, and its primary requirements (usually called assumptions). Then we show how to perform the analysis for each type of study.

2.5.2 Linear Regression Model

A linear regression model includes a response, model parameters, variables, and error term. A main effects model with two factors and a two-factor interaction is written as shown below.

$$y = \beta_0 + \beta_1 z_1 + \beta_2 z_2 + \beta_{12} z_1 z_2 + \varepsilon$$

In this equation, the response is denoted by y, the model parameters (an intercept, two slopes, and a plane) by β_0, β_1, β_2, and β_{12}, the coded factors by z_1 and z_2, and the error term by ε. First notice that the response is an additive function of each of these terms. You'll also notice that the parameters and error are denoted by Greek letters, which is standard notation. The letters from the English alphabet represent constants for each run and are considered to be measured without error. The parameters are estimated by finding the regression line that minimizes the sum of squared deviations between the observed data and the predicted values. Perhaps this can best be illustrated through an example of a poorly fitting regression line. Figure 2.9 demonstrates a linear regression fit by least squares that clearly misses the observed data. But what this figure also demonstrates is that the regression line is positioned to minimize the squared residuals, and thus provides a fit that splits the difference between the observed values at its

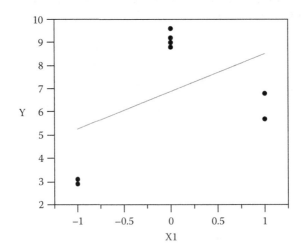

FIGURE 2.9
Linear regression fit by least squares without needed quadratic term.

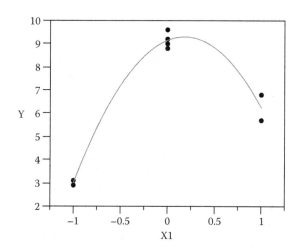

FIGURE 2.10
Linear regression fit by least squares with quadratic term.

three levels. Figure 2.10 shows the fit when a quadratic term is added to the model and the equation now passes through the center of the points at each level. The model results are valid when the residuals are independent, normally distributed, and have constant variance across the value of each factor, but also assume that the correct model has been chosen.

For designed experiments, the variables z_1 and z_2 are the coded variables as described in Section 2.3.3. Because the coded variables subtract the midpoint of the factor range, the intercept (β_0) represents the mean response at the center point. The parameters of the main effects represent the change in the response for every one unit increase in the *coded variables* when the other variables are held constant. For example, if we are trying to predict the viable cell density (VCD) as a function of temperature (z_1; range 31–35°C with a midpoint of 33°C) and culture day (z_2; range 4–10 days with a midpoint of 7 days), β_1 represents the change in VCD as the temperature is increased from 31 to 33°C or 33 to 35°C, which are both one unit increases in the coded variables. Similarly, β_2 represents the change in VCD as the culture day is increased from four to seven days or from seven to ten days. When the observed data are collected and analyzed, the parameters will be estimated and their standard error and p-value will be calculated. When the model assumptions are met, estimates of regression parameters follow a t-distribution with degrees of freedom obtained from the error term.

2.5.3 Model Fitting

Linear regression models are fit using ordinary least squares. As already described, this method minimizes the squared distances between the observed data points and the predicted model. The default output from a regression model is an analysis of variance table that shows the partitioning of variability into the variation attributed to the model terms and the variation generically called the error term. As we'll show later, the error term is composed of different terms. In addition, estimates for the model parameters are calculated that can be used to create a predictive model for each response. While this approach is mathematically optimal with normally distributed data, outliers or extreme points can cause misleading estimates of the parameters. For this reason we next discuss the assumptions made by the model and how to evaluate these assumptions.

2.5.4 Model Assumptions

As stated above, all models are wrong in the sense that the empirical model is an approximation of the unknown (and perhaps unknowable) mechanistic model. It is therefore critical to ensure that the chosen model fits the observed data adequately to act as a surrogate for a mechanistic model. If the model does not properly fit the observed data, inferences from the data will be misleading. The critical assumption for the model described in Section 2.5.2 involves the error term. The model requires the errors to be independent and normally distributed with a mean of 0 and constant variance of σ^2. These requirements mean that data points should be roughly balanced above and below the regression line with equal spread along the entire length of the line.

Of these assumptions, violations of independence and constant variance have a greater impact on statistical inference than data that are not perfectly normally distributed. The assumption of independence is best verified at the design execution. Experimental runs should be randomized and design features that would introduce correlation—the likelihood of getting similar responses for some runs—should be eliminated. Sometimes correlation is inevitable—such as when certain runs are performed in a homogeneous environment but other runs are not—and then a different type of experimental design is needed. Examples of these designs are randomized complete block designs and split-plot designs. Constant variance is most often verified using a plot of the residuals vs. predicted values from the model. The plot should show an absence of a pattern. Fan-shaped patterns in which the spread of the residuals is larger for larger values of the predicted values indicate that the variance is not constant over the range of one or more factors. Often, a transformation of the response will provide the solution to make the model fit the observed data better. A logarithmic transformation is the most common method of transformation. Figures 2.11 and 2.12 show examples of residual plots that indicate satisfactory agreement with model assumptions. Although not perfect, the spread of residuals for each predicted value in Figure 2.11 is an example of a common pattern that indicates that variances are generally homogeneous. In Figure 2.12 the residuals follow closely the line of normality and all are contained within the confidence intervals and thus agree with the normality assumption.

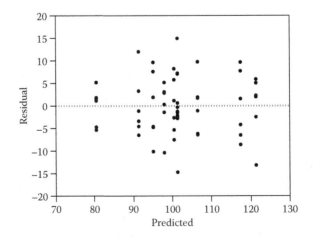

FIGURE 2.11
Plot of residuals vs. predicted values.

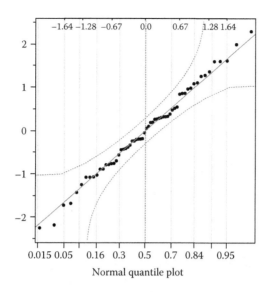

FIGURE 2.12
Normal probability plot of residuals.

If best practices have been followed and the experiment has been designed with replication, the error is composed of two terms, pure (or replication) error and lack-of-fit error. Pure error is the variability from replicates. Lack-of-fit error refers to the variability from terms that could be included in the model but weren't because they were judged to not be important. Lack-of-fit for these terms can be tested using the sums of squares from the pure error. We'll show an example of this later. Another source of error is the variability in the response due to unmeasured variables. We will not cover this topic here but the reader should note that a poorly fitting model can be due to variables that have not been measured.

2.5.5 Statistical Analysis for Screening Experiments

In screening experiments the focus is on identifying the main effects that influence the process. A normal probability plot is often the first tool used to identify statistically relevant effects. This is primarily due to its ability to identify effects without needing p-values. Screening designs often have low numbers of replicates, and so there may be low power to detect effects. The normal probability plot can identify potential effects without a statistical test.

We begin with an intuitive description of a normal probability plot. Imagine a hypothetical, large screening study of a pretend process with 100 factors, of which only four are statistically significant. Now imagine running the experiment, calculating the main effects for each factor, and then creating a histogram. If the actual experiment produced results that were true to the theoretical nature of the process, 96 of the effects would constitute noise and would lie in a symmetric pattern within approximately plus or minus two standard deviations of zero. These "noise effects" indicate no difference between the high and low levels of the factor. Four of the effects would lie more than two standard deviations from 0 and these could be clearly seen as outliers in the histogram. A probability plot takes this concept of a normally distributed histogram of the effects and puts it onto a linear

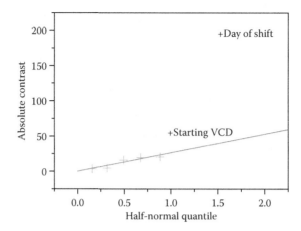

FIGURE 2.13
Half-normal probability plot from screening study.

scale. It plots the effect of each term in the statistical model on the y-axis and the expected random variation from a normal distribution without any effects on the x-axis. A straight line is applied to the plot to indicate where the observed effects should fall if they come from a normal distribution due to only random variation. In other words, effects that lie on the line are assumed to not be statistically relevant because they follow a normal distribution while effects that lie off the line may be important because they are aberrations from a theoretical normal distribution, and constitute a statistically relevant departure. The degree of departure is a subjective evaluation without a statistical criterion.

There are two types of these plots. A normal probability plot graphs effects based on their actual value while a half-normal plot conveys the same information by graphing the absolute value of the effects. Figure 2.13 shows an example of such a plot. The "+" symbols that deviate far from the line represent terms in the model that may be statistically relevant. Those that lie on the line are no different than random variation.

This plot is especially useful in situations where there is no replicate variability. Without replication, statistical hypothesis testing cannot be performed and thus p-values for the main effects cannot be generated. Because the effects that lie on the line are considered noise, it is possible to remove those terms from the model and add them to the error term. Although no-replication designs have been used successfully, replicate variability is always preferred over this so-called lack-of-fit error because it gives a better estimate.

After determining relevant effects from the probability plot, these effects can be added to a statistical model to estimate the magnitude of the effect and get p-values. Fundamentals of the linear regression analysis were covered in Sections 2.5.2 through 2.5.4.

CONTINUATION OF CASE STUDY 2.1: SCREENING DESIGN FOR POTENCY ASSAY METHOD DEVELOPMENT

In Section 2.4.1 we designed a Resolution III 2^{6-3} fractional factorial with two center points. Each condition was replicated in duplicate on each of three days. After running the experiment it's time to analyze the data.

First, let's look more in-depth at how the projection property of fractional factorials works so we can understand why we might want to remove all irrelevant terms in the model. Recall the six factors that were listed in order of priority: Cell density, sample incubation time, substrate concentration, substrate incubation time, biotinylation concentration, and biotinylation incubation time. Let's say we represent these factors using the letters A–F, respectively. Table 2.7 shows the eight-run Resolution III screening study that the team designed using the coded levels that we introduced earlier, shown here as + for 1 and – for –1. The center points are not shown but they are denoted by 0 for each factor. The design generators, or how the fractional factorial is created for D, E, and F, are also shown in the column heading. Because the levels of D, E, and F are a function of the levels of other factors, we have introduced aliasing. In particular, the main effect D is aliased with the two-factor interaction A*B, E is aliased with A*C, and F with B*C. Note that in addition to D being aliased with A*B, A is also aliased with B*D and B is aliased with A*D.

If the main effects and interactions for particular factors are determined not to be scientifically or statistically relevant to the experimental objectives after data has been analyzed, these factors can be removed from the analysis. If the irrelevant factors have been strategically designated at the end of the alphabetical list, the initial design will have fewer factors but with the same number of runs. This allows the design to be "projected" into a design of higher resolution.

For example, let's assume that after the experimental data are analyzed only the first three factors denoted A, B, and C are statistically and scientifically relevant. If we cover the last three columns from the table we see that the remaining design is a full factorial in the remaining three factors. Thus, the Resolution III design has been projected into Resolution V with interactions and main effects completely unaliased. Similarly, if A, B, C, and D are found to be relevant but E and F are not, the remaining design is a Resolution IV 2^{4-1} ½ fractional factorial.

With this background, let's look at the statistical analysis. This screening design is unusual because there is substantial replication. Although we could have used a normal probability plot, we'll jump right into a statistical model.

Because we tested nine unique combinations, the model can have up to nine terms. We'll start by adding the six main effects which leaves us with the ability to add three more terms. One of the nine terms is reserved to estimate lack-of-fit of a linear

TABLE 2.7

Screening Design for Case Study 2.1

A	B	C	D = AB	E = AC	F = BC
–	–	–	+	+	+
+	–	–	–	–	+
–	+	–	–	+	–
+	+	–	+	–	–
–	–	+	+	–	–
+	–	+	–	+	–
–	+	+	–	–	+
+	+	+	+	+	+

TABLE 2.8

Parameter Estimates from Initial Model for Case Study 2.1

Model Term	Estimate	*p*-value
Intercept	101.3	<0.0001
Cell density	7.3	<0.0001
Sample incubation time	9.5	<0.0001
Substrate concentration	3.6	0.0004
Substrate incubation time	1.3	0.17
Biotinylation concentration	−1.3	0.19
Biotinylation incubation time	−0.5	0.62
Substrate concentration * Substrate incubation time	0.1	0.89

model while another is used for the intercept. After this accounting, this means we can include one other model term. We'll add any two-factor interaction that is not aliased. In this case, we choose substrate concentration × substrate incubation time.

The coefficients of each factor and *p*-value are shown in Table 2.8. Three main effects were found to have small *p*-values: cell density, sample incubation time, and substrate concentration. Notice that the larger estimates have the smallest *p*-values. This pattern will always be the case: The larger the estimate, the greater the effect, and the smaller the *p*-value. Recall that the estimate is the mean difference in %RP for a one-unit increase in the coded variables. This increase is equivalent to moving from the low level to the center point or the center point to the high level. In this case, the coefficient (estimate and coefficient are often used interchangeably) of 9.5 for sample incubation time means that the %RP increased 9.5% as sample incubation time was increased from its center point to its high level (equivalently, the low level to the center point). The value of 9.5 is the largest coefficient of the main effects, which means that sample incubation time has the largest effect across its studied levels of the six factors within the tested ranges. This large effect means that the allowable sample incubation time for the assay will need to be tightened to ensure that different times do not provide vastly different %RP results for the same sample. The other coefficients can be interpreted in a similar fashion. Notice that the model coefficient for substrate concentration is statistically significant but its effect of 3.6 is about 40% of the largest effect. After discussion, the team decided that such a small difference in the %RP may not be practically important. The significance for this main effect is due to having six replicates of each condition. As the number of replicates increases, there is increased statistical power to find significant effects that may not be scientifically relevant. It is ideal to choose the number of replicates based on a statistical power analysis, but this requires an a priori estimate of the replicate variability, which can be difficult to estimate in screening experiments. In cases where a power analysis cannot be performed, we recommend using statistical significance as a guide to selecting meaningful main effects and using the magnitude of the coefficients and their confidence intervals as the primary way to determine meaningful effects.

Recall, however, that the screening design in this case study is a Resolution III fractional factorial in which main effects are aliased with two-factor interactions.

This means that the main effects identified by the linear regression model may not actually be causing the observed effect and may be caused by two-factor interactions. Because three of the main effects were not significant, dropping these from the analysis and analyzing a full factorial in the three significant main effects could help us unalias the interactions, but it's only recommended if the team has confidence that those interactions are unlikely to occur. Let's now create a new model that includes the three significant main effects of cell density, sample incubation time, and substrate concentration, and add their two- and three-factor interactions. The estimates and *p*-values for this model are shown in Table 2.9.

Notice that the estimates and the *p*-values are exactly the same as Table 2.8! The only difference is the model term. This is what happens when two model terms are aliased—due to the experimental design, the formulas to calculate the estimates are exactly the same so we can't determine which is causing the effect. So the effect we previously attributed to substrate incubation time is equivalent to that due to the cell density*sample incubation time interaction. Which one is causing the effect. Similarly, the strong main effect we attributed to sample incubation time could be due to the two-factor interaction of cell density and substrate incubation time. Which one is it? Due to aliasing, we can't tell for sure, and it actually could be a combination of the two. Some statisticians assume—which is not 100% reliable but a good rule-of-thumb—that a significant interaction has at least one significant main effect. This example highlights the advantages and disadvantages of screening designs. We have learned which main effects appear to be relevant—but we can't have absolute certainty due to the aliasing. If we make strong assumptions about the absence of three main effects and all their interactions, we can project the design into a higher resolution and gain valuable information. But that information comes at the cost of not further considering potentially aliased effects. The subject matter expertise of the team will be crucial in this stage. After huddling together and considering the mechanism of action of the molecule and other assay properties, the team decided that an interaction between cell density and substrate incubation time was unlikely, and decided to assume that the results they observed were due solely to the main effects in Table 2.9. If the aliasing with this type of design leaves you troubled, you will want to use either other designs that do not have aliasing.

TABLE 2.9

Parameter Estimates from Final Model for Case Study 2.1

Model Term	Estimate	*p*-value
Intercept	101.3	<0.0001
Cell density	7.3	<0.0001
Sample incubation time	9.5	<0.0001
Substrate concentration	3.6	0.0004
Cell density*sample incubation time	1.3	0.17
Cell density*substrate concentration	−1.3	0.19
Sample incubation time*substrate concentration	−0.5	0.62
Cell density*sample incubation time*substrate concentration	0.1	0.89

Before we leave this example, we should examine the curvature. As described in Sections 2.1.1 and 2.5.4, lack-of-fit error is the variability attributed to terms that could be added to the model but were not. These lack-of-fit terms can be evaluated in aggregate to determine if one or more should be added to the model. So, for example, if we had decided to leave out cell density and its interactions, those terms would be considered lack-of-fit error terms. We could test these terms against the residual variability to determine if they needed to be included in the model. In this example, the design included two center points on each of six plates for a total of twelve replicated center points. The model thus allows us to estimate a quadratic effect, what is commonly called curvature. Because the center point is at the mid-point of all factors, we can't tell which factor(s) is causing the curvature. So the curvature test is whether the center point does not fall along the linear pattern defined by the means at the high and low levels of each factor. In this case, Table 2.10 contains the lack-of-fit p-value of 0.88, which indicates that the model does not have significant curvature because it is much greater than the default significance level of 0.05. This result means that we will not need to use an optimization design to explore the response surface because the optimal region will be between the high and low levels of the factors. Figure 2.14 shows the %RP on the y-axis vs. cell density on the x-axis. In this example, there is no lack-of-fit because the regression line passes through the center of each level of cell density. Lack-of-fit would have been demonstrated by a regression line that did not pass through the average of the center points.

TABLE 2.10

Lack-of-Fit for Curvature

Source	DF	Sums of Squares	Mean Squares	F Ratio	p-value
Lack of Fit	1	1.05	1.05	0.024	0.88
Pure Error	51	2253.39	44.18		
Total Error	52	2254.44			

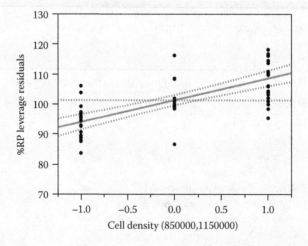

FIGURE 2.14
No lack-of-fit in regression.

2.5.6 Statistical Analysis for Characterization Experiments

After determining important factors in the screening phase, we move to characterization experiments to learn about their interactions. These characterization experiments differ from those for screening in at least two important ways: (1) They should include replication, preferably with three to five replicates, so experimental variability can be estimated, and (2) the designs are Resolution V, so there is no aliasing of main effects or two-way interactions with other lower-order terms. Because of these differences, the normal probability plot typically is not used because analysis can be performed using a statistical model. While the basics of running a linear regression model for characterization designs are the same as for screening designs, we'll provide some additional insight. Importantly, the effects in the statistical model can be interpreted as a causal effect for those very terms—no need to worry about potential aliasing. As we've already pointed out, these characterization experiments can either be designed as a stand-alone experiment or from a fortuitous screening study. We'll now present an example of an analysis of a screening experiment that turns into a characterization experiment.

CONTINUATION OF CASE STUDY 2.2: CELL CULTURE ROBUSTNESS DESIGN

In Case Study 2.2, a 2^{4-1} fractional factorial design was created to assess the robustness on titer of four factors. The experiment was subsequently executed and data were generated from ten runs, including the eight factorial runs and two center points to provide replicate variability. With ten runs there are ten estimable quantities. Because there are two replicate points of the center point, one of the estimable quantities is the replicate variability, or also sometimes called *pure error*. Nine other effects are estimable: An intercept, the four main effects, three two-factor interactions, and a curvature term. Recall that two-factor interactions are aliased with other two-factor interactions in this Resolution IV design.

The design of this study is a Resolution IV screening design in which main effects are aliased with three-factor interactions, terms that we often assume are negligible unless there is a strong reason to suspect otherwise. Although having replicates allows us to calculate p-values, there are only two so our estimate may not be robust, and we decide to begin the analysis using a normal probability plot, shown in Figure 2.15. In this case, three effects are highlighted: Temperature, viable cell density, and pH, although the departure from the line of normality for the latter two is very slight. Because no interactions are visible, this plot clearly shows that our focus should be on the three main effects.

After looking at the clear evidence that only three main effects appear to be relevant, we move to an analysis from a linear regression model. For illustration purposes, we'll first keep all the estimable factors in the model. The estimates are shown in Table 2.11. You'll first notice that the lack-of-fit is not significant, with a p-value of 0.52. It appears that a linear relationship is sufficient to describe all of the main effects and interactions in the model. Notice that all three two-factor interactions have large p-values, which is what we expected from the normal probability plot. In addition, the estimates of these interactions are essentially 0. This is strong evidence that there are no interactions with these four factors. Because none of these interactions is significant—and recall these are aliased with other two-factor interactions—we'll assume the three- and

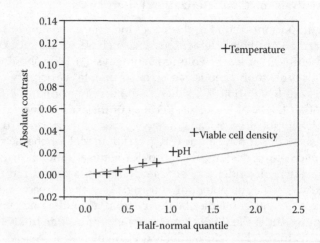

FIGURE 2.15
Half-normal probability plot for robustness design.

TABLE 2.11

Parameter Estimates from Initial Model of Case Study 2.2

Model Term	Estimate	*p*-value
Intercept	1.90	<0.0001
Temperature	0.13	0.009
Viable Cell Density	−0.044	0.069
pH	0.024	0.19
Vol Feed Media	−0.004	0.79
Temp*VCD#	0.001	0.93
Temp*pH#	−0.001	0.93
Temp*Vol Feed Media#	0.1	0.89
Lack of Fit	–	0.52

#—Aliased with another two-factor interaction.

four-factor interactions are also not significant. This leaves us with four main effects. Temperature—as the team suspected—is clearly significant and has an estimate of 0.13. This means that moving from the center point to the highest temperature resulted in an increase in titer of 0.13 g/mL. This small increase is expected and does not concern the team. If the bioreactor fluctuates on the higher end more than expected but within the upper range of 38°C, they will get slightly higher titer, but even if temperatures tends to be on the low end, the titer is sufficient to supply the clinical program.

We'll remove the model terms with large *p*-values, which results in removing all interactions and the volume of feed media main effect. This action leaves us with a Resolution V design, or a characterization experiment. Let's examine this process more carefully. First, in removing the four terms we are left with four estimable quantities in the model: an intercept and three main effects. Recall that we could estimate up to nine model terms. What happens to the four terms that we've removed? The answer is that they go into the error term. The error term is now made up of pure error (or replicate variability), these additional four terms, and the curvature term. Note that this is only appropriate if the interaction and curvature terms are essentially 0—mimicking the noise of the process. Sometimes we call the terms thrown into the error lack-of-fit, a term that we introduced earlier when testing for curvature. The same principle applies—we can test the appropriateness of this decision by testing all the terms put into the residual against the pure error. With only one degree of freedom for the pure error, our estimates are likely not that robust. Hopefully you can see from this discussion the value of replicates!

After removing the interactions and feed media main effect, the lack-of-fit p-value is 0.90 with five degrees of freedom (see Table 2.12). Assuming that the error variability is representative of what truly would happen with more replicates, this p-value provides clear evidence that none of these terms is needed in our model. The model estimates for the main effects are shown in Table 2.12. Notice that the estimates are identical to those in the previous table but the p-values are not. Why did this happen? Recall that we ran the center points at the exact center level of each factor. Recall also that we designed the experiment with an equal number of low and high levels for each factor in a systematic pattern. Although it wasn't apparent then, because of these two facts the model terms in the design we created are orthogonal to each other. This means that regardless of the terms in the model, we'll get the same estimates. The p-values, however, are different. This occurs because we took the interaction terms and one main effect and put them into the error term. In this case, the p-values all decreased. This decrease can be attributed to these four additional terms providing less variation than the pure error, and thus decreasing the total estimate of replicate variability. A rule of thumb is that variability cannot be estimated well until a minimum of six replicates are observed. The engineer went back to her estimate of pure error from previous experiments and determined that it was 0.00065, only slightly higher than the 0.00054 from the estimate of residual variability from this experiment, but considerably lower than the 0.0013 estimate of pure error from the two replicates in this experiment. Experience across many decades has shown the value of three to five replicates in an industrial setting to estimate experimental variability.

In this case, temperature, viable cell density, and pH are all shown to be statistically significant. What the engineer learns is that although she has three significant main effects, the difference in titer between the low and high levels is low enough that she feels confident that she can run the process with the proposed ranges and get sufficient titer to supply clinical trials. It's important to note that the estimates from the model are the mean estimates and individual batches could be outside of the confidence interval of the mean.

TABLE 2.12

Parameter Estimates from Final Model of Case Study 2.2

Model Term	Estimate	p-value
Intercept	1.90	<0.0001
Temperature	0.13	<0.0001
Viable Cell Density	−0.044	0.0012
pH	0.024	0.021
Lack of Fit	–	0.90

2.5.7 Statistical Analysis for Optimization Experiments

The statistical analysis for optimization experiments depends entirely on a statistical model. In these Resolution V or greater experiments, no aliasing is present but curvature needs to be estimated for each factor. The correct modeling of the curvature depends on having a quadratic term for each term (or rarely, an even higher order polynomial term) in the model. Whereas characterization experiments employ only linear terms, finding the optimal point with curvature requires a polynomial term. The general form of determining the correct model follows the same process as that for a characterization study.

**CONTINUATION OF CASE STUDY 2.3: ANTIBODY
PURIFICATION OPTIMIZATION DESIGN**

Case Study 2.3 was introduced in Section 2.4.3. In that experiment, a screening study showed that three factors (pH, concentration of NaCl in the elution buffer, and conductivity) were important. After removing unimportant factors, the resulting design was a full factorial in the three factors. The experimenters also discovered that curvature was present, so they augmented the initial design to include axial points to determine from which factor the curvature was coming. They included center points as suggested by the statistical software to ensure that this second block of experiments would be orthogonal to the first. In this section we present the combined analysis of both sets of experiments.

The statistical model for the combined data set allows main effects for each factor, their two-factor interactions, a quadratic effect for each factor, and other higher-order interaction terms. These latter interactions, such as a linear effect for pH as a function of a quadratic effect for NaCl elution, are assumed to be negligible and are typically put into the error term by default and tested for relevance using a lack-of-fit test. The estimates from the analysis of yield are shown in Table 2.13. The quadratic terms for NaCl concentration and conductivity are both statistically significant so optimization requires us to understand the curvature of these two factors. In addition, the interactions between pH and conductivity and pH and NaCl elution have p-values less than the significance level. Usually the objective of optimization experiments is

TABLE 2.13

Parameter Estimates for Yield, Case Study 2.3

Model Term	Estimate	Std. Error	p-value
Intercept	178.6	35.22	0.0009
pH	−9.7	5.60	0.12
NaCl Elution	0.4	0.09	0.002
pH*NaCl Elution	−0.9	0.31	0.022
Conductivity	−9.1	0.91	<.0001
pH*Conductivity	−17.7	3.13	0.0004
NaCl Elution*Conductivity	0.1	0.05	0.31
pH^2	−38.2	44.11	0.41
$NaCl\ Elution^2$	0.1	0.03	0.039
$Conductivity^2$	−10.8	2.71	0.0039

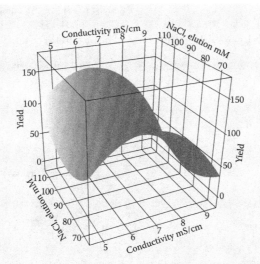

FIGURE 2.16
Response surface fit for yield as function of NaCl elution and conductivity. pH is constant at 6.

to find the best combinations of the factors. Figure 2.16 shows the response surface diagrams for yield as a function of the two significant quadratic factors. It becomes clear when looking at this figure that a linear model would misrepresent the effects and would cause the scientists to miss the sweet spot. Based on the figure the highest yield can be achieved with a pH near the low end, conductivity at the center point, and NaCl elution at the high end of its range. The prediction profiler in JMP can be used to determine the mathematical optimum, as shown in Section 2.6.

2.6 Analyzing Multiple Responses Simultaneously

Multiple responses are usually measured in every experiment and methods for analyzing all responses simultaneously can be employed. While each response can be analyzed separately as described in Section 2.5, this section presents the methods for analyzing all responses simultaneously.

The first method for analyzing multiple responses is to perform the univariate analysis of each response and overlay contour plots of each response. This process allows the creation of a simultaneous region of best operability for all responses. Most statistical software will create these overlay plots for the mean response and some will create the plots for the distribution of the data (for example, an appropriate region for 95% of the predicted responses). In this way the region that satisfies the optimal conditions for all responses can be discovered. Predictions and confidence intervals within this region can be calculated. An example is shown in Figure 2.17. The solid line in the middle of the figure indicates the combination of NaCl elution and pH that is predicted on average to result in an HMW of 1%. Similarly, the solid line at the top of the figure is indicative of yield of 95%. The dots on one side of these solid lines indicate the direction of higher values of either yield or HMW. The plot indicates that higher NaCl elution leads to higher yield and higher HMW.

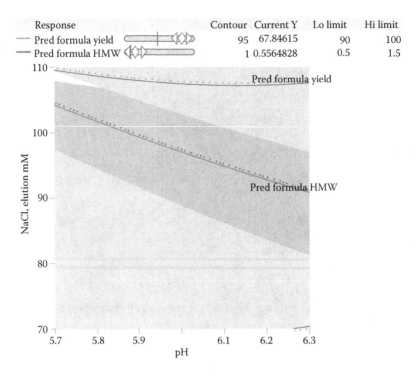

FIGURE 2.17
Overlaid contour plots for yield and HMW.

The shaded area below the solid line in the middle of the figure is an area where the average HMW is predicted to be between 0.5% and 1%; likewise, the shaded area above its solid line is indicative of average HMW values of 1–1.5%. The region in the middle of the figure predicts yield between 90–95%.

Another method for analyzing multiple responses simultaneously involves the use of desirability functions. Desirability functions are simple in concept: the value of each experimental run for each response is normalized on a 0 to 1 scale and then the scores across all responses are aggregated using the geometric mean. On this scale, 1 and 0 represent the ideal response and unacceptable response, respectively. This scale is used because it makes combining responses easy. The difficulty in this approach is that the actual responses are changed into a subjective scale. Because of the subjectivity, different desirability functions may result in different conclusions. However, discussion with subject matter experts and careful thought have led to this approach being successful for half a century. We now continue Case Study 2.3 and show how to use desirability functions.

CONTINUATION OF CASE STUDY 2.3: ANTIBODY PURIFICATION OPTIMIZATION DESIGN

In Section 2.5.7 we analyzed yield data from an experiment in antibody purification. The scientists also measured aggregate levels and we now desire to simultaneously analyze both responses. Although not required, we will begin by first analyzing

TABLE 2.14

Parameter Estimates for Aggregate, Case Study 2.3

Model Term	Estimate	Std. Error	*p*-value
Intercept	−19.19	3.80	0.0007
pH	2.15	0.60	0.0061
NaCl Elution	0.05	0.01	0.0006
pH*NaCl Elution	0.05	0.034	0.1487
Conductivity	0.45	0.10	0.0013
pH*Conductivity	0.41	0.34	0.2524
pH^2	−0.11	4.76	0.9827
NaCl Elution^2	0.02	0.003	0.5504
Conductivity^2	0.01	0.29	0.9808

aggregate levels to better aid our interpretation of the desirability functions. Table 2.14 has the coefficients and standard errors of the terms in the statistical model for aggregate. Note that all three main effects are again statistically significant but neither the interactions nor quadratic effects are needed.

To implement the simultaneous analysis we will convert the observed yield and aggregate levels for each run into a desirable score that ranges from 0 to 1, where 0 is unacceptable and 1 is an ideal response. There are many ways to set this score but the scientists on this project worked together as a team and determined that a level of 0.5% aggregate was ideal while anything above 1.5% was completely unacceptable. Levels between 0.5% and 1.5% were judged to decrease linearly in desirability. Thus, observed aggregate levels less than or equal to 0.5% were changed into a desirability score of 1, levels above 1.5% into a score of 0, and the in-between levels as a linear function between 0 and 1, with each 0.1% increase corresponding to a 0.1 decrease in desirability. Likewise, the process was repeated for yield. In this case, yields above 80 were assigned a score of 1, below 50 of 0, and a quadratic function in desirability for observed yields between 50 and 80. Then the yield and aggregate desirability scores were multiplied and a square root taken to calculate an overall desirability score. The range of desirability scores makes it apparent that a handful of runs yielded very high scores. Under the conditions we determined, these runs are considered the best at producing both high yields and low aggregate levels. This overall score can then be analyzed using the response surface model that was used for both yield and aggregate. In this case, the prediction profiler in Figure 2.18 shows that the best scores are achieved with pH at 6.13, a NaCl concentration of 70 MM, and conductivity at 5 mS/cm. The yield at this combination is predicted to be 91.5%, the HMW 0.31%, and the overall desirability greater than 0.99. Because this combination was not tested during the response surface experimentation, the sweet spot found using the desirability scores should be verified with further experiments to ensure that the predicted results agree with the actual. The residual-by-predicted plots show no obvious lack-of-fit, but predicted results should always be verified because we want to ensure that this is a useful model.

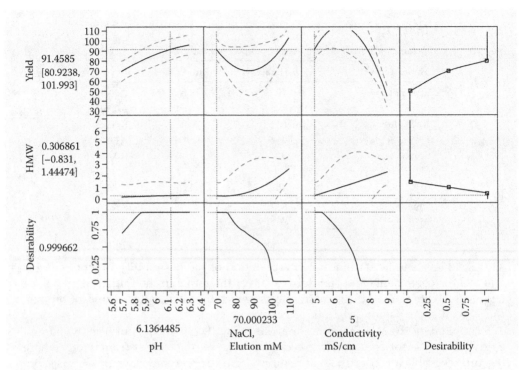

FIGURE 2.18
Model predicted results for both responses with desirability functions.

2.7 Summary

In this chapter we presented the critical elements to performing classical DOE, including two-level fractional and full factorials and response surface designs. These designs have been used for decades with great success. We outlined successful strategies using the projection property and sparsity-of-effects principle to design experiments in an efficient manner. We explained the fundamentals of linear regression and showed how to analyze each type of design. Finally, using three case studies, we illustrated all of these principles. While classical DOE has been and continues to be an invaluable tool, these designs have limitations. In the next chapter we will discuss modern and alternative methods in the context of formulation development that address these limitations.

References

Box, G.E.P. and Draper, N. (1987). *Empirical Model-Building and Response Surfaces*, 1st edition. John Wiley & Sons. See page 424.

Box, G.E.P. and Wilson, K.B. (1951). On the experimental attainment of optimum conditions (with discussion). *Journal of the Royal Statistical Society Series B* 13(1):1–45.

Branning, R. and Torbeck, L. (2009). QbD: Convincing the skeptics, BioPharm International, May 2009.

Fisher, R.A. (1926). The arrangement of field experiments. *Journal of the Ministry of Agriculture of Great Britain* 33, 503–513.

Jones, B. and Nachtsheim, C. (2011). A class of three-level designs for definitive screening in the presence of second-order effects. *Journal of Quality Technology* 43, 1–15.

Myers, R.H., Montgomery, D.C., and Anderson-Cook, C.M. (2016). *Response Surface Methodology: Process and Product Optimization Using Deigned Experiments*, 4th edition. Wiley.

3

Quality by Design Applied in Formulation Development and Robustness

Pierre Lebrun, Perceval Sondag, Xavier Lories,
Jean-François Michiels, Eric Rozet, and Bruno Boulanger

CONTENTS

3.1 Introduction

Optimizing a formulation buffer for biological products, such as vaccines or monoclonal antibodies, is a complex task for several reasons: First, the degradation pathways of such products are difficult to apprehend, and the stabilizing impact of a formulation buffer is hard to measure and understand. Second, the formulation ingredients might be numerous, leading to potentially costly experiments to study them all (Yu, 2015).

From a quality by design (QbD) perspective, the FDA's Process Validation (PV) initiative makes clear that industries have an urgent need to gain a comprehensive understanding of their manufacturing processes (FDA, 2011a). Extensive process design and characterization can thus be primarily carried out in order to succeed in the process performance qualification phase and implement an optimal control strategy, protecting the patient and the business. For development and characterization studies, a systematic QbD initiative has been described for the pharmaceutical industry in documents such as the International Conference on Harmonization (ICH), which established the overall methodology to achieve these expectations. For instance, the ICH Q8 guideline on pharmaceutical development emphasizes the QbD concept, stating that quality should not be tested into products, but should be built in (ICH, 2005, 2008, 2009; FDA, 2011b). The design space (DS) concept is also introduced in this guideline and defined as "the multidimensional combination and interaction of input variables (e.g., materials attributes) and process parameters that have been demonstrated to provide assurance of quality." The concept of assurance of quality refers to the guarantees that the process will show multiple critical quality attributes (CQA)—being reported measures of the output—within some predetermined specifications related to safety, efficacy, and economic reasons, such as material cost and process yield. Ideally, all these considerations and specifications are mentioned in the quality target product profile (QTPP), the main description of the objectives that the product must achieve.

Of particular interest to the industry, ICH indicates that as long as the process and formulation parameters are kept within the factor ranges of quality (the DS), no regulatory post-approval change is needed. To cope with the natural variability of the process parameters and material attributes, changes can then be implemented without any burden, within a properly demonstrated DS.

Thus, the DS of a process must clearly guarantee its reliability and robustness to ensure this nice property. In order to report the DS more easily, the parameter settings on which the process will rely, namely the maximum and normal operating ranges (MOR and NOR), will be chosen as convenient ranges within the DS.

3.2 Design Space Definition and Visualization

In the context of the investigation of multiple formulation factors, design of experiments (DoE) is perfectly adapted to gather data and translate how the combination of these factors (namely, the critical process parameters [CPP]) affects the product CQAs. Eventually, this will help defining the combinations of CPPs that will guarantee that the products CQAs will remain within specifications in the future use of the process. This combination of CPPs defines the design space (DS) (ICH, 2009). In this context, the DS is identified as a region of reliable robustness in the experimental design. To provide guarantees of future quality, DS can be defined in a risk-based framework. In this way, the approach finally would be compliant with QbD expectations.

3.2.1 Quality Target Product Profile and Critical Quality Attributes

When considering optimizing a formulation, or assessing its robustness, several options exist. In a quality by design framework, it is now well recognized that when a formulation is designed to deliver robust quality of the drug product, most problems of stability and out-of-specification results can be avoided. Applied to formulation, QbD guidance documents emphasize a systematic approach for the development based on clear and predefined objectives clearly stated in the quality target product profile (QTPP). For instance, a formulation scientist would want to develop a formulation that will provide guarantees that product stability will be preserved during at least the envisaged shelf-life. Particularly, the investigator should keep in mind that the risk that the drug product will or will not fulfill this quality requirement is paramount in the decision to qualify a formulation as satisfactory or not.

In order to define the quality of a formulation buffer, it is important to realize that most of its promises are about the qualities which will be successfully preserved during the shelf-life of the drug substance and drug product. With this in mind, probably the most important CQA is the degradations during the manufacturing process and the shelf-life. A small total degradation is desirable.

Of course, the need to obtain experimental data quickly will make it mandatory to use accelerated stability studies such as repeated freeze-thaw, room temperature and high temperature degradation, and agitation. When possible, the link between those stresses, and the time they are likely to occur during the normal manufacturing process, should be recorded. For instance, during routine use of the product, the latter might stay at room temperature for more than half a day.

Finally, other CQAs could be derived from bioanalytical specificity, verifying that a particular buffer does not create a particular matrix effect (i.e., does not interact with the assay), as it could lead to unforeseen analytical issues.

In general, it is enviable to rank the CQAs given their impact on final product quality (say, on efficacy and safety), and the analytical process with which they will be analyzed during the formulation study and the future routine should be highlighted: Assay qualification or validation (ICH, 1995), including bias, precision, whenever possible the total error (Hubert et al., 2004), the reportable result format, the limits of detection and quantifications, and so on. This will improve the understanding of the results of the experiments and their applicability in routine.

3.2.2 Critical Process Parameters

Similar to the aforementioned ranking of the CQAs, a thorough analysis of what is known on the CPP is generally made to gather relevant prior knowledge. This will help in constructing an experimental design with the required properties.

To do so, it is classically advocated to analyze what is known from earlier developments of the formulation or similar formulations. The Ishikawa diagram (Ishikawa, 1968) and failure mode and effects analysis (FMEA) (Cohen et al., 1994) are obvious methodologies that can be used to identify factors impacting the CQAs and leading to results outside the QTPP.

3.2.3 Design of Experiments

With that information, and depending on the stage of development, screening, optimization, or robustness designs can be selected. Screening designs such as fractional factorial designs, Plackett and Burman designs, or D-optimal designs might be chosen for their quality of expressing the main effects of CPP onto the CQAs. Orthogonality of the parameter estimates is a necessary property to allow the individual evaluation of main effects and possibly interactions from the designed experiments. Then, optimization/response surface designs such as the rotatable central composite design or I-optimal design are powerful choices when the number of critical factors is lower though their effects and interactions can be quite intricate. In that respect, it is noted that the I-optimal designs that maximize the quality of prediction generally beneficiate from a good D-optimality (Goos et al., 2016). The opposite is design dependent and thus it seems consistent at this stage to advocate for I-optimal designs. This also allows I-optimal designs to be well-suited for a proper identification of effects and interactions, although some efficiency can be lost in parameter estimation. Finally, in the robustness stage, a careful design selection can be made from the information gathered at the screening and optimization phases. Because the aim is usually to provide prediction of the guarantees of success of the formulation and identify the DS, designs built for prediction, such as I-optimal designs, are an obvious choice. Also, smaller ranges for the CPP can be preferred, as CPP combinations leading to failure should have already been identified during screening and optimization.

Obviously a lot of formulation experiments can be written under the form of a mixture of CPP. In this case, I-optimality is also the preferred choice in order to handle mixture and non-mixture CPP, and possibly other constraints that must be fulfilled to avoid the designs being out of the edge of failure.

If knowledge on the possible CPP and interactions is weak, hence preventing the experimenter from building an optimal design or choosing among simpler textbook designs (based on the necessary rationale), a new class of design is available, called *definitive screening designs* (Jones and Nachtsheim, 2011). Those designs are built on the CPP sparsity principle and are meant to be robust against model choice errors. These slightly augmented screening designs offer, at less cost, the possibility to estimate the main effects independently from second-order effects (interaction and quadratic effects) and the ability to estimate all quadratic effects (one by one). Despite some correlations, the confounding is not complete between all second-order effects. When the number of active parameters is not higher than three, all quadratic models can be estimated jointly. It is noted that estimating significant second-order effects might be spurious due to partial aliasing of the parameters, and a design augmentation with the objective to remove confounding could be privileged to further study high-order effects.

Then the final word of the analysis of those designs often requires the use of statistical techniques, such as stepwise regression, to allow identification of the most significant effects and sort them out from noisy factors. These stepwise techniques have various pitfalls, one of the prominent ones being that a selected model is chosen based on the previously selected model. This may commonly prevent the stepwise algorithm from reaching a global optimal effects selection. Model averaging techniques can nowadays be easily implemented in the Bayesian framework using, for example, a spike-and-slab linear regression model (Mitchell and Beauchamp, 1988; Ishwaran and Rao, 2005; freely available through the R package BoomSpikeSlab [Scotts]) or a regularized horseshoe prior linear regression model (Piironen and Vehtari, 2017). These techniques are promising and are being currently evaluated by the authors. Those are however out of the scope of this chapter.

Eventually, the most important point regarding model building is to confirm the model selection with a scientific rationale in terms of understanding of the formulation. In that respect, an option that has been found to be valuable is to select effects that potentially make a CQA reach its specification limits (even if the effect is only partially "significant"), instead of selecting very "significant" parameters (with, say, a p-value < 0.05), but for which the CQA might stay comfortably within the specification limits, as illustrated in Figure 3.1.

A last class of design widely applied in formulation is referred to as *space-filling designs*. They are generally used in early formulation and rely on a random, yet systematic exploration of many qualitative factors being continuous descriptors of the properties of buffers and excipients (Benazzouz, 2013). Interestingly, the authors will come back to these space-filling designs in Sections 3.2.9 and 3.3 to explore a high-dimensional space of factor during prediction to identify a DS.

A last point concerning DoE is its applicability in multi-response experiments. Briefly, and as shown in the next section, degrees of freedom are lost for the estimation of the parameters, as classically, but also with the number of responses/CQA to be considered jointly in a model (see parameter v in Equation 3.1). To our knowledge, no software allows accounting optimally and automatically for the multivariate degrees of freedom. In this

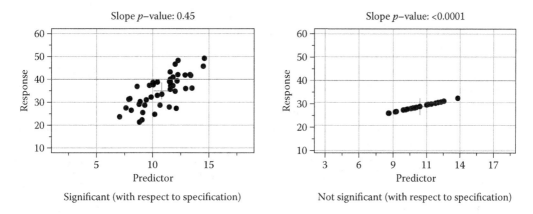

FIGURE 3.1
Parameter selection beyond the *p*-value. (Horizontal line) Upper specification limit. Left: *A* nonsignificant factor (*p*-value > 0.05) with a strong effect on the CQA, which would not be picked by *a* stepwise model. Right: A very significant factor (*p*-value < 0.05) with low to no effect on the CQA, which would be picked by stepwise model. *p*-Values are indicated for illustration only.

case, the designs often lead to the singularity of multivariate multiple linear models, with a poorly definite residual covariance matrix.

3.2.4 Model

To estimate the effects, interaction, and the CPPs, as well as the correlations that will be observed between the responses, a multivariate multiple linear regression (MMLR) can be adopted. As mentioned previously, other statistical models are possible but MMLR allows for a closed-form identification of its predictive distribution. This model is fitted for every response jointly. Let the following model be applied:

$$\mathbf{Y} = \mathbf{XB} + \mathbf{E}, \text{ with } \varepsilon_n \sim \mathbf{N}(0, \Sigma),$$

With ε_n, the *n*th line of $\mathbf{E}$, the $(N \times M)$ matrix of residuals, $\mathbf{Y}$ being a $(N \times M)$ matrix containing M responses during the N experiments, X being the $(N \times F)$ design matrix, and B being the $(F \times M)$ matrix containing the F parameters estimated for each of the M responses. In order to account for the variability of the parameters B and Σ, the $(M \times M)$ residual covariance matrix, a predictive density of new predicted responses, can be obtained in the Bayesian framework, considering in the following a noninformative prior distribution $p(\mathbf{B}, \Sigma) = |\Sigma|^{-(M+1)/2}$ (Box and Tiao, 1973; Peterson, 2004). In this context, the predictive posterior density of a new predicted set of responses $\left(\tilde{y}|\mathbf{X} = \mathbf{x}_0, \text{ data}\right)$ at a new operating condition $\mathbf{x}_0 \in \chi$, is identified as a multivariate Student's *t* distribution, defined as

$$\left(\tilde{y}|\mathbf{X} = \mathbf{x}_0, \text{ data}\right) \sim T_M\left(\mathbf{x}_0\hat{\mathbf{B}}, \frac{\mathbf{A}}{v}\left(1 + \mathbf{x}_0(\mathbf{X}'\mathbf{X})^{-1}\mathbf{x}_0'\right), v\right), \tag{3.1}$$

where $\hat{\mathbf{B}}$ is the least squares estimate of B, $\hat{\mathbf{B}} = (\mathbf{X}'\mathbf{X})^{-1}\mathbf{X}'\mathbf{Y}$; $\mathbf{A} = (\mathbf{Y} - \mathbf{X}\tilde{\mathbf{B}})'(\mathbf{Y} - \mathbf{X}\tilde{\mathbf{B}})$ is a scale matrix and $v = N - (M + F) + 1$ is the degrees of freedom.

Thanks to this predictive distribution, it is easy to verify the model adjustment to the data by visually comparing the marginal prediction intervals taken as quantiles of the T distribution in Equation 3.1.

3.2.5 Probability of Success

This risk analysis imposes a significant shift from traditional optimization techniques based on overlapping mean responses surface or desirability functions. Indeed, these two techniques suffer from two unpleasant gaps. First, providing "assurance of quality" for future manufacturing implies the need to make predictions about the future quality, given the past evidence (prior knowledge) and data. This uncertainty also implies making use of the correlation structure that may exist between various CQAs assessed simultaneously. Sadly, the uncertainty of what may happen in the future is generally poorly assessed by practitioners, and this is unfortunate given the number of papers written on the subject (Peterson, 2008; Peterson and Yahah, 2009; Peterson and Lief, 2010; Lebrun et al., 2012 and 2013). It is noted that desirability functions (Harrington, 1965) suffer from the same issues, but it must be recognized that (1) they are still valuable in very early development, when no specific QTPP and specification exists and one must rank the candidate formulations given what the CQAs can achieve in term of quality; and (2) some work has been done to attempt propagating models and measurements error up to the Global Desirability Index (Steuer, 2000; Le Bailly and Govaerts, 2005; Lebrun et al., 2008). Still, in more advanced phases of formulation in a regulated environment, desirability functions still lose track of the fixed specifications that must be met through the compromise they allow.

To overcome these issues, a simple solution has been defined first by Peterson (2008), making use of the posterior probability to meet specifications for all CQAs jointly. This posterior probability is named *probability of success* (PoS), and is defined as

$$\text{PoS} = \left(\tilde{y} \in \Lambda \middle| \mathbf{x}_0, \text{ data} \right) \approx \frac{1}{n^*} \sum_{n=1}^{n^*} I(\tilde{y}^s \in \Lambda), \qquad (3.2)$$

with $\tilde{y}^s$ being on random draw from Equation 3.1 on a total of n^* Monte-Carlo simulations and Λ being a set of specifications, for instance $\Lambda = \{\lambda_{11} \le \tilde{y}_1 \le \lambda_{21}, \ldots, \lambda_{M1} \le \tilde{y}_M \le \lambda_{M2}\}$. This is elegant in that (1) this PoS is a very specific form of a global desirability index, achieving exact multicriteria decisions (Lebrun, 2012b, Chapter 5); (2) this PoS accounts for correlation between responses within each $\tilde{y}^s$ draw; and (3) this PoS is computed from a posterior predictive distribution (see Equation 3.1), thus it fully takes into account the model and measurement uncertainties. As shown here, for a simple model such as the MMLR, a closed-form solution exists (Equation 3.1), which is directly related to the definition of classical prediction intervals (quantiles of the T distribution in Equation 3.1 are beta-expectation intervals, more generally referred to as prediction intervals). However, mathematical developments (Bayesian or Frequentist) do not allow the computation of an exact closed-form for the predictive distribution when complex correlation structures exist, such as in mixed-effect models or when normality assumptions are not met, as with generalized linear models. In this case, the Bayesian setting has found an appropriate unified framework to deliver such a probability, using the Markov Chain Monte Carlo techniques to adjust the model, and Monte Carlo error propagation to compute the final outcome from a sampled predictive distribution.

3.2.6 Visualization of the Results

Typically, in formulation it is common to carry out an optimization or a robustness analysis over more than seven formulation factors. Several techniques have been proposed in order to represent a design space. When the space of a factor is limited, an obvious solution is to represent the results as a trellis of bivariate contour plots in the same way as the mean response surfaces are presented. Instead of the mean response, however, the posterior probability of success is used. This presents generally well, but has the disadvantage that each graph is made conditionally to values of other factors. Hence, the view is quite incomplete and does not help much in identifying normal operating ranges (NOR) within the design space. A non-visual approach to deal with more complex surfaces in a space of factors with a large number of dimensions has been proposed as electronic sortable spreadsheets. Indeed, a computer system can easily answer if an experimental condition belongs to the design space or not, by storing either the probability values on a grid of conditions or by computing them on the fly (Peterson and Yahyah, 2009). A powerful and effective visualization of the results is obtained by projecting the multidimensional prediction made on a random exploration of the experimental domain, to a bivariate pairs plot arranged as a scatterplot matrix.

This graph is obtained as follows:

- A space-filling design is created to explore a random selection of factor conditions covering the experimental domain.
- For each condition, the PoS is computed as explained previously.
- The computed PoS are color-coded for a probability range between 0 and 1.
- All the points are projected on a two-dimensional plane, defined by a combination of two factors of the design.
- This projection is carried out for all possible two-factor combinations.
- The resulting graph is a squared scatterplot matrix with F rows and columns (where F is the number of factors).

An illustration of this projection process is provided in Figure 3.2 for three points selected in a three-factor experimental space. Typically, it is shown that the three points of this computer experiment aiming at covering the complete experimental domain are presented on each of the subpair plots being the projections. All information is always represented in each bivariate graph.

This graph could easily be mistaken for classical contour plots as provided by classical software, including JMP®, MODDE®, Design-Expert®, or Minitab®. The projection plot presented here shows simulations made on the complete experimental space in a single graph, and allows a relatively easy determination of the design space limits, as will be shown in the example in Section 3.3.

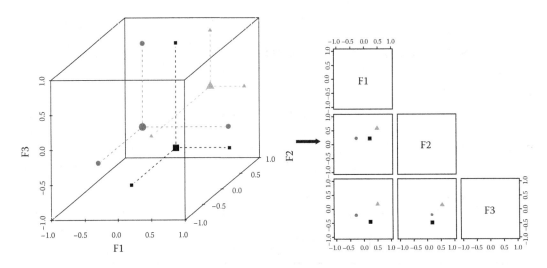

FIGURE 3.2
Illustration of the visualization of the design space. Left: Points within the three-dimension experimental space. Right: Pairs plot presenting the projected points on the different faces of the cube.

3.2.7 Determining and Reporting the Design Space

Determining "the multidimensional combination and interaction of input variables" comes down to defining the multivariate area in which the PoS is greater or equal to the predefined acceptance value.

The relationship between the factors and the PoS can be complicated to identify and to report. Most commonly, maximum or normal operating ranges are defined on each factor, leading to a reported design space having the shape of a hyperrectangle and having a hypervolume inferior or equal to the actual design space. Determination of the different ranges can be done by successively trimming the factor ranges or by using appropriate algorithms.

Note that reporting a design space as a hyperrectangle is not a regulatory requirement, but it eases reporting as a simple, convenient table of the ranges. Any way of reporting a region with a PoS greater or equal to the predefined value is acceptable.

For a complex design space shape, several sets of MOR could be identified, among which one should be chosen and inside which the NOR can be defined. This decision can be based on different criteria, such as

- Maximizing the ranges for hard-to-control factors.
- Maximizing the global hypervolume of the resulting space.
- Finding a robustness region where a nominal setting of interest is found.

Again, in ICH Q8:

> Moving within the design space is not considered as a change. Movement out of the design space is considered to be a change and would normally initiate a regulatory post approval change process.

This should be considered when choosing how the design space is reported from a regulatory point of view; the reported DS (here, this would be the MOR) is the only final and valid DS.

3.2.8 Design Space vs. PAR

The design space, reported as the hyperrectangle resulting from the combination of the MOR, *is not* equivalent to the combination of proven acceptance ranges (PAR).

A proven accepted range is defined as

> A characterized range of a process parameter for which operation within this range while keeping other parameter constant will result in producing a material meeting relevant quality criteria.

Based on this definition, the PAR is assumed to have been established based on univariate, or historical, nonsystematic experiments, and is therefore to be avoided as factor interactions are likely not included—hence, they are missing the design space definition.

3.2.9 Illustration

As an illustration, a circular design space (corresponding to the area within the dotted circle in Figure 3.3) can be reported as a combination of included MOR (see plain rectangle), but not as the combination of PAR (dashed rectangle), which includes points outside the design space, because multivariate aspects are not accounted for in the modeling (the reader can also imagine the dramatic impact factor interactions would have). The reporting of the design space (MOR) can therefore be made as follows in Table 3.1.

Notice that, in this case, the exact relationship is relatively easy and the design space could also be reported as the sets of points for which

$$Factor_1^2 + Factor_2^2 \leq 0.5.$$

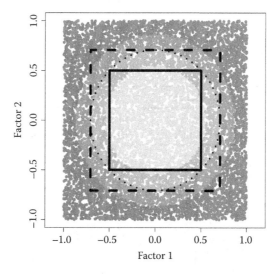

FIGURE 3.3
Illustration of a design space defined over a two-factor experimental space.

TABLE 3.1

Illustrative Representation of the MOR inside the DS

CPP	MOR Lower Boundary	MOR Upper Boundary
Factor$_1$	−0.5	0.5
Factor$_2$	−0.5	0.5

Note: Inside the reported MOR, regulatory flexibility regarding factor settings is maximal.

3.3 Example

In this example, the idea is to identify the design space to guarantee the long-term stability of a new vaccine formulation. The vaccine is planned to be stored for a maximum of twelve months (shelf-life) at 5°C. The critical quality attributes of this stability study are the difference in potency and in virus titer between the release and the twelve-month time point. The acceptance criteria are listed in Table 3.2. The objective of this study is to find a combination of the four identified critical process parameters (pH, slat concentration, surfactant concentration and product target titer) leading to a stable product. Note that, in practice, the number of CQAs and CPPs is usually higher, but are reduced here for the sake of clarity.

The target, low levels, and high levels of each CPP is presented in Table 3.3. According to these, a full factorial design of experiments would require 54 experiments. This is usually not possible in practice, due to experimental set up, budget, and time constraints. Therefore, a 20-experiment I-optimal design is conducted. A possible randomized design, as well as the measured responses, are presented in Table 3.4.

TABLE 3.2

Critical Quality Attributes

Assay	Response	Acceptance Criteria
QPA	Potency	Δ Potency limit = −0.2 log IU/mL
Vp-qPCR	Virus titer	Δ Titer limit = −0.2 log vp/mL

TABLE 3.3

Experimental Design

Formulation Factor		Target	Low Level	High Level
Buffer composition	pH	6.6	6.35	6.85
	Salt (mM)	75	50	100
	Surfactant (%w/w)	0.02	0.01	0.03
Concentration	Titer (vp/mL)	NA	10^{-1}	10^{1}

TABLE 3.4

I-Optimal Design

Run	pH	Salt (mM)	Surfactant (%w/w)	Titer (vp/mL)	Δ Potency (log IU/mL)	Δ Virus Titer (log vp/mL)
1	6.85	100	0.03	0.1	−0.049	−0.074
2	6.35	100	0.03	10	−0.188	−0.182
3	6.85	75	0.03	10	−0.08	−0.081
4	6.6	75	0.02	1	−0.023	−0.021
5	6.35	50	0.02	10	−0.206	−0.241
6	6.6	100	0.01	10	−0.221	−0.221
7	6.6	75	0.02	1	−0.021	−0.036
8	6.35	75	0.01	10	−0.264	−0.259
9	6.6	50	0.03	10	−0.067	−0.071
10	6.85	100	0.01	1	−0.131	−0.103
11	6.85	50	0.03	1	−0.066	−0.058
12	6.35	75	0.03	0.1	−0.117	−0.141
13	6.85	50	0.02	0.1	−0.04	−0.079
14	6.85	100	0.02	10	−0.166	−0.198
15	6.85	75	0.01	0.1	−0.068	−0.064
16	6.35	100	0.01	0.1	−0.244	−0.212
17	6.35	50	0.01	0.1	−0.249	−0.203
18	6.6	75	0.02	1	−0.027	−0.048
19	6.6	75	0.02	1	−0.01	−0.026
20	6.85	50	0.01	10	−0.257	−0.216

A MMLR is fitted on both responses jointly:

$$
\begin{aligned}
Y = {} & \beta_0 + \beta_1 * pH + \beta_{11} * pH^2 + \beta_2 * Salt + \beta_{22} * Salt^2 + \beta_3 * Surfactant \\
& + \beta_{33} * Surfactant^2 + \beta_4 * Titer + \beta_{44} * Titer^2 + \beta_{14} * pH * Titer \\
& + \beta_{34} * Surfactant * Titer + \mathbf{E}
\end{aligned}
\tag{3.3}
$$

This model can be written in matrix form as

$$ \mathbf{Y} = \mathbf{XB} + \mathbf{E}, $$

with ε_n, the nth line of $\mathbf{E}$, assumed to follow a multivariate normal distribution, $\varepsilon_n \sim N(\mathbf{O}, \Sigma)$, $n = 1,\ldots, 20$. $\mathbf{X}$ is then the (20×11) centered and reduced design matrix and $\mathbf{B}$ is the (11×2) matrix containing the 11 effects for each of the 2 responses. The modeled effects have been chosen so that the model has the best properties for each response, jointly.

Once the model is fitted, the predictive distribution of a new observation for a known set of formulation factors can be observed according to the formula presented in Equation 3.1 in Section 3.2.4.

Once the model is fitted, a simple way to evaluate it is to compare the posterior predictive distribution at each row of the design with the observed responses. Figure 3.4 shows the observed data along with the prediction intervals at 95% coverage. One can see that the variability of the replicates at the center of the design (diamonds) is well expressed by the prediction intervals, and that these ones capture well most of the data at about their centers.

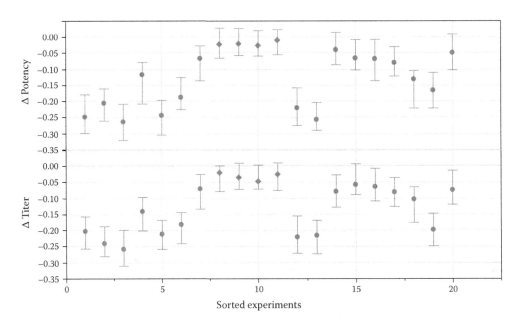

FIGURE 3.4
Observed data (point) and prediction intervals (95% expected coverage). The diamonds are independent replicates at the center of the design.

This gives enough confidence in the model fit, but appropriate residuals graphs and other model summaries shouldn't be overlooked (not presented here, for brevity's sake).

Monte Carlo (MC) simulations can then be used to draw a large number (n^*) of new observations (Metropolis and Ulam, 1949), and the MC estimate of the posterior probability to meet specifications is

$$P\left(\widetilde{CQA} \in \Lambda \big| \tilde{x}, data\right) \cong \frac{1}{n^*} \sum_{s=1}^{n^*} I\left(\widetilde{CQA}^{(s)} \in \Lambda\right)$$

Where $\widetilde{CQA}$ is the ($2 \times n^*$) matrix of predicted observations, Λ is the set of specifications, and $\tilde{x}$ is the set of formulation factors (CPP). Then, the PoS is calculated at each possible combination of formulation factors following a space-filling design. The design space is identified as all the possible combinations of formulation factors within the experimental design that ensure that

$$P\left(\widetilde{CQA} \in \Lambda \big| \tilde{x}, data\right) \geq \pi,$$

where π is the minimum acceptable probability of success for all CQAs, jointly.

To identify the design space, one should ideally estimate $P\left(\widetilde{CQA} \in \Lambda \big| \tilde{x}, data\right)$ at every possible combination of the formulation factors using the space-filling design. The latter is created using simple random uniform draws for each factor and this is the most basic equivalent of DoE in the case of computer simulation experiments. Better suited space-filling designs exists, but the uniform design has the advantage of being simple while providing good coverage of the space. Figure 3.5 shows an example of 500 simulations for a random exploration of three formulation factors.

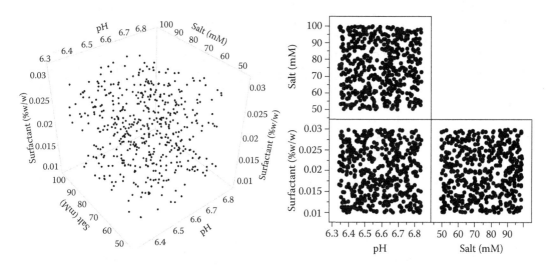

FIGURE 3.5
Example of exploration grid for three factors. Left: 3D representation. Right: Pairs plot representation.

On each point, the posterior probability of meeting specifications for both CQAs jointly can be calculated. To visualize the data, bivariate pair plots can then be recreated by coloring the dots with respect to the PoS, as explained in Section 3.2.6.

Figure 3.6 presents the probabilities of success for the different combinations of formulation factors. The points can be presented in gray when the probability of success is higher than a predefined minimal quality level, say, 99% for both CQA jointly; and in black,

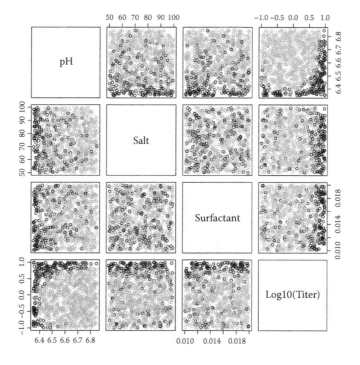

FIGURE 3.6
Probabilities of success for all factor combinations. Points in gray: PoS >= 99%; Points in black: PoS < 99%.

when the probability of success is below that quality level (continuous scale can be implemented as easily). This visualization allows an overview of the CPP impacts, for example, the pH and the titer have a critical effect on the probability to meet specifications. The salt concentration doesn't seem to have a critical effect on the PoS, either because the CQA is always far from the specification within the experimental domain of those CPPs (see Figure 3.1), or because the model, measurement systems, and factor control are excellent on the experimental range. A small interaction seems present between the surfactant and the titer. However, avoiding low pH and high titer is sufficient to identify the DS/MOR in order to guarantee a high probability of success (see Figure 3.7, in which pH levels have been reduced to 6.5 to 6.85, and titer levels have been reduced to 10^{-1} to $10^{.75}$).

Final formulation DS/MOR can then be expressed in simple tabular format, as shown in Table 3.5.

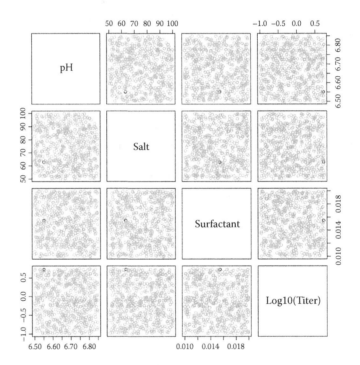

FIGURE 3.7
Probabilities of success after reducing the ranges (MOR) for low pH and high titers. Points in gray: PoS >= 99%; Points in black: PoS < 99%.

TABLE 3.5

DS Presented as MOR for the Formulation Factors

Factor	MOR Lower Bound	MOR Upper Bound
pH	6.5	6.85
Salt (mM)	50	100
Surfactant (%w/w)	0.02	0.03
Titer (vp/mL)	10^{-1}	$10^{.75}$

3.4 Conclusion

The QbB paradigm implies that the quality of future formulated drugs is the result of the way that the formulation was developed. The design space for formulation is a tool that is built over design of experiments. However, it remains clear today that often only the mean responses are taken into account. This approach doesn't provide any clue on future process capabilities, and fails to give any information on how the process will perform in the future. Scientists that rely on a mean-based design space certainly will be disappointed by the future results, because the risk is high to fail to meet their specifications more often than planned. In the opinion of the authors, using mean responses also fail at answering the regulatory requirements to demonstrate the assurance of quality (and not what would only happen to quality on average).

The approach that consists in using the joint posterior predictive distribution of CQAs fully takes into account all uncertainties and dependencies to make sure that the decision and its associated risks are controlled. This risk-based method allows improvement and control of the drug formulation to obtain satisfying stability results, given predefined specifications. When the dimensionality becomes too high, as is often the case with formulation development and robustness studies, bivariate projection of the results into pairs plots with random exploration of the experimental domain can be useful to determine the factors that have a critical effect on the probability of success.

References

Benazzouz, A., Moity, L., Pierlot, C., Sergent, M., Molinier, V., and Aubry, J.-M. 2013. Selection of a greener set of solvents evenly spread in the Hansen space by space-filling design. *Industrial & Engineering Chemistry Research* 52(47), 16585–16597.

Box, G.E.P., Tiao, G.C. 1973. *Bayesian Inference in Statistical Analysis*. Wiley, New York.

Cohen, M.R., Senders, J., Davis, N.M. 1994. Failure mode and effects analysis: Dealing with human error. *Nursing* 94, 24(2), 40–42.

Eglajs, V., Audze P. 1977. New approach to the design of multifactor experiments, in *Problems of Dynamics and Strengths*, pp. 104–107. 35. Riga: Zinatne Publishing House.

Food and Drug Administration (FDA). 2011a. Guidance for Industry Process Validation: General Principles and Practices. Current Good Manufacturing Practices (CGMP). Revision 1.

Food and Drug Administration (FDA). 2011b. Applying ICH Q8(R2), Q9, and Q10 Principles to CMC Review. Chapter 5000. Pharmaceutical Sciences, 5016.1.

Goos, P., Jones, B., and Syafitri, U. 2016. I-optimal design of mixture experiments. *Journal of the American Statistical Association* 111(514), 899–911.

Harrington, E.C. 1965. The desirability function. *Industrial Quality Control* 21, 494–498.

Hubert, P., Nguyen-Huu, J.-J., Boulanger, B., Chapuzet, E., Chiap, P., Cohen, N., Compagnon, P.-A., Dewé, W., Feinberg, M., Lallier, M. et al. 2004. Harmonization of strategies for the validation of quantitative analytical procedures: A SFSTP proposal—Part I. *Journal of Pharmaceutical and Biomedical Analysis* 36(3), 579–586.

International Conference on Harmonization (ICH) of Technical Requirements for Registration of Pharmaceuticals for Human Use. 1995. Topic Q2(R1): Validation of Analytical Procedures: Text and Methodology. Geneva.

International Conference on Harmonization (ICH) of Technical Requirements for Registration of Pharmaceuticals for Human Use. 2005. Topic Q9: Quality Risk Management. Geneva.

International Conference on Harmonization (ICH) of Technical Requirements for Registration of Pharmaceuticals for Human Use. 2008. Topic Q10: Pharmaceutical Quality System. Geneva.

International Conference on Harmonization (ICH) of Technical Requirements for Registration of Pharmaceuticals for Human Use. 2009. Topic Q8(R2): Pharmaceutical Development. Geneva.

Ishikawa, K. 1968. *Guide to Quality Control*. Tokyo: JUSE.

Ishwaran, H., Rao, J.S. 2005. Spike and slab variable selection: Frequentist and Bayesian strategies. *The Annals of Statistics* 33(2), 730–773.

Jones, B., Nachtsheim, C.J. 2011. A class of three-level designs for definitive screening in the presence of second-order effects. *Journal of Quality Technology* 43(1):1.

Le Bailly de Tilleghem, C., Govaerts, B. 2005. Uncertainty propagation in multiresponse optimization using a desirability index. Technical Report 0532, Université catholique de Louvain, Louvain-la-Neuve.

Lebrun, P. 2012. A Bayesian Design Space Applied to Pharmaceutical Development. PhD dissertation, University of Liège, Belgium. See http://bictel.ulg.ac.be/ETD-db/collection/available/ULgetd-12192012-155142.

Lebrun, P., Boulanger, B., Debrus, B., Lambert, P., Hubert, P. 2013. A Bayesian design space for analytical methods based on multivariate models and predictions. *Journal of Biopharmaceutical Statistics* 23(6), 1330–51.

Lebrun, P., Govaerts, B., Debrus, B., Ceccato, A., Caliaro, G., Hubert, P., Boulanger, B. 2008. Development of a new predictive modelling technique to find with confidence equivalence zone and design space of chromatographic analytical methods. *Chemometrics and Intelligent Laboratory Systems* 91, 4–16.

Lebrun, P., Krier, F., Mantanus, J., Grohganz, H., Yang, M., Rozet, E., Boulanger, B., Evrard, B., Rantanen, J., Hubert, P. 2012. Design space approach in the optimization of the spray-drying process. *European Journal of Pharmaceutics and Biopharmaceutics* 80(1), 226–234.

McKay, M.D., Beckman, R.J., Conover, W.J. 1979. A comparison of three methods for selecting values of input variables in the analysis of output from a computer code. Technometrics (JSTOR Abstract). *American Statistical Association* 21 (2), 239–245.

Metropolis, N., Ulam, S. 1949. The Monte Carlo method. *Journal of the American Statistical Association* 44(247), 335–341.

Mitchell, T.J., Beauchamp, J.J. 1988. Bayesian variable selection in linear regression. *Journal of the American Statistical Association* 83(N404), 1023–1032.

Peterson, J.J. 2004. A posterior predictive approach to multiple response surface optimization. *Journal of Quality Technology* 36(2), 139–153.

Peterson, J.J. 2008. A Bayesian approach to the ICH Q8 definition of design space. *Journal of Biopharmaceutical Statistics* 18, 959–975.

Peterson, J.J., Lief, K. 2008. The ICH Q8 definition of design space: A comparison of the overlapping means and the Bayesian predictive approaches. *Statistics in Biopharmaceutical Research* 2, 249–259.

Peterson, J.J., Yahyah, M. 2009. A Bayesian design space approach to robustness and system suitability for pharmaceutical assays and other processes. *Statistics in Biopharmaceutical Research* 1(4).

Piironen, J., Vehtari, A. 2017. Sparsity information and regularization in the horseshoe and other shrinkage priors. Preprint arXiv: 1707.01694.

Steuer, D. 2000. An improved optimisation procedure for desirability indices. Technical Report 27/00, SFB 475, Dortmund University.

Yu, L. 2008. Pharmaceutical quality by design: Product and process development, understanding, and control. *Pharmaceutical Research* 25, 781–791.

4

Analytical Procedure Development and Qualification

Richard K. Burdick

CONTENTS

4.1 Introduction

Analytical chemistry is used across the pharmaceutical industry to quantify and identify the components in drug substances, drug products, and raw materials to ensure that the final dosage form remains safe and efficacious from lot release throughout the product's shelf life. To understand any potential shifts in the components impacting safety and efficacy, laboratories require analytical procedures that are reliable, fit for use, and executed consistently over time. Analytical procedures provide the instructions that ensure consistent use of laboratory equipment, solution preparation, measurement recording, and documentation. As such, analytical procedures form a critical component in any quality system. This chapter considers statistical methods that ensure that these procedures are fit for their intended purposes.

4.1.1 Description of an Analytical Procedure

Analytical procedures must be clearly defined in order to perform the appropriate statistical analysis. Descriptors such as "replicates" or "preparations" without further explanation often lead to confusion. Table 4.1 reports terminology used in this chapter to describe the stages of an analytical procedure.

TABLE 4.1

Stages of an Analytical Procedure

Stage	Description of Stage
Decision Unit	The material from which a sample is collected. A decision is made for this unit. For example, if sampled material from a drug product lot is used to make a disposition decision, the decision unit is the drug product lot.
Laboratory Sample	The material sample from the decision unit that is received by the laboratory.
Analytical Sample	Material created by any manipulation of the laboratory sample, such as crushing or grinding.
Test Portion	The quantity of material taken from the analytical sample for testing.
Test Solution	The solution resulting from dissolving the test portion.
Reading (Individual Determination)	A single measured numerical value from the test solution.
Reportable Value	A numerical value that summarizes one or more readings.

Not all analytical procedures have all stages shown in Table 4.1. For example, liquid laboratory samples that require no further manipulations immediately progress to the test solution stage.

Replication can occur at any stage in the process and should be performed in the stages that contribute the greatest variability. A replication strategy that addresses both the number of replications and the stages at which replication is performed should be determined prior to the official qualification (validation) study.

The reportable value is the value obtained from one whole completion of the procedure incorporating the specified replication strategy. The reportable value defined in this manner will be used for making a decision concerning the decision unit.

Table 4.2 provides an example of the stages defined in Table 4.1 for a solid dosage product.

Since relatively large variations associated with the test portion and reading stages were discovered in prequalification analytical work, replications were made at each of these two stages.

TABLE 4.2

Stages for Solid Dosage Coated Pills

Stage	Description of Stage			
Decision Unit	Lot of drug product, coated pills			
Laboratory Sample	100 coated pills			
Analytical Sample	20 pills are removed from the laboratory sample and are crushed with a mortar and pestle			
Test Portion	Replicate 1: 1 gram crushed powder aliquot from analytical sample		Replicate 2: 1 gram crushed powder aliquot from analytical sample	
Test Solution	Replicate 1: Test portion is dissolved in 1 L solvent		Replicate 2: Test portion is dissolved in 1 L solvent	
Reading (Individual Determination)	Reading 1 of replicate 1: Test solution	Reading 2 of replicate 1: Test solution	Reading 1 of replicate 2: Test solution	Reading 2 of replicate 2: Test solution
Reportable Value	Average value of four readings			

4.1.2 Description of Life Cycle Approach

Martin et al. (2013) describe a holistic view of the analytical procedure life cycle using concepts consistent with quality by design (QbD), ICH Q8 (2009), and the FDA process validation guidance (2011). The performance requirements of a procedure are defined by the analytical target profile (ATP). The ATP defines the analyte to be measured, the concentration range, procedure performance criteria, and product specifications. The criteria and specifications are established to define the purpose of the analytical procedure.

To be fit for its intended use, the analytical procedure should produce reportable values that meet the requirements of the decision. The use of the reportable value should be clearly defined in a decision rule, which includes the acceptable probability of making a wrong decision. An analytical procedure is considered to be fit for its intended use if the reportable values meet the requirements of the decision rule with the acceptable probability of being wrong. All this information is included in the ATP.

An analytical procedure can be considered to have a life cycle with three stages:

1. Stage 1: Procedure Design. This stage includes the activities of selecting an appropriate technology and deciding upon the method parameters. Potential sources of variation are identified in this stage, as well as a replication strategy.

2. Stage 2: Procedure Performance Qualification. This stage demonstrates the analytical procedure is fit for its intended use. This process is described in USP <1225> as method validation. In the new life cycle paradigm, experiments are used to demonstrate that uncertainty meets the requirements specified in the ATP. Performance parameters that may need to be established during this stage under <1225> include accuracy, precision, specificity, detection limit (limit of detection [LOD]), quantitation limit (LOQ), linearity, and range. In some situations (e.g., biological assay), relative accuracy takes the place of accuracy. This chapter focuses on how to establish the analytical performance characteristics of accuracy and precision. USP <1210> provides more information on validation under <1225>. Throughout the rest of this chapter, we will use the term *qualification* as opposed to validation to reference the Stage 2 experiment.

3. Stage 3: Continued Procedure Performance Verification. This final stage provides ongoing assurance that the analytical procedure continues to operate as required. This includes activities such as the routine use of the procedure, transfer of the procedure between laboratories, and adoption of a control strategy.

4.1.3 Measurement Error Models

A useful model for representing a reportable value is

$$Y = \tau + \beta + E \qquad (4.1)$$

where Y is a reportable value, τ is the true or accepted reference value, β is the systematic bias of the procedure, and E is a random measurement error. Both τ and β are fixed statistical parameters, and E is a normal random variable with an assumed mean of zero and standard deviation σ. The magnitude of σ depends on the replication strategy used to produce the reportable value. Under Equation 4.1, the reportable value is a normal random variable with mean $\tau + \beta$ and standard deviation σ.

- Accuracy

    Accuracy of an analytical procedure as defined in USP <1225> is the closeness of agreement between τ and Y. Closeness is expressed as the long-run average of $(Y - \tau)$. This long-run average is called *systematic bias* and is represented by the term β. To estimate β, it is necessary to know the true value, τ. USP <1225> notes that a reference standard or a well-characterized orthogonal procedure can be used to assign the value of τ. Accuracy should be established across the required range of the procedure.

    The definition of accuracy provided by the International Organization for Standardization (ISO) is different than the USP definition. In ISO, accuracy combines the systematic bias (termed trueness) and precision. In this chapter we adhere to the USP definition.

- Precision

    Precision of an analytical procedure is defined in USP <1225> as the degree of agreement among reportable values when the procedure is applied repeatedly (possibly under different conditions) to multiple samples of a given test solution. For many analytical procedures, precision can be assessed even if accuracy cannot be defined due to lack of knowledge concerning τ. The most common precision metric is the standard deviation, σ. The square of the standard deviation, σ^2, is called the variance. Precision improves as σ decreases. Many commonly used statistical procedures rely on the assumption of the normal distribution, for which σ is a natural descriptor of variability.

    One other measure commonly used in the industry is the percent relative standard deviation (%RSD). It is expressed as $\sigma/\mu \times 100\%$ where μ is the mean for the population described by σ. Burdick et al. (2017) and Torbeck (2010) provide more discussion on this metric.

4.2 Stage 1: Procedure Design

Stage 1 includes the activities of selecting an appropriate technology and deciding upon the procedure parameters. Potential sources of significant variation are identified in this stage. Martin et al. (2013) note that experiments conducted in Stage 1 can be leveraged to support the Stage 2 qualification experiment. A lack of work in Stage 1 will often lead to a failed qualification in Stage 2.

The following series of questions provided in USP <1210> should be considered in Stage 1 in order to ensure a successful procedure performance qualification in Stage 2.

1. What are the allowable ranges for operational parameters such as temperature and time that impact the performance of the analytical procedure?
    a. Robustness of these ranges can be determined using statistical design of experiments (DoE; see Chapters 2 and 3).
2. Are there ruggedness factors that impact precision?
    a. Factors such as analyst, day, and instrument that vary in routine use and impact the precision of a test procedure are called *ruggedness factors*. When ruggedness factors impact precision, reportable values within the same ruggedness

grouping (e.g., analyst) are correlated. Depending on the strength of the correlation, this may necessitate a statistical analysis that appropriately accounts for this dependence. Ruggedness factors should be identified and their magnitude assessed during Stage 1. Incorporation of ruggedness factors in the Stage 2 analysis is discussed in Section 4.3.2.

3. Are statistical assumptions for data analysis reasonably satisfied?

   a. These assumptions typically include normality, homogeneity of variance, and independence of reportable values. It is useful during Stage 1 to employ statistical tests or visual representations to help answer these questions. USP <1010> provides information on this topic.

4. What is the required analytical range for the procedure?

5. Do accepted reference values or results from an established procedure exist for determination of τ?

   a. If not, ICH Q2 (2005) states accuracy may be inferred once precision, linearity, and specificity have been established.

6. What is the replication strategy?

   a. To answer this question, it is necessary to understand the contributors to the procedure variance and the procedure's ultimate purpose. Estimation of variance components during Stage 1 provides useful information for making this decision. As noted earlier, one should replicate against the sources representing the largest components of procedure variation.

7. What are appropriate acceptance criteria for the qualification in Stage 2?

   a. We provide discussion on this topic in Section 4.3.

8. How large a qualification experiment is necessary in Stage 2?

   a. Qualification experiments should be properly powered to ensure that if accuracy and precision truly meet prespecified acceptance criteria, the result of the statistical test supports this position. Computer simulation is a useful tool for performing power calculations as discussed in Section 4.3.3.

4.3 Stage 2: Procedure Performance Qualification

4.3.1 Individual Qualification for Accuracy and Precision

We begin with an example reported by Weitzel (2012) in which a drug substance (DS) procedure is to be qualified in accordance with USP <1225>. The DS is a USP compendial substance, and there is a monograph that describes a test procedure that uses high-performance liquid chromatography (HPLC) to determine the assay. The reportable value is the mass fraction of DS in the drug substance, and the specification is ≥ 980 and ≤ 1020 mg/g.

- Accuracy

   In accordance with <1225>, accuracy was determined by applying the test procedure to a reference standard. Accuracy for the assay is to be described by a confidence interval on the difference between the mean reportable value and the accepted true value (τ). ICH documents recommend that accuracy be assessed using a minimum of nine determinations over a minimum of three concentration levels, covering the specified range.

Recovery of the assay is calculated using the concentration of the DS in the reference standard which is 100%. Three different quantities of reference standard were weighted to correspond to three different percentages of the test concentrations, 50%, 100%, and 150%. The resulting data are reported in Table 4.3 and graphed in Figure 4.1. The true value for all three concentrations is $\tau = 1000$ mg/g.

Figure 4.1 suggests that the average difference between $\tau = 1000$ and the reportable value changes as a function of the concentration. Weitzel (2012) notes this is unimportant because in practice, material will be close to 100% concentration. Thus, only the 100%

TABLE 4.3

Qualification Experiment

Replicate	Concentration		
	50%	**100%**	**150%**
1	1004	998	987
2	1006	999	993
3	1008	998	992
4		996	
5		999	
6		994	
Average	$\bar{Y}_{50} = 1006.0$	$\bar{Y}_{100} = 997.33$	$\bar{Y}_{150} = 990.7$
Standard deviation	$S_{50} = 2.00$	$S_{100} = 1.97$	$S_{150} = 3.21$
Sample size	$n_{50} = 3$	$n_{100} = 6$	$n_{150} = 3$

Note: Reportable value is mg/g.

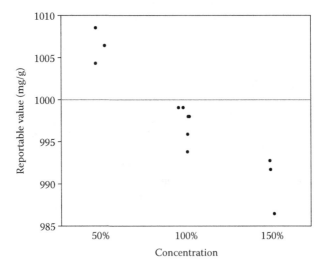

FIGURE 4.1
Plot of accuracy data.

concentration values will be used for the remaining analysis. To simplify notation, define $\bar{Y} = \bar{Y}_{100} = 997.33$, $S = S_{100} = 1.97$, and $n = n_{100} = 6$. (Note: Figure 4.1 suggests there is no difference in the spread of the values across the concentration levels. This would allow the pooling of variances across the three levels even if only the mean of the 100% concentration is of interest. However, we will work with the standard deviation estimate based only on the 100% concentration data in the example).

A formula to construct a $100 \, (1 - \alpha)\%$ confidence interval on the bias, β, for the 100% concentration is

$$(\bar{Y} - \tau) \pm t_{1-\alpha/2:n-1} \times \frac{S}{\sqrt{n}} \tag{4.2}$$

where $t_{1-\alpha/2:n-1}$ is the quanitle of a t-distribution with area $1 - \alpha/2$ to the left and degrees of freedom $n - 1$

From Equation 4.2, the 95% confidence interval ($\alpha = 0.05$) for β is

$$(997.33 - 1000) \pm t_{0.975:5} \times \frac{1.97}{\sqrt{6}}$$

$$(997.33 - 1000) \pm 2.57 \times \frac{1.97}{\sqrt{6}} \tag{4.3}$$

$$L = -4.7 \, \text{mg/g}$$

$$U = -0.6 \, \text{mg/g}.$$

At this point, the estimated bias between -4.7 mg/g to -0.6 mg/g would be compared to an appropriate qualification criterion. This process is described later in this section.

- Precision

  ICH documents recommend that repeatability be assessed using a minimum of nine determinations covering the specified range or using a minimum of six determinations at 100% of the test. Thus, the data in Table 4.3 can be used to assess repeatability. Precision as described by the standard deviation is estimated with the sample standard deviation, S. A $100 \, (1 - \alpha)\%$ upper bound on the repeatability standard deviation is

$$U = \sqrt{\frac{(n-1) \times S^2}{\chi^2_{\alpha:n-1}}} \tag{4.4}$$

where $\chi^2_{\alpha:n-1}$ represents the percentile from the chi-squared distribution with area α to the left, and degrees of freedom $n - 1$. For the present example, the computed 95% upper bound

$$U = \sqrt{\frac{5 \times 1.97^2}{\chi^2_{0.05:5}}}$$

$$U = \sqrt{\frac{5 \times 1.97^2}{1.145}} \tag{4.5}$$

$$U = 4.1 \, \text{mg/g}.$$

Typically, only the upper bound on the standard deviation is of interest. If a lower bound (l) is desired, one can use Equation 4.4 by replacing α with $1 - \alpha$.

- Qualification Criteria for Accuracy and Precision

    It is hard to determine if a procedure is fit for use when accuracy and precision are considered independently. Many companies use criteria for each component separately based on historical norms. As an example, suppose the accuracy criterion is that the bias must be less than 1% of τ in absolute value, and the repeatability standard deviation must be less than 2% of τ. The test for accuracy is performed by comparing the computed interval in Equation 4.3 to the acceptance criterion $0.01 \times \tau = 0.01 \times 1000 = 10$ mg/g. Since all values in the interval from $L = -4.7$ to $U = -0.6$ are in absolute value less than 10 mg/g, the criterion is satisfied and the required level of accuracy is demonstrated. For precision, the upper bound in Equation 4.5 is $U = 4.1$ mg/g, which is less than the criterion of $0.02 \times \tau = 0.02 \times 1000 = 20$ mg/g. Thus, the desired level of precision is also demonstrated for this procedure. The problem with such criteria is that they don't demonstrate that a procedure is fit for use in the context of an ATP. This problem is attacked directly in the next section.

- A Holistic Qualification of Accuracy and Precision

    As noted in the previous section, meaningful validation criteria for individual tests of accuracy and precision that are consistent with a given ATP are hard to develop. Use of an ATP requires criterion that focuses on the combined impact of both properties. A procedure with a relatively small standard deviation can allow more bias than a procedure with a relatively large standard deviation. This inherent trade-off between accuracy and precision requires a holistic qualification of the procedure performance.

    Hubert et al. (2004, 2007a, 2007b) proposed a criterion that can be used to simultaneously qualify accuracy and precision. Using this criterion, a method is fit for use if

$$Pr(-\lambda < Y - \tau < \lambda) \geq P \tag{4.6}$$

where $\lambda > 0$ is an acceptable limit defined a priori to be consistent with the ATP. The term P is a desired probability value (e.g., $P = 0.90$). In other words, a method is fit for use if the probability is at least P that the absolute value of the difference between the reportable value and the true value is less than λ.

- Qualification Using a Holistic Criterion

    Equation 4.6 can be rewritten as

$$
\begin{aligned}
Pr(-\lambda < Y - \tau < \lambda) &\geq P \\
Pr(-\lambda + \tau < Y < \lambda + \tau) &\geq P \\
1 - Pr(-\lambda + \tau < Y < \lambda + \tau) &\leq 1 - P \\
\pi &\leq 1 - P
\end{aligned}
\tag{4.7}
$$

where $\pi = 1 - Pr(-\lambda + \tau < Y < \lambda + \tau)$ is the probability that the reportable value will fall outside the interval from $-\lambda + \tau$ to $\lambda + \tau$. Recall from Equation 4.1 that the reportable value Y has a normal distribution with mean $\tau + \beta$ and standard deviation σ.

Mee (1988) provides a confidence interval for π that can be used to test the following set of hypotheses:

$$H_0 : \pi \geq 1 - P$$
$$H_1 : \pi < 1 - P. \tag{4.8}$$

In particular, the null hypothesis H_0 is rejected and the procedure satisfies Equation 4.6 if the 100 (1 − α)% upper bound on π is less than 1 − P. This approach provides a statistical test with a Type 1 error rate of α. The following algorithm can be used to compute the desired 100 (1 − α)% upper bound on π:

1. Compute

$$K_L = \left(\frac{\bar{Y} - (-\lambda + \tau)}{S} \right)$$
$$K_U = \left(\frac{(\lambda + \tau) - \bar{Y}}{S} \right). \tag{4.9}$$

2. If either K_L or K_U exceeds $(n-1)/\sqrt{n}$, set $K^* = \min(K_L, K_U)$, go to Step 5. Otherwise, compute the maximum likelihood point estimator (MLE) of π using the formula

$$\hat{\pi} = \Phi\left(-\sqrt{\frac{n}{n-1}} \times K_L \right) + \Phi\left(-\sqrt{\frac{n}{n-1}} \times K_U \right). \tag{4.10}$$

where $\Phi(\cdot)$ is the area in a standard normal curve to the left of ($\cdot$).

3. Determine the $100\hat{\pi}\%$ percentile of a beta distribution with parameters $(n - 2)/2$ and $(n - 2)/2$ using the inverse cumulative distribution function (Excel, Minitab, and SAS all have this function). Denote this value as b.

4. Compute

$$K^* = \frac{(1 - 2 \times b) \times (n - 1)}{\sqrt{n}}. \tag{4.11}$$

5. Solve the equation

$$Pr\left[t_{\lambda:n-1} \leq \sqrt{n} \times K^* \right] = 1 - \alpha, \text{ to get } \lambda. \tag{4.12}$$

where $t_{\lambda:n-1}$ is a noncentral t-variate with noncentrality parameter λ and degrees of freedom $n - 1$. Unfortunately, this function cannot be solved in Excel since it does not have information for a noncentral t-distribution. There are functions in JMP®, Minitab®, SAS®, and R® that can be used to solve Equation 4.12. After solving for λ, the upper bound on π is

$$U = 1 - \Phi\left(\frac{\lambda}{\sqrt{n}}\right) \tag{4.13}$$

This upper bound is approximate, and hence the probability of a Type 1 error is not exactly α.

An alternative approach is performed using the following steps:

1. Compute a 100 $(1 - 2\alpha)$% tolerance interval that contains 100 P% of the population of future reportable values of Y. This tolerance interval can be computed using the formula

$$
\begin{aligned}
L &= \bar{Y} - K \times S \\
U &= \bar{Y} + K \times S \\
K &= \sqrt{\frac{\left(1 + \dfrac{1}{n}\right) Z_{(1+P)/2}^2 \times (n - 1)}{\chi_{2\alpha:n-1}^2}}
\end{aligned}
\tag{4.14}
$$

where $\chi_{2\alpha:n-1}^2$ is the chi-squared percentile with $n - 1$ degrees of freedom and area 2α to the left, and $Z_{(1+P)/2}$ is a standard normal percentile with area $(1 + P)/2$ to the left.

The value of K is based on an approximation, but exact values are provided in some software packages or can be found in statistical tables (see, e.g., Meeker et al., 2017).

2. If the computed tolerance interval falls completely in the range from $-\lambda + \tau$ to $\lambda + \tau$, reject the null hypothesis in Equation 4.8 and conclude the procedure has been qualified for both accuracy and precision.

Apart from differences due to approximations applied for both approaches, the two methods perform comparably. (In fact, for situations where bounds are on only one side, the two methods are exact and can be shown to be algebraically equivalent.)

To demonstrate these calculations, consider the example presented earlier where $\bar{Y} = 997.33$, $S = 1.97$, $n = 6$ and assume $\lambda = 10$ mg/g, $\tau = 1000$ mg/g, $\alpha = 0.10$, and $P = 0.95$. Steps of the Mee approach are shown in the following.

Step 1:

$$
\begin{aligned}
K_L &= \left(\frac{\bar{Y} - (-\lambda + \tau)}{S}\right) = \left(\frac{997.33 - (-10 + 1000)}{1.97}\right) = 3.72 \\
K_U &= \left(\frac{(\lambda + \tau) - \bar{Y}}{S}\right) = \left(\frac{(10 + 1000) - 997.33}{1.97}\right) = 6.43
\end{aligned}
\tag{4.15}
$$

Step 2: Since both these values exceed $(n-1)/\sqrt{n} = 5/\sqrt{6} = 2.04$, then set $K^* = \min(K_L, K_U) = (3.72, 6.43) = 3.72$ and go to Step 5.

Step 5: Solve the equation

$$
\begin{aligned}
Pr\left[t_{\lambda:n-1} \leq \sqrt{n} \times K^*\right] &= 1-\alpha \\
Pr\left[t_{\lambda:6-1} \leq \sqrt{6} \times 3.72\right] &= 1-0.10 \\
Pr\left[t_{\lambda:5} \leq 9.11\right] &= 0.90.
\end{aligned}
\tag{4.16}
$$

Using the SAS function "tnonct," the noncentrality parameter that satisfies Equation 4.16 is $\lambda = 4.946$. The 90% upper confidence bound on π is then

$$
\begin{aligned}
U = 1-\Phi\left(\frac{4.946}{\sqrt{6}}\right) &= 1-\Phi(2.019) \\
U = 1-0.978 &= 0.022.
\end{aligned}
\tag{4.17}
$$

Since the upper bound in Equation 4.17 is less than $1 - P = 1 - 0.95 = 0.05$, the null hypothesis in Equation 4.8 is rejected, and the procedure is qualified with respect to the criterion.

The computed tolerance interval defined in Equation 4.14 is

$$
\begin{aligned}
K &= \sqrt{\frac{\left(1+\dfrac{1}{n}\right)Z_{(1+P)/2}^2 \times (n-1)}{\chi_{2\alpha:n-1}^2}} \\[2ex]
K &= \sqrt{\frac{\left(1+\dfrac{1}{6}\right)Z_{(1+0.95)/2}^2 \times 5}{\chi_{0.20:5}^2}} \\[2ex]
K &= \sqrt{\frac{\left(1+\dfrac{1}{6}\right)1.96^2 \times 5}{2.343}} = 3.093 \\[2ex]
L &= \bar{Y} - K \times S \\
L &= 997.33 - 3.093 \times 1.97 = 991.2\,\text{mg/g} \\
U &= \bar{Y} + K\sqrt{S^2} \\
U &= 997.33 + 3.093 \times 1.97 = 1003.4\,\text{mg/g}
\end{aligned}
\tag{4.18}
$$

Since this entire interval fits in the range from $-\lambda + \tau = 990$ mg/g to $\lambda + \tau = 1010$ mg/g, the procedure has been shown to be fit for use.

The choice of a Type 1 error rate of 0.10 for this example is made because accuracy and precision are being simultaneously qualified. When accuracy and precision are qualified individually, the traditional value of 0.05 is used for each qualification. However, the Type 1 error rate for the two tests taken as a set can be as high as 0.10. For this reason, the Type 1 error rate of 0.10 seems justified.

It is also possible to estimate $Pr(-\lambda + \tau < Y < \lambda + \tau)$ in Equation 4.6 directly using a Bayesian approach. These methods use a framework different than the frequentist hypothesis testing paradigm and focus on the predictive probability that any future reportable value will fall within predefined limits $-\lambda + \tau$ and $\lambda + \tau$, given past data and knowledge. A good overview of this approach is provided by Sondag et al. (2016).

4.3.2 Incorporation of a Ruggedness Factor

Suppose that research in Stage 1 discovered significant variation in reportable values made on different days when all other conditions were held constant. For this reason, a qualification experiment performed in Stage 2 consisted of three reportable values made on four different days at the 100% concentration level. There are $d = 4$ days and all days have $r = 3$ reportable values. The data are presented in Table 4.4 and plotted in Figure 4.2. The overall average of the $n = d \times r = 4 \times 3 = 12$ measurements is $\bar{Y} = 999.0$.

Figure 4.2 reveals two sources of variation in the data. In addition to the variation among the three measurements taken on a given day (repeatability), there are also differences in the levels across days. In particular, Day 4 seems high and Day 3 seems low relative to the first two days. Symbolically, this day-to-day variation is denoted as σ_D^2 and the repeatability is denoted as σ_R^2. The sum of these two sources of variability is called the *intermediate precision* (IP) variance. That is,

$$\sigma_{IP}^2 = \sigma_D^2 + \sigma_R^2. \tag{4.19}$$

The square root of the IP variance is called the *IP standard deviation*.

The term "day" is referred to as a ruggedness factor. Ruggedness factors such as day, analyst, column, or equipment cause variation in a reportable value beyond the level represented by repeatability. Impactful ruggedness factors should be identified during Stage 1 so that they can be included in the Stage 2 qualification experiment.

TABLE 4.4

Qualification Experiment with Ruggedness Factor

Reportable Value	Day 1	Day 2	Day 3	Day 4
1	999	997	994	1002
2	998	1002	989	1003
3	1000	1002	997	1005
Average	$\bar{Y}_{D1} = 999.0$	$\bar{Y}_{D2} = 1000.3$	$\bar{Y}_{D3} = 993.3$	$\bar{Y}_{D4} = 1003.3$
Standard Deviation	$S_{D1} = 1.00$	$S_{D2} = 2.89$	$S_{D3} = 4.04$	$S_{D4} = 1.53$

Note: Response in mg/g at 100% concentration.

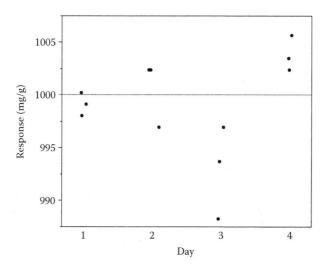

FIGURE 4.2
Plot of measurements for ruggedness study.

The data in Table 4.4 are now used to estimate the intermediate precision standard deviation. Once this is estimated, it can be used to qualify the procedure using the holistic approach described previously.

The estimation of the repeatability variance is done by averaging the within-day variances across the four days. Since all four standard deviations are based on $r = 3$ measurements, the estimate is simply the arithmetic average of the variances for each day. Thus, the estimate for σ_R^2 is

$$S_R^2 = \frac{S_{D1}^2 + S_{D2}^2 + S_{D3}^2 + S_{D4}^2}{4}$$

$$S_R^2 = \frac{1.00^2 + 2.89^2 + 4.04^2 + 1.53^2}{4} \tag{4.20}$$

$$S_R^2 = 7.00.$$

Estimation of σ_D^2 requires calculating the variance of the four day averages, and subtracting out the variation within days. An appropriate estimator for σ_D^2 is

$$S_D^2 = \frac{\sum_{i=1}^{d}\left(\bar{Y}_{Di} - \bar{Y}\right)^2}{(d-1)} - \frac{S_R^2}{r}$$

$$S_D^2 = \frac{\left[(999.0 - 999.0)^2 + \ldots + (1003.3 - 999.0)^2\right]}{(4-1)} - \frac{7.00}{3} \tag{4.21}$$

$$S_D^2 = \frac{52.67}{3} - \frac{7.00}{3}$$

$$S_D^2 = 15.22.$$

The estimated IP variance is

$$S_{IP}^2 = S_D^2 + S_R^2$$
$$S_{IP}^2 = 15.22 + 7.00 \tag{4.22}$$
$$S_{IP}^2 = 22.22$$

The estimated IP standard deviation is $S_{IP} = \sqrt{22.22} = 4.71 \text{ mg/g}$.

When a ruggedness factor is a major contributor to intermediate precision, it is important to go through this two-step process of estimating the repeatability and within-day variances separately and then summing to get the intermediate precision variance. If one merely estimates the intermediate precision variance by computing the sample variance of the combined set of twelve observations in Table 4.4, σ_{IP}^2 will be underestimated. In this present example, the computed standard deviation of the combined data set of twelve measurements is 4.41 mg/g which is less than the standard deviation of 4.71 mg/g computed using the two-step process.

The proportion of total IP variance due to the ruggedness factor is expressed as the ratio

$$\rho = \frac{\sigma_D^2}{\sigma_D^2 + \sigma_R^2}. \tag{4.23}$$

As general rule, one should use the two-step process to estimate σ_{IP}^2 if $\rho \geq 0.30$. If $\rho < 0.3$, the variation from the ruggedness factor can remain in the repeatability variance, and the degree of underestimation is not too severe. For this example, the estimated value of ρ is

$$\hat{\rho} = \frac{S_D^2}{S_D^2 + S_R^2} = \frac{15.22}{15.22 + 7.0} = 0.68 \tag{4.24}$$

and the two-stage process is warranted.

A ruggedness factor must be described as either a fixed effect or a random effect in order to perform the appropriate qualification test. In the present example, "day" is described as a random effect. This is because the four days are conceptually viewed as a representative sample from an infinitely large number of days in which the procedure will be executed. Contrast this with a ruggedness effect such as analyst. Most labs might have only two or three analysts who will perform the procedure. This set of analysts forms a finite set, all of which will be used to perform the qualification experiment. A factor such as an analyst with a finite set of levels is called a *fixed effect*. As will be shown, the probability of passing the qualification (i.e., the power) depends on whether a factor is fixed or random.

A statistical tolerance interval can now be used to qualify the procedure against the criteria in Equation 4.6 with $\tau = 1000 \text{ mg/g}$ and $\lambda = 20 \text{ mg/g}$. Appropriate adjustments to

Equation 4.14 to incorporate the ruggedness factor "day" provides the 100 $(1 - 2\alpha)\%$ tolerance interval that contains 100 $P\%$ of the population:

$$L = \bar{Y} - K \times S_{IP}$$

$$U = \bar{Y} + K \times S_{IP}$$

$$K = \sqrt{\frac{\left(1 + \dfrac{1}{d \times r}\right) Z_{(1+P)/2}^2 \times df}{\chi_{2\alpha:df}^2}}$$

$$df = \frac{S_{IP}^4}{\dfrac{\left[\displaystyle\sum_{i=1}^{d}\left(\bar{Y}_{Di} - \bar{Y}\right)^2\right]^2}{C \times (d-1)^2} + \dfrac{(r-1) \times S_R^4}{r^2 \times d}}$$

$$C = \begin{cases} (d-1) & \text{if the ruggedness factor is random} \\ \dfrac{[d-1+2\theta]^2}{d-1+4\theta} & \text{if the ruggedness factor is fixed} \end{cases}$$

$$\theta = \max\left[0, \ \frac{r \displaystyle\sum_{i=1}^{d}\left(\bar{Y}_{Di} - \bar{Y}\right)^2}{2S_R^2} \times \left(\frac{d(r-1)-2}{d(r-1)}\right) - \frac{d-1}{2}\right].$$

(4.25)

With P = .96 and assuming day to be a random factor so that $C = d - 1$, the computed 80% two-sided tolerance interval is

$$df = \frac{S_{IP}^4}{\dfrac{\left[\displaystyle\sum_{i=1}^{d}\left(\bar{Y}_{Di} - \bar{Y}\right)^2\right]^2}{(d-1)^3} + \dfrac{(r-1) \times S_R^4}{r^2 \times d}}$$

$$df = \frac{22.22^2}{\dfrac{[52.67]^2}{(4-1)^3} + \dfrac{(3-1) \times 7.0^2}{3^2 \times 4}} = 4.7 = 5 \text{ (rounded)}$$

(4.26)

$$K = \sqrt{\frac{\left(1 + \dfrac{1}{d \times r}\right) Z_{(1+P)/2}^2 \times df}{\chi_{1-2\alpha:df}^2}} = \sqrt{\frac{\left(1 + \dfrac{1}{4 \times 3}\right)(2.05)^2 \times 5}{2.34}} = 3.12$$

$$L = 999.0 - 3.12\sqrt{22.22} = 984.3 \,\text{mg/g}$$

$$U = 999.0 + 3.12\sqrt{22.22} = 1013.7 \,\text{mg/g}$$

This interval qualifies the procedure since it falls between $-\lambda + \tau = 980$ and $\lambda + \tau = 1020$ mg/g.

For purposes of illustration, suppose the $d = 4$ levels of the ruggedness factor represented the only four analysts who would perform the procedure for the foreseeable future. In this case, "analyst" would be a fixed effect so that

$$\theta = \max\left[0, \frac{r\sum_{i=1}^{d}(\bar{Y}_{Di} - \bar{Y})^2}{2S_R^2} \times \left(\frac{d(r-1)-2}{d(r-1)} \right) - \frac{d-1}{2} \right]$$

$$\theta = \max\left[0, \frac{3 \times 52.67}{2 \times 7.00} \times \left(\frac{4(3-1)-2}{4(3-1)} \right) - \frac{4-1}{2} \right] = \max[0, 6.96] = 6.96$$

$$C = \frac{[d-1+2\theta]^2}{d-1+4\theta}$$

$$C = \frac{[4-1+2 \times 6.96]^2}{4-1+4 \times 6.96} = 9.28$$

$$df = \frac{S_{IP}^4}{\left[\dfrac{\left[\sum_{i=1}^{d}(\bar{Y}_{Di} - \bar{Y})^2 \right]^2}{C \times (d-1)^2} + \dfrac{(n-1) \times S_R^4}{n^2 \times d} \right]}$$ (4.27)

$$df = \frac{(22.22)^2}{\dfrac{[52.67]^2}{9.28 \times (4-1)^2} + \dfrac{(3-1) \times (7.00)^2}{3^2 \times 4}} = 13.7 = 14 \text{ (rounded)}$$

$$K = \sqrt{\frac{\left(1 + \dfrac{1}{d \times r}\right) Z_{1+P/2}^2 \times df}{\chi_{1-2\alpha:df}^2}} = \sqrt{\frac{\left(1 + \dfrac{1}{4 \times 3}\right)(2.05)^2 \times 14}{9.47}} = 2.60$$

$$L = 999.0 - 2.60\sqrt{22.22} = 986.7 \text{ mg/g, and}$$

$$U = 999.0 + 2.60\sqrt{22.22} = 1011.3 \text{ mg/g.}$$

When the ruggedness factor is fixed, the value for df will be greater than it is for the random case. This has the effect of decreasing the width of the tolerance interval, and increasing the power of the test. In the present example, df has increased from 5 to 14. The resulting 80% tolerance interval that contains 96% of the population is from 986.7 to 1011.3, which is shorter than the corresponding random effects interval from 984.3 to 1013.7.

Hoffman and Kringle (2005) propose an alternative tolerance interval to Equation 4.25 for the random effects model. It is described by the USP Statistics Expert Team (2014). As demonstrated in the next section, Equation 4.25 provides a Type 1 error rate close to the desired level for all situations considered for the fixed model, and for the random model when $d > 2$.

To reemphasize points made earlier, discovery of impactful ruggedness factors must be made during Stage 1. This knowledge allows the analyst to design a qualification experiment that recognizes likely causes of variability and powers the experiment to ensure a procedure that is fit for use will pass the qualification.

One other important concept concerns the sample size taken for a random ruggedness factor. A sample size of $d = 4$ days was selected for the design reported in Table 4.4. The choice of sample size greatly impacts the ability to pass the qualification tests described in this chapter. As d increases, the probability of passing the qualification increases. To determine an appropriate sample size, one performs a statistical power calculation. This is the topic of the next section.

4.3.3 Power Considerations

The size of the qualification experiment has an impact on the ability to satisfy the testing criterion. This is particularly true when the experiment contains a ruggedness factor that is defined to be random. In general, select at least four samples ($d \geq 4$) from any random ruggedness factor that accounts for at least 30% of the total intermediate precision. Designs that employ only two levels of a random factor ($d = 2$) simply do not have sufficient power to ensure a procedure will meet the qualification criterion.

The easiest way to determine power for an experimental design is to use statistical simulation. Statistical power is defined as the probability of satisfying the test criterion for a given true value of the parameter of interest. Table 4.5 reports powers for three values of d where day is a random effect and there are $r = 3$ measurements per day. The qualification is based on an 80% tolerance interval with $P = 0.96$, $\tau = 1000$ mg/g, and $\lambda = 20$ mg/g. The parameter π is the true probability that a reportable value will fall outside the range from $-\lambda + \tau$ and $\lambda + \tau$. The simulated power in the shaded rows where $\pi = 1 - P = 0.04$ represents the Type 1 error rate for the hypotheses in Equation 4.8.

Examination of Table 4.5 provides the following observations:

1. A sample of size $d = 2$ does not supply acceptable power for any case shown in the table.

2. It is desirable for the Type 1 error rate to be as close as possible to 0.10 without going over. The simulated Type 1 error rate is less than 0.10 when $\rho = 0.3$ for all three designs, but is greater than 0.10 when $\rho = 0.6$, and $d = 2$ or 4.

3. Power generally decreases as ρ increases.

TABLE 4.5

Power of Several Ruggedness Designs Using Tolerance Interval with Random Effects and Desired Type 1 Error Rate of 0.10 ($r = 3$)

σ_{IP}	π	ρ	$d = 2$	$d = 4$	$d = 6$
4.71	0.0000315	0.3	0.62	0.91	0.99
6.00	0.001	0.3	0.41	0.67	0.83
7.71	0.01	0.3	0.21	0.30	0.39
9.69	0.04	0.3	0.09	0.08	0.08
4.71	0.0000315	0.6	0.55	0.81	0.95
6.00	0.001	0.6	0.42	0.57	0.72
7.71	0.01	0.6	0.26	0.30	0.35
9.69	0.04	0.6	0.13	0.11	0.10

TABLE 4.6

Power of Several Ruggedness Designs Using Tolerance Interval with Fixed Effects and Desired Type 1 Error Rate of 0.10 ($d = 2$)

σ_{IP}	π	ρ	$r = 3$ Random	$r = 3$ Fixed	$r = 6$ Random	$r = 6$ Fixed
4.71	0.0000315	0.3	0.62	0.72	0.77	0.97
6.00	0.001	0.3	0.41	0.47	0.60	0.74
7.71	0.01	0.3	0.21	0.23	0.31	0.35
9.69	0.04	0.3	0.09	0.10	0.10	0.10
4.71	0.0000315	0.6	0.55	0.75	0.63	0.99
6.00	0.001	0.6	0.42	0.45	0.51	0.82
7.71	0.01	0.6	0.26	0.21	0.35	0.35
9.69	0.04	0.6	0.13	0.09	0.18	0.09

Table 4.6 demonstrates that power is greater when a ruggedness factor is fixed as opposed to random. In this table, $d = 2$ and the qualification is again based on an 80% tolerance interval with $P = 0.96$, $\tau = 1000$ mg/g, and $\lambda = 20$ mg/g. As with the previous table, the shaded rows provide the simulated Type 1 error rate.

Examination of Table 4.6 provides the following observations:

1. A random effects model of size $d = 2$ does not maintain the Type 1 error rate as ρ and r increase.

2. The fixed effects model provides greater power than the random effects model, and the difference increases as ρ and r increase.

3. The fixed effects model maintains the desired Type 1 error rate.

In summary, proper recognition of the nature of a ruggedness factor is imperative in order to design a qualification experiment with adequate statistical power.

4.3.4 Holistic Qualification of a Bioassay Method

This section describes a holistic qualification for a bioassay method. Table 4.7 provides an analysis of variance summary table for data from qualification of a bioassay procedure described in USP Chapter <1033>.

The design consists of eight independent runs across five known potency values, with two recorded values for each potency value on each run. The factor "Run" is a random effect with $d = 8$ levels with $r = 10$ replicates for each level across five fixed values of

TABLE 4.7

ANOVA for <1033> Bioassay Data

Source	df	MS	F Ratio	Prob > F
Known potency	4	5.21836	3083.6	<.0001
Run	7	$S^2_{Run} = 0.03406$	20.1	<.0001
Repeatability	$\nu = 68$	$S^2_R = 0.00169$		

"Known potency." In total, there are $n = d \times r = 8 \times 10 = 80$ recorded relative potency values, with error degrees of freedom $\nu = 68$. Before computing Table 4.7, the logarithm was taken of each relative potency value because the log–normal model is traditionally employed for modeling relative potency data. The average of all 80 log-transformed potency values is 0.0407. (Note: The eight runs reported in <1033> were formed by combinations of two ruggedness factors. However, each of these factors contributed less than 30% of the total intermediate precision variance and are combined with the repeatability.) Figure 4.3 provides a plot of the data.

There are two sources of variability in the data attributed to the analytical procedure: Run-to-run variability (denoted σ^2_{Run}) and repeatability (denoted σ^2_R). The intermediate precision variance is accordingly defined as $\sigma^2_{IP} = \sigma^2_{Run} + \sigma^2_R$.

A useful metric for defining "fit for use" for a bioassay is based on the probability of an out of specification (OOS) signal when the process is in a state of control. Note that by setting $-\lambda + \tau = LSL$ and $\lambda + \tau = USL$ where LSL and USL are lower and upper specifications, respectively, Equation 4.6 becomes

$$Pr(LSL < Y < USL) \geq P. \tag{4.28}$$

The probability of an OOS signal is defined as $\pi = 1 - Pr(LSL < Y < USL)$ and to pass qualification, it is required to show that $\pi \leq 1 - P$. For this example, the specification limits are stated to be $LSL = 0.71$ and $USL = 1.41$ (in the original scale).

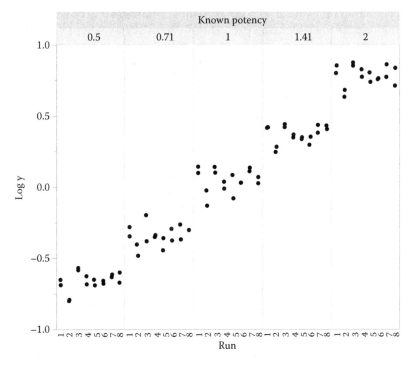

FIGURE 4.3
Plot of <1033> data.

To qualify the bioassay, we employ the tolerance interval procedure described in Equation 4.14. In particular,

1. The desired Type 1 error rate is set at $\alpha = 0.10$.
2. A $100\,(1 - 2\alpha)\% = 80\%$ two-sided tolerance interval that contains $100\,P\%$ of the population is computed using the log-transformed data.
3. If the back-transformed tolerance interval in Step 2 falls entirely in the range between *LSL* and *USL*, then one concludes that the analytical procedure satisfies the qualification criterion and is fit for use. Based on the company risk profile, it is decided to select $P = 0.99$ which allows an OOS rate no greater than 0.01.

Before computing the tolerance interval in Step 2, it is important to account for the process variability that must also be contained within the specification limits. To do this, define

$$\rho^* = \frac{\sigma_P^2}{\sigma_P^2 + \sigma_{IP}^2} \qquad (4.29)$$

where σ_P^2 represents the expected process variation. If an estimate of σ_P^2 is not available, one can select ρ^* based on historic performance for similar assays. For a bioassay, a reasonable value for ρ^* is 0.20 since bioassay procedures typically have more variability than the process being monitored.

The random effects form of the tolerance interval in Equation 4.25 is used to compute a tolerance interval for this example because it involves two mean squares. This equation is adjusted to account for ρ^* and provides the $100\,(1 - 2\alpha)\%$ tolerance interval to contain $100P\%$ of the population:

$$L = \bar{Y} - K \times S_{IP}\sqrt{\frac{1}{1-\rho^*}}$$

$$U = \bar{Y} + K \times S_{IP}\sqrt{\frac{1}{1-\rho^*}}$$

$$K = \sqrt{\frac{\left(1 + \dfrac{1}{d \times r}\right) Z_{(1+P)/2}^2 \times df}{\chi_{2\alpha;df}^2}} \qquad (4.30)$$

$$S_{IP}^2 = \frac{S_{Run}^2}{r} + \frac{(r-1) \times S_R^2}{r}$$

$$df = \frac{S_{IP}^4}{\dfrac{S_{Run}^4}{r^2 \times (d-1)} + \dfrac{(r-1)^2 \times S_R^4}{r^2 \times v}}$$

Using the data from Table 4.7,

$$S_{IP}^2 = \frac{0.03406}{10} + \frac{(10-1) \times 0.00169}{10} = 0.004927$$

$$df = \frac{(0.004927)^2}{\dfrac{0.03406^2}{10^2 \times (8-1)} + \dfrac{(10-1)^2 \times 0.00169^2}{10^2 \times 68}} = 14.4 = 14 \text{ (rounded)}$$

$$K = \sqrt{\frac{\left(1 + \dfrac{1}{80}\right) Z_{(1+0.99)/2}^2 \times 14}{\chi_{0.20:df}^2}} = \sqrt{\frac{\left(1 + \dfrac{1}{80}\right) 2.576^2 \times 14}{9.467}} = 3.152 \quad (4.31)$$

$$L = 0.0407 - 3.152 \times \sqrt{\frac{0.004927}{1-0.2}} = -0.207, \text{ and}$$

$$U = 0.0407 + 3.152 \sqrt{\frac{0.004927}{1-0.2}} = 0.288.$$

The back-transformed bounds of the tolerance interval to the original scale are $L = \exp(-0.207) = 0.813$ and $U = \exp(0.288) = 1.33$. Since this interval falls entirely within the range from $LSL = 0.71$ to $USL = 1.41$, the procedure meets the qualification criterion.

4.3.5 Holistic Qualification of a Relative Purity Method

This example concerns a relative purity assay obtained from chromatographic peak integration. Using the normalization procedure, measurements represent the percentage of peak area in relation to the total area of a curve defined by absorbance on the vertical axis and time on the horizontal axis. The measurement for a given peak is typically represented as "% of total area under the curve." Since there is generally no acknowledged "true value," qualification is focused on the precision of the procedure.

Consider a reverse phase (RP) chromatography procedure where the platform lower specification limit (LSL) for the main peak is 95%, with an expected process mean of $\mu = 98\%$. The procedure will be used for lot disposition using a decision rule that the measured value of "% of total area under main peak" must exceed $LSL = 95\%$ for lot release. Thus, a reasonable criterion for qualification is to demonstrate that when the process is in control,

$$\Pr(LSL \leq Y) \geq P$$
$$1 - \Pr(LSL \leq Y) \leq 1 - P$$
$$1 - \Pr\left(\frac{LSL - \mu}{\sqrt{\sigma_{IP}^2 + \sigma_P^2}} \leq Z\right) \leq 1 - P \quad (4.32)$$

where $1 - P$ represents an acceptable proportion of out-of-specification (OOS) signals, σ_{IP}^2 is the intermediate precision variance of the RP procedure, σ_P^2 is the manufacturing process variance, and Z is a standard normal random variable.

Equation 4.32 is true if

$$\sqrt{\sigma_{IP}^2 + \sigma_P^2} < \frac{\mu - LSL}{Z_P} \tag{4.33}$$

where Z_P is the standard normal quantile with area P to the left. Now expressing Equation 4.33 in terms of σ_{IP}, it is required that

$$\sigma_{IP} < \frac{\mu - LSL}{Z_P} \times \sqrt{(1 - \rho^*)} = C \tag{4.34}$$

where ρ^* is the proportion of total variation due to the manufacturing process as defined in Equation 4.29.

To qualify the procedure, one must reject the null hypothesis in the following set

$$\begin{aligned} H_0 &: \sigma_{IP} \geq C \\ H_1 &: \sigma_{IP} < C \end{aligned} \tag{4.35}$$

where K is defined in Equation 4.34. The null hypothesis in Equation 4.35 is rejected with a Type 1 error rate of α if the $100\,(1 - \alpha)\%$ upper confidence bound on σ_{IP} is less than C.

For a sample of n independent observations, the sample variance S^2 is the estimator for σ_{IP}^2. The $100\,(1 - \alpha)\%$ upper confidence bound on σ_{IP} is therefore Equation 4.4, which is

$$U = \sqrt{\frac{(n-1)S^2}{\chi_{\alpha:n-1}^2}}. \tag{4.36}$$

If the design contains a ruggedness factor, σ_{IP}^2 can be estimated using Equation 4.30, and $(n - 1)$ in Equation 4.36 is replaced with df in Equation 4.30.

For the qualification experiment of the RP chromatography procedure in this example, $LSL = 95\%$ and $\mu = 98\%$. The procedure is known to be precise relative to the manufacturing process, so the value $\rho^* = 0.8$ is used in establishing the qualification criterion. Based on the company risk profile, the value $1 - P = 0.03$ is deemed an acceptable false OOS rate. Using this information, the qualification criterion is

$$\begin{aligned} C &= \frac{\mu - LSL}{Z_P} \times \sqrt{(1 - \rho^*)} \\ C &= \frac{98 - 95}{Z_{0.97}} \times \sqrt{(1 - 0.8)} = \frac{98 - 95}{1.88} \times \sqrt{(1 - 0.8)} = 0.71. \end{aligned} \tag{4.37}$$

The qualification experiment provides twelve independent measurements of % main peak. The sample variance is $S^2 = 0.15$. Thus, the 95% upper confidence bound ($\alpha = 0.05$) is

$$U = \sqrt{\frac{(n-1)S^2}{\chi_{\alpha:n-1}^2}} = \sqrt{\frac{(12-1)0.15}{4.57}} = 0.60. \tag{4.38}$$

Since $U = 0.60$ is less than $C = 0.71$, the qualification criterion is satisfied and the procedure is qualified as fit for use.

4.3.6 Limit of Detection (LOD) and Linearity

The limit of detection (LOD) is the minimum amount of an analyte that can be reliably detected. In the previously described relative purity procedure, it answers the question, "How high should a curve be (measured as absorbance) before one begins integration?" Conventionally, the LOD is defined as

$$LOD = \mu + 3.3 \times \sigma_{IP} \qquad (4.39)$$

In the present example, μ is the true baseline value (i.e., the point of no signal) on the absorbance axis. Typically, μ and σ_{IP} are estimated from a collected sample of data.

Definition is more complex when the horizontal axis rather than the vertical axis is the scale for which the LOD is of interest, because back-transformations are required. As an example, for data such as Table 4.3, it is typically of interest to define LOD on the concentration scale as opposed to the signal scale. Chapter <1210> of the USP guidance (2017) provides definitions and formulas that can be used for this situation.

In situations where back-transformed data are necessary, the issue of calibration linearity becomes an important consideration. LeBlond, Tan, and Yang (2013) offer a full discussion of this topic.

4.4 Step 3: Continued Procedure Performance Verification

The final step in the life cycle is continued monitoring of the procedure. System suitability tests to monitor procedure performance are an integral part of any ongoing procedure verification. System suitability tests are needed to ensure a qualified procedure is still operating as it was during the qualification testing. Failure to implement system suitability tests before an application could provide reportable values that are not fit for use. Depending on the type of procedure, system suitability tests can be based on any number of attributes including retention time, LOD, resolution, tailing factor, precision, or accuracy.

One attribute often used in a system suitability test is the standard deviation of n measurements from a test sample made prior to the actual measurement. If the standard deviation is less than some fixed value, then the system suitability criterion is met and the procedure can be used to make the desired measurements. In order to establish the criterion for a system suitability test, one should answer the question, "How large might a standard deviation be for a new sample of n measurements made on a single day if the procedure is operating at the same level it was during qualification?" This question can be answered by computing the 95% upper prediction bound

$$U = S_{IP} \sqrt{F_{1-\alpha:n-1,df}} \qquad (4.40)$$

where n is the sample size used in the future system suitability test, S_{IP} is the standard deviation of the IP in the qualification study, and df are the degrees of freedom for the IP estimate in the qualification study (see, e.g., Meeker et al., 2017).

To demonstrate, assume the procedure qualified in Section 4.3.2 for the ruggedness study will be monitored using a suitability test where $n = 6$ random replicates are tested for a given test sample prior to measurement of the samples of interest. The estimated IP standard deviation from the qualification experiment is $S_{IP} = 4.71$ based on $df = 5$ degrees of freedom. Using these data,

$$U = S_{IP}\sqrt{F_{1-\alpha:n-1,df}}$$
$$U = 4.71\sqrt{F_{0.95:6-1,5}} = 4.71\sqrt{5.05} = 10.6\,\text{mg/g}. \tag{4.41}$$

Thus, a reasonable system suitability test is to collect $n = 6$ independent measurements of a test material and compute the standard deviation. If the standard deviation is less than $U = 10.6$ mg/g, the criterion is met and the procedure can be applied to make the desired measurements.

Control charting of reference material is another form of system suitability testing. If outcomes of the parameter of interest can be represented with a normal probability model, and sufficient data are available from past applications of the procedure, one might employ the three-sigma rule used on control charts to describe expected behavior. For example, an interval for expected retention time values might be represented as

$$\bar{Y} \pm 3 \times S \tag{4.42}$$

where $\bar{Y}$ is a sample mean of measured values from data collected during qualification or prior work, and S is the sample standard deviation of the same data set. If retention time for the suitability test falls in this range, the procedure can be used to make measurements.

There is a large body of material on statistical control charts that can be used to monitor procedures and to make sure they remain operating as intended. Recent pharmaceutical applications are provided in Section 5.2 of Burdick et al. (2017) and in Altan, Hare, and Strickland (2016). ASTM E2587 (2016) provides more information on the topic of control charts.

References

Altan S, Hare L, Strickland H (2016). Process capability and statistical process control, in *Nonclinical Statistics for Pharmaceutical and Biotechnology Industries*, ed. Zhang L, pp. 549–573. Springer, Heidelberg.

ASTM E2587 (2016). Standard practice for use of control charts in statistical process control. ASTM International, West Conshohocken, PA.

Burdick RK, LeBlond DJ, Pfahler LB, Quiroz J, Sidor L, Vukovinsky K, Zhang L (2017). *Statistical Applications for Chemistry, Manufacturing and Controls (CMC) in the Pharmaceutical Industry*. Springer, Heidelberg.

FDA (2011). Process validation: General principles and practices, guidance for industry. CDER.

Hoffman D, Kringle R (2005). Two-sided tolerance intervals for balanced and unbalanced random effects models. *Journal of Biopharmaceutical Statistics* 15, 283–293.

Hubert Ph, Nguyen-Huu J-J, Boulanger B, Chapuzet E, Chiap P, Cohen N, Compagnon P-A, Dewe W, Feinberg M, Lallier M, Laurentie M, Mercier N, Muzard G, Nivet C, Valat L (2004). Harmonization of strategies for the validation of quantitative analytical procedures: A SFSTP proposal—Part I. *Journal of Pharmaceutical and Biomedical Analysis* 36, 579–586.

Hubert Ph, Nguyen-Huu J-J, Boulanger B, Chapuzet E, Chiap P, Cohen N, Compagnon P-A, Dewe W, Feinberg M, Lallier M, Laurentie M, Mercier N, Muzard G, Nivet C, Valat L, Rozet E (2007a). Harmonization of strategies for the validation of quantitative analytical procedures: A SFSTP proposal—Part II. *Journal of Pharmaceutical and Biomedical Analysis* 45, 70–81.

Hubert Ph, Nguyen-Huu J-J, Boulanger B, Chapuzet E, Cohen N, Compagnon P-A, Dewe W, Feinberg M, Laurentie M, Mercier N, Muzard G, Valat L, Rozet E (2007b). Harmonization of strategies for the validation of quantitative analytical procedures: A SFSTP proposal—Part III. *Journal of Pharmaceutical and Biomedical Analysis* 45, 82–96.

International Conference on Harmonization (ICH) (2005). Q2 (R1) Validation of analytical procedures: Text and methodology.

International Conference on Harmonization (ICH) (2009). Q8 (R2) Pharmaceutical development.

LeBlond D, Tan CY, Yang H (2013). Stimuli to the revision process: Confirmation of analytical method calibration linearity. *Pharmacopeial Forum* 39(3).

Martin GP, Barnett KL, Burgess C, Curry PD, Ermer J, Gratzl GS, Hammond JP, Herrmann J, Kovacs E, LeBlond DJ, LoBrutto R, McCasland-Keller AK, McGregor PL, Nethercote P, Templeton AC, Thomas DP, Weitzel J (2013). Stimuli to the revision process: Lifecycle management of analytical procedures: Method development, procedure performance qualification, and procedure performance verification. *Pharmacopeial Forum* 39(5).

Mee RW (1988). Estimation of the percentage of a normal distribution lying outside a specified interval. *Communications in Statistics—Theory and Methods* 17(5), 1465–1479.

Meeker WQ, Hahn GJ, Escobar LA (2017). *Statistical Intervals: A Guide for Practitioners and Researchers.* Wiley, New Jersey.

Sondag P, Lebrun P, Rozet E, Boulanger B (2016). Assay validation, in *Nonclinical Statistics for Pharmaceutical and Biotechnology Industries,* ed. Zhang L, pp. 415–432. Springer, Heidelberg.

Torbeck LD (2010). %RSD: Friend or foe? *Pharmaceutical Technology* 34(1), 37–38.

USP 41-NF 36 General Chapter <1010> (2017). Analytical data—Interpretation and treatment. U.S. Pharmacopeial Convention, Rockville, MD.

USP 41-NF 36 General Chapter <1033> (2017). Biological assay validation. U.S. Pharmacopeial Convention, Rockville, MD.

USP 41-NF 36 General Chapter <1210> (2017). Statistical tools for procedure validation. U.S. Pharmacopeial Convention, Rockville, MD.

USP 41-NF 36 General Chapter <1225> (2017). Validation of compendial procedures. U.S. Pharmacopeial Convention, Rockville, MD.

USP Statistics Expert Team In-Process Revision: <1210> (2014). Statistical tools for procedure validation. *Pharmacopeial Forum* 40(5).

Weitzel MLJ (2012). The estimation and use of measurement uncertainty for a drug substance test procedure validated according to USP <1225>. *Accreditation and Quality Assurance* 17, 139–146.

5

Strategic Bioassay Design, Development, Analysis, and Validation*

David Lansky

CONTENTS

5.1 Introduction

5.1.1 Supporting a Biotechnology Product

Bioassays are used to support development, clinical trials, licensing, and manufacturing of biotechnology products. Because these activities span years to decades, it is important to use strategies for design, management, analysis, and maintenance that are initially robust and will continue to deliver potency measurements that have consistent meaning over long

---

* This chapter is © David Lansky. Reprinted with permission.

periods of time. This chapter will focus on statistical design and analysis strategies that help ensure that bioassays deliver high-quality measurements of potency (with low bias and high precision) and more. Among other things, good design and analysis strategies help protect bioassays against location and sequence or order effects (within the assay); provide robustness against changes in critical reagents; support monitoring of location, sequence, and other effects with production assay data; and, by using modular designs, are relatively easy to adapt to changing performance requirements. Other management issues that are important to ensure that a bioassay continues to perform well include demonstrating robust broadly, and including using at least two established suppliers for each reagent.

5.1.2 Product Specifications Ensure Efficacy and Safety

Ideally, product specifications are based on knowledge of a range of product activity (potency) that has been shown (via clinical trials) to be both safe and effective. To support a claim that product from the production process is represented by clinical experience, it is reasonable to set the product specification by using the inner 95% confidence intervals of the most extreme lots that have been shown to be safe and effective (Figure 5.1). With clinical experience based on a relatively small number of lots, it is important to demonstrate safety and efficacy over a deliberately widened range of activity levels (for instance, the open points in Figure 5.1 that represent clinical lots used at high and low doses). When little is known about the safety or efficacy of a product, the product specifications may be negotiated with regulatory agencies based on other similar products or general knowledge about a related class of products. It is useful to think of product specifications as an "operating window" that must contain whatever amount of product degradation is allowed over the product's shelf life, variation in the product due to manufacturing, as well as uncertainty about the product due to both bias and variation in the bioassay. This idea leads to a "release specification" that is narrowed from the product specifications by the upper confidence limit on the amount of loss of potency during the shelf life of the product (Figure 5.1). Because assay bias (from all

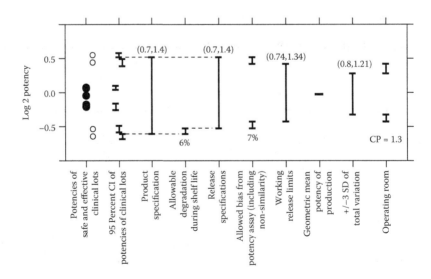

FIGURE 5.1
For a typical protein product, combining production experience, clinical experience, degradation, and assay capability into a manufacturing system. The open circles near the left side of the plot represent clinical lots (black solid circles) that were used in the clinic at high or low doses.

sources combined) is systematic, it is sensible to further narrow the release specifications to "working release limits" by an upper confidence interval endpoint of the total amount of bias allowed to ensure that the actual potency of the released material is within the release specifications while the measured potency is within the working release limits (Figure 5.1).

Broadly speaking, it is clear that the bioassay performance requirements are driven by the product specifications (which are based on what is medically appropriate) as well as consideration of degradation and process variation. Mature manufacturing and quality control systems production variation plus measurement variation will have a process capability of 1.3 or more (see Chapter 8 for more on this topic), with process control limits at ±3 standard deviations (SD) of total variation (production variation plus measurement variation) at least 1 SD inside release specifications (assuming that there is no bias from the bioassay) (see Figure 5.1 and [23]). It is important to note that it is a substantial challenge to build a system with a process capability (Cpk) of 1.3 that can accommodate manufacturing variation, clinical experience, degradation limits, bias, and precision performance of the assay. To achieve a Cpk of 1.3 typically requires clinical experience that is much broader than what would be observed from manufacturing variation alone, narrow bounds on degradation, narrow bounds on assay bias, high precision from the assay, and replicate assays. It is especially important to recognize that these ambitious requirements are needed whether the goal is to support a typical protein product or vaccine product. A hypothetical protein product is illustrated with seven simulated lots having a percent geometric standard deviation (PGSD, which is %GCV in [21]) among lots of 7%, a PGSD among assays of 3.5%, where four assays are used for a reported value; further, the total bias (as percent geometric bias) is limited to 7% and the loss of potency during storage is limited to 6% (Figure 5.1). Note that there are also clinical results shown for this protein product at shifted target potencies of 1/2 and 2. While it is not necessary to meet all these performance targets, it is important that the system as a whole achieve reasonable process capability. A hypothetical vaccine product is also shown with 30 simulated lots having a PGSD among lots of 60% and a PGSD among assays of 15%, where four assays are used for a reported value; further, the total

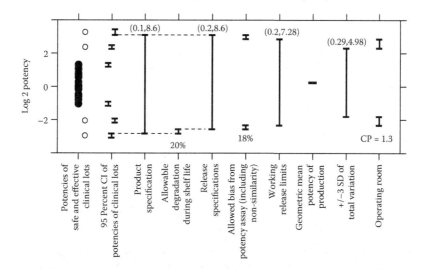

FIGURE 5.2
For a typical vaccine product, combining production experience, clinical experience, degradation, and assay capability into a manufacturing system. The open circles near the left side of the plot represent clinical lots (black solid circles) that were used in the clinic at high or low doses.

bias (as percent geometric bias) is limited to 18% and the loss of potency during storage is limited to 20% (Figure 5.2). Again, for the vaccine product, clinical results are shown at shifted target potencies, here at 1/16th and 16. Note that the figures that illustrate these two cases are visually very similar; they differ only in the scaling of the log potency axis. Other methods for assessing product specifications are described in Chapter 6.

5.2 Statistical and Strategic Introduction

Biological assay design and analysis are often presented using the simplest of statistical designs, a completely randomized design (CRD) [10,25]. This is helpful because it keeps the focus on how bioassays are different from other analytic technologies that are typically analyzed using calibration based methods. Unfortunately, most practical biological assays have a more complex design than a CRD; blocks are usually present while split-unit and strip-unit statistical designs are common [22]. Assays where each dilution of each sample appears on each of several plates can be described as "blocked by plate" or as "having plate blocks" and should have an analysis that allows different curve shapes for each block (for each plate). Assays where samples are assigned to plate rows and dilutions are assigned to plate columns (or vice versa) are strip-unit designs; the rows and columns are important groups in the assay design and it is often important to recognize these groups in the analysis (Figures 5.3 and 5.4 and [22]). When a bioassay with a complex design structure such as a randomized complete block design (RCBD) or a strip-unit design has important variation associated with blocks, rows, or columns in the design and these important sources of variation do not appear in the analysis model, the resulting estimates of residual error are completely unreliable (because the estimate of residual error will increase or decrease as the variation associated with blocks and other elements of the design increase and decrease). Analysis of bioassays involves data-based decisions, with many based on error estimates derived largely from the residual error

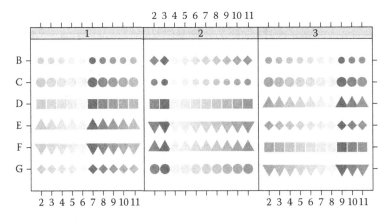

FIGURE 5.3
A strip-unit design, with one row for each of six samples on each of three plates. The panel headers indicate the plate number, the symbol indicates the sample, and the shading intensity indicates the dilution. Note that the assignments of samples to row within plate, column for the starting dilution, and dilution direction are assigned at random for each plate. The highest concentrations are in columns 7, 3, and 9 (for plates 1, 2, and 3) with dilution to the right on plates 1 and 3, while dilution is to the left on plate 2. This very restricted randomization is, at least for some labs, practical by hand.

estimate(s). Decisions such as which observations are outliers, whether the assay passes assay acceptance criteria, and whether samples pass sample acceptance criteria (typically similarity) all depend on the residual error estimate; additionally, estimates of the variation of potency or confidence intervals on potency are often based on within-assay estimates of variation. Because statements about the expected precision performance of an assay are fundamentally based on the precision of the assay, it is not possible to make realistic forecasts of assay performance without good estimates of the variation associated with each important source of variation in the assay design. Hence, for a bioassay to exhibit reliably reproducible behavior, it must have an analysis that respects the design of the assay.

It can sometimes be helpful to place strategically chosen dilutions on the edges of the plate where they may be ignored in order to increase the chances that there will be good data from both asymptotes for all samples and several observations on the steep portion of the response curve for each sample. While it is not particularly convenient in the illustrated assay design (for plates 1 and 3), it is often find helpful to use a twelve-point dilution series with dilutions three and ten on the edges; this is illustrated in Figure 5.4.

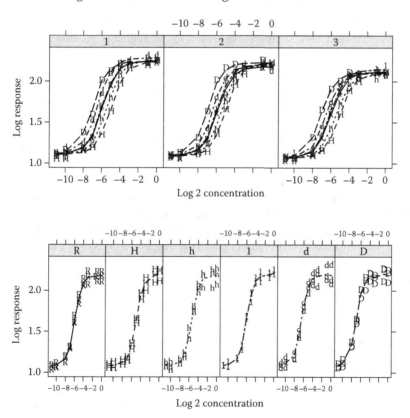

FIGURE 5.4
Data from the strip-unit design in Figure 5.3 fit with a four parameter logistic strip-unit model (upper panels) and a four parameter logistic completely randomized design (CRD) model (lower panels). There is one panel for each plate of the strip-unit model and one panel for each sample of the CRD model. The variation around the fitted curves is clearly larger with the CRD model which ignores the structure of the assay. The samples are labeled as D (long-dashed lines, with potency 2), d (dash-dot lines with potency 1.41), R (solid lines, with potency 1), 1 (long-dash with dot, with potency 1), h (short-dashed line, with potency 0.71), and H (dashed line, with potency 0.5). Note that the dilution series is a twelve-point two-fold dilution series with dilutions 3 and 10 omitted; this is intentional so the series spans a wider concentration range.

Biological assay design and analysis draws upon a collection of statistical tools; these include blocking, recognition of experimental units, regression (linear or nonlinear) models, equivalence testing, outlier detection methods (potentially using nonparametric regression, and methods for detecting multiple outliers), as well as methods for dealing with nonconstant variance and possibly non-normally distributed data [21,22]. The core concepts that distinguish bioassay design and analysis from what is familiar to many, namely calibration-based analytic methods, are

- A bioassay measures activity in the bioassay relative to a reference sample that is assumed to contain the same active analyte (hence the bioassay is a measure of function rather than a measure of concentration or amount).
- The design of the bioassay includes multiple dilutions of each of the reference and test samples.
- As a check that it is reasonable to assume that the reference and test contain the same active analyte, bioassays contain a preliminary test of similarity (of the concentration–response relationship) between reference and test samples.
- The reference and test samples are tested close together in time, in space, and using the same group of organisms.

The last item on this list turns each bioassay into a statistical block, where comparisons between reference and test (whether for similarity or potency) are within-assay (or within-block) comparisons; note that there may be multiple levels of blocking.

This chapter focuses on the properties, design, and analysis of bioassays that are indirect (with fixed dilutions) with quantitative response. Most of the statistical ideas, design strategies, and analysis methods presented here will transfer to blocked bioassays whether they are direct or indirect, have quantitative or discrete responses, use cells or animals, and so on. Further, the design and analysis strategies presented here may be useful for ELISA and other calibration-based analytic methods.

It is fairly common to check during development and validation that there are no important location or sequence (or time order) effects. Monitoring an assay system to ensure that location or sequence effects have not become important is rare; in many assays this monitoring is not practical because the assay design has location or sequence effects confounded with sample, dilution, or both. Assays do change over time; experience has shown that assay problems appear (all too often) as out of specification batches of product. These assay problems are (usually) eventually traced to changes in assay (critical reagents) that increase the impact of location or sequence effects; in assays where these are confounded with sample or dilution, they cause bias in potency. An important part of assay life cycle management is monitoring location and sequence effects. This monitoring is difficult unless the design allows separate estimates of location, sequence, sample, and dilution effects. Good designs make it relatively easy to monitor location, sequence, dilution, and other potential contaminating effects.

5.2.1 Common Properties of Bioassays

Most quantitative response bioassays display increasing variation with increasing responses (as is common in many biological systems); for most of these bioassays a log or square root transformation is at least a good candidate transformation to stabilize the variance. Additionally, in most of these bioassays the distribution of responses (within dose by sample combinations) is skewed; a good choice of a transformation will also yield near-symmetric distributions. In practice, the designs used in bioassay laboratories are at least blocked and more commonly split- or strip-unit designs (or close to these); assays with a simple completely randomized design are rare. The variation observed in bioassays is rarely only additive on the response or transformed response scale; in most cases much of the variation in response can be associated with how the EC50 or asymptote of maximum response (or response range) varies from block to block (Figure 5.4).

For assays that have a completely randomized design, a simple linear means model (with a mean response for each combination of sample and dilution) is an excellent way to estimate experimental error, σ^2, from the ε_{ijk} in

$$y_{ijk} = \mu_{ij} + \varepsilon_{ijk},$$

where

- y is the (possibly transformed) response,
- i is the sample index,
- j is the dilution index,
- k is the replicate index,
- μ_{ij} is the mean response for sample i at dilution j, and
- ε_{ijk} are the errors or residuals around the fitted means; these residuals are assumed to be normally distributed, independent, and have constant additive variance (σ^2).

If the ε_{ijk} are indeed independent, normally distributed, and have constant variance (σ^2), the analysis is relatively easy; much of the bioassay literature and regulatory guidance assumes this simple, but rarely realistic, case. For assays that have a blocked design and additive error the model changes only slightly to

$$y_{ijk} = \mu_{ij} + \beta_k + \varepsilon_{ijk}, \tag{5.1}$$

where β_k is the additive block effect (note that the replicates are now "by block").

When important variation in the assay can be well described by block (or other grouping in the assay design) specific curve parameters, the variation in the assay is likely to be poorly fit by models that assume that all variation is additive in the response (as in Equation 5.1). An important consequence of nonadditive variation is that nonlinear mixed models (which can often be approximated by simply fitting the nonlinear model separately in each block) may yield appreciably better fits than a blocked means model. When nonlinear mixed models typically yield better fits than means models, this provides evidence that the variation in many bioassay systems is not additive in the response.

What is particularly striking is that in many bioassay systems variation that is not simply additive in the response appears only after prolonged use of the system and can sometimes be attributed to subtle effects of changes in critical reagents. An interesting implication of this is that when monitoring assays with models that only allow variation that is additive in the response it is likely that certain important sources of variation will be difficult to detect.

In many bioassays variation in curves across blocks is clearly associated with variation in logEC50 or response range. Two particularly important findings from simulation studies that examine the impact of variation in bioassay curve parameters associated with blocks and other elements of bioassay design structure (such as experimental units of rows and columns on cell culture plates) are that (1) when important variation in curve parameters associated with design structure is omitted from the analysis model, the analyses substantially overestimate the error (making it much harder to pass equivalence tests for similarity), and (2) if the analysis model includes important sources of variation in the assay design structure, the driver of the precision of potency is the size of the residual variation around sample-specific within-block response curves (Figure 5.4). Further, using assay designs that provide some protection against location effects and including the important parts of the design structure of the assay in the analysis models combine to provide protection from variation associated with design structure factors.

5.2.2 Issues with Common Analysis Strategies

Almost all outlier detection methods assume normally distributed data; hence, bioassays with skewed data typically require transformation before outlier detection. A common approach to outlier detection is to use Dixon's method (see Chapter 1) on small numbers of replicates (which may be pseudo-replicates or from separate blocks). Using Dixon's is appropriate if the data (perhaps after transformation) are nearly normal in distribution, the number of outliers is known, and the data set is small (between 3 and 40 observations) [9]. Performing outlier detection on subgroups of observations that are from a common sample at a common dilution is a poor strategy because it fails to use information about expected response from nearby dilutions and hence has lower power than alternative methods.

An analysis method that is widely used for radioimmunoassays involves fitting nonlinear models with (optionally iteratively re-) weighted least squares [3,7,8,19]. It is important to note that radioimmunoassays tend to have appreciably less variance than bioassays, and in particular tend to have variation that is much more nearly additive (in the response). It is because so much of the variation in bioassays is not additive that nonlinear models with (optionally iteratively re-) weighted least squares are, in general, a poor choice for bioassay analysis; there are hints of these issues in [8].

There are better choices than the commonly used parameterization of the four parameter logistic model:

$$y = \frac{A - D}{1 + \exp(-B \times (x - C))} + D + \varepsilon,$$

where

- y is the response,
- A is the "upper" asymptote,
- B is the shape,
- C is the natural log of the EC50,
- D is the "lower" asymptote,
- x is the log concentration of the sample, and
- ε are the errors or residuals around the fitted values; these residuals are assumed to be normally distributed, and independent [17].

Because there is often appreciable correlation between the asymptotes an alternative form has better properties:

$$y = \frac{A}{1 + \exp(-B \times (x - C))} + D + \varepsilon,$$ (5.2)

where

- A is the response range (the difference between asymptotes),
- B is the shape,
- C is the natural log of the EC50,
- D is the no-dose asymptote [17].

Some abstract concepts (such as intrinsic and parameter effect curvature) have important practical consequences for nonlinear models; these considerations lead to strong recommendations against five parameter logistic models [16] because of both parameter effects and intrinsic curvature [3,19]. Further, the common form of the five-parameter logistic model has additional important inherent problems, namely, a lack of identifiability and insufficient flexibility; an alternative five-parameter model addresses some of these issues [20].

While similarity testing via equivalence tests is becoming common, it is rare that equivalence test bounds are linked to performance properties of the assay (for example; bias of estimated potency). In many cases the equivalence bounds are set based on methods 1, 2, or 3 of [22,24] which have a known critical flaw. These methods are all sensitive to the size (number of observations in) and precision of the assay. It is important that the equivalence bounds be set based on either subject matter knowledge (an understanding of the impact of a given shift in the response range or curve shape) or on a more general understanding of the impact of various shifts in (perhaps scaled) changes in curve parameters on critical properties of potency (such as bias). While knowledge of the importance of various sizes of a shift in a curve parameter may be limited and knowledge of the impact of such shifts on the critical properties of potency may also be limited, it is important to move beyond the simple starting methods proposed in [22]. A useful starting point for equivalence bounds for some products that limits the bias in potency to 10% requires that 90% confidence intervals for shifts in no-dose asymptote, range (difference in asymptotes), and the sum of no-dose asymptote plus range to be entirely within ±10% while shifts in the curve shape parameter have 90% confidence intervals entirely within ±50%. For products that can tolerate more bias in potency due to undetected nonsimilarity, wider similarity equivalence bounds are appropriate. For many products potency bias limits near or even under 5% will be valuable, for these products equivalence bounds will need to be appreciably narrower.

5.3 A Recommended Bioassay Analysis Strategy

Any sound analysis strategy must begin with a good understanding of the assay process. This should include identification of all blocking factors and experimental units in the assay, capturing these in an "assay design structure model." While this is easy to say, it is easy to make mistakes here; experienced analysts will check and recheck their understanding of the assay procedure by repeatedly reviewing the assay protocol and repeated discussions with the team that performs the assay.

5.3.1 Transformation

Bioassay assay analyses make several assumptions when fitting the statistical models. It is important to understand how to assess whether each of these is reasonable and how to address potential violations of these assumptions. The statistical assumptions behind most bioassay models are that the residuals (differences between the observed values and the values predicted by the model) are independent, have constant variance, and are normally distributed. In some bioassays these assumptions are clearly not reasonable and different models may be much more appropriate; for example, in a mouse survival bioassay a logit–log or survival analysis model may be used. In many assays with quantitative (not discrete) responses, the residual variation around the fitted model is often nonconstant and non-normal; for these assays a transformation of the response that yields nearly constant variation and near normally distributed residuals is an appropriate first step. A Box–Cox (or Power Law) analysis, residual plots, subject matter knowledge about the biological and chemical processes in the assay, and experience are all valuable tools when choosing a transformation [4,26]. Ensuring independence of residuals requires use of a sound statistical design for the bioassay and recognition of the design in the analysis model.

5.3.2 Outlier Management

In many bioassay systems it is important to check for and possibly remove unusual observations. It is important that there be a managed process that uses good statistical methods to detect unusual observations as candidate outliers along with good record-keeping of the outlier management process. Elements of good outlier management include records showing what observations were investigated, by whom, in what ways; what analyses were performed with and without suspect observations; which observations were ultimately removed; and what is revealed by periodic summaries of the frequency and contributing systematic causes of unusual observations. Potentially important systematic causes of problems in the assay may be detected as increased frequencies of outliers associated with location, timing, laboratory, analyst, or batch of reagent. Statistical methods for outlier detection that are often particularly useful include Grubbs' test (also known as the extreme Studentized deviates or ESD test) to detect a single outlier (with versions for detecting other known numbers of outliers) [2]. Rosner's test (also known as the generalized extreme Studentized deviates or GESD) does well at detecting multiple outliers when the number of outliers is not known but a maximum number of outliers can be set [2]. Most outlier detection methods assume normally distributed observations [2]. For small groups of data many are comfortable with Dixon's test. Rather than apply Dixon's to many small subsets of the data, it is far more effective to transform the observations to near-constant variance and near-normality then fit a smooth curve to the concentration-response curve for each sample, using a (possibly mixed) smoothing model that includes the important sources of variation in the design structure of the assay, and use the ESD or GESD methods [2]. These smooth curves should not be the same function as will be used to assess similarity or estimate potency to avoid having the outlier detection method force the data to fit the shape of the selected model function. It is also important that any models used to assess outliers also include the important elements of the assay design structure such as blocks, rows, or columns.

5.3.3 Assay Acceptance Criteria

To avoid rejecting more than a few percent of good assays it is wise to use a minimal collection of assay acceptance criteria, each with fairly wide ranges. For example, there may be limits set at ±3 or more standard deviations around their means for several parameters of the reference standard curve fit by an unrestricted nonlinear mixed model. Experience shows that reference range, reference shape (the B parameter), and the log of the residual standard deviation are useful. Additional important practical assay acceptance criteria include limits on the number of outliers, not only overall, but also for various subgroups. It is usually considered reasonable to omit an entire sample or dilution from a block if there are more than a few outliers in the sample or dilution within the block. Similarly, it is sensible to limit the number of observations, samples, and dilutions that may be removed from a block before the entire block is considered suspect.

It is sensible to include limits on the numbers of various types of outliers as part of the assay acceptance criteria. With data that has a near-constant residual variance, perform outlier detection on the residuals from a (possibly simplified) mixed model (that captures the design structure) and that fits sample-specific smooth curves across dilutions using a generalized extreme Studentized deviates test (GESD; [18] and Chapter 1); note that this is one way to satisfy the recommendations in [22]. Because the number of outliers in a well-managed assay system should be small, it is sensible to set the outlier detection critical *p*-value so that the expected or average number of falsely detected outliers is near 1/2 per assay. Performing a search for a modest number of observations (perhaps 5–10) unusual observations per assay may also be reasonable. While it is also sensible to check for unusual observations at the level of each random effect (such as sample in block, dilution in block, block, etc.), it is not yet clear how to effectively and reliably combine this multilevel outlier detection with the multiround outlier detection of the GESD procedure. As mentioned above, it is also sensible to set bounds on the numbers of outliers allowed from each of the various groups in the assay simply because a group that contains several unusual observations makes the entire group suspect.

5.3.4 Mixed Models

Using (possibly) transformed and (possibly) outlier removed data, it is sensible to fit an unrestricted nonlinear mixed model that uses fixed effect terms for sample and dilution (or sample-specific fixed effect curve parameters) and random effects associated with the groups (blocks) and experimental units in the assay. Because there may be random effects for multiple curve parameters associated with each random factor (blocks and each experimental unit), it is often necessary to perform some selection of models to find those that fit well without including many random effects that have near-zero variance or covariance terms. This selection process is a bit of an art because these complex nonlinear mixed models can be quite sensitive to starting values. It is often helpful to fit models with only a few random effects and then use the estimates from these fits as starting values for fits of models with more complex sets of random effects. After fitting a collection of mixed-effect models with unrestricted fixed effects, it is sensible to assess similarity for each (mixed effect) model; equivalence tests are recognized as the most appropriate strategy [6,12,22].

5.3.5 Equivalence Testing for Similarity

Equivalence testing is now well established as more appropriate than difference tests for assessing similarity. There is still debate about how to measure nonsimilarity and set equivalence bounds. For four parameter logistic models of the form shown in Equation 5.2, comparisons among composite and parameter-specific measures of nonsimilarity show appreciable benefits to some combinations of these two approaches. Ratio estimates (such as $\frac{A_{\text{Test}}}{A_{\text{Ref}}}$) have bias and variance that increase more rapidly with residual variance than scaled shifts of the form:

- $\%\Delta_A = 100 \times (A_{\text{Test}} - A_{\text{Ref}}) \overline{A_{\text{Ref}}^*}$,

- $\%\Delta_D = 100 \times (D_{\text{Test}} - D_{\text{Ref}}) \overline{A_{\text{Ref}}^*}$ (not a typo), and

- $\%\Delta_B = 100 \times (B_{\text{Test}} - B_{\text{Ref}}) \overline{B_{\text{Ref}}^*}$

where * indicates long-term averages (unpublished results).

Composite measures of nonsimilarity such as F ratios for evaluating the restricted or reduced model compared to the unrestricted or full model or the χ^2 (the numerator from the F test for model reduction) are sensitive to the response scale, and (for F) the residual. Scaled shifts are largely insensitive to the response scale for the assay. It is useful to include a bound on the sum of the scaled shifts in range (A) and no-dose asymptote (D). With equivalence bounds set at ±10% for range, no-dose asymptote, and the sum of range and no-dose asymptote plus a separate bound at ±50% for the B parameter (sometimes called slope or shape), the median bias of potency for samples that pass similarity will be under 10% (unpublished results).

While there may be other important criteria that lead to yet narrower equivalence bounds, it seems unreasonable to set equivalence bounds that do not at least control bias in potency. For many assay systems a sensible starting point for equivalence test bounds are those that limit the median bias in potency to 10%. While many assays are initially unable to reliably pass equivalence tests with these bounds, after a suitable transformation, a sensible outlier detection process, extending the dilution range, recognizing the blocks (and other elements of the design structure), performing the analysis using all samples together, and possibly increasing the number of blocks (or replicates) in the assay, this set of equivalence bounds will be practical. It is clear that for some biotechnology products different bias limits are appropriate (for example, many vaccines have very wide specification limits and can tolerate more bias in potency while other products have narrow specification limits and will require narrower bias limits for potency). Equivalence bounds that control median bias are a first practical step toward sensitivity-based equivalence bounds. Likely next steps include equivalence bounds based on tolerance intervals rather than median bias and additional sensitivity-based considerations ensuring other desirable properties of potency.

5.3.6 Model Selection

Associated with each candidate random effect model, there is a (possibly partially) reduced model where all test sample-specific parameters that have been shown to be equivalent to reference sample parameters are fit as common parameters. While many labs routinely compare each reference–test sample pair via a separate pair of unrestricted and restricted models, fitting all samples in the assay simultaneously is preferable because this approach yields better estimates of all random effects (variance and covariance terms). Akaike's information criterion (AIC), Bayes information criterion (BIC), and a small-sample version of AIC, sometimes known as AICc are all reasonable criteria for random effects model selection. There is an important strategic choice: whether the random effect model should be selected based on the unrestricted model fits or based on comparisons of the restricted model fits. Using AICc to choose the random effect model based on the restricted models yields lower bias and higher precision estimates of potency (unpublished results largely based on ideas developed by Carrie Wager) from both simulated assay data and multiple validation experiments, as well as [1,5]. Mixed models are very helpful for bioassays and are at times challenging to fit for nonlinear models with many of the statistically complex designs that are used for practical bioassays. It is reasonable to impose some constraints on the collections of random effects that may be included in a model; for example, it is sensible to require that when a model includes a random effect associated with a unit that is nested in another random factor (for example, row nested in plate) for a parameter, the parameter must also have a random effect associated with the enclosing unit (the plate). It can be important to consider covariances among random effects. In practice it is necessary to remove unimportant random effects through a model selection process; AIC and BIC are good tools for guiding model selection [5,15]. Because nonlinear mixed models are quite sensitive to starting values, it is helpful to fit simpler models (with fewer random effects) first and use the parameter estimates from fits of models as starting values for more complex models.

For bioassays that are performed in split-unit or strip-unit designs where there are important random effects on these parameters associated with experimental units used for samples, dilutions, or both, nonlinear mixed models have even larger advantages compared with models that assume additive variation or are fit with weights where the weights are intended to address nonconstant variation. This is partly because there are particularly useful interpretations of variation associated with some combinations of parameters and sources. For example:

- Large or increased variation in log EC50 associated with blocks may be a signal more care is needed when making initial dilutions.

- Large or increased variation in log EC50 associated with units assigned different dilutions within-block may be a signal that there are problems with insufficient mixing, poorly sealed tips, or other issues in the dilution process.

- Variation in the no-dose asymptote among samples or blocks is not about the drug product, it may indicate problems with uniformity of cell preparations, cell handling, or culture of blocks.

- Variation in the range among blocks may indicate issues with cell preparation, cell handling, or culture conditions.

It can be particularly effective to monitor these interpretable measures of specific types of variation.

5.3.7 Bioassay Analysis Summary

To summarize, effective analyses of data from cell-based assay systems can use the following sequence of steps:

- Transform the response data to eliminate most if not all of any systematic nonconstant variance around the concentration–response curve.

- After transformation, use a nonparametric regression mixed model (typically a smoothing spline) to detect unusual observations; these are usually managed by analyzing the assay with and without these suspect observations.

- The assay analysis includes limits on the number of outliers that may be removed in each of several relevant groups (for example, a sample on a plate), if there are too many outliers in a group the entire group is removed. Note that this can lead to removal of a plate or failure of the entire assay.

- The transformed data without outliers is fit with a collection of full (unconstrained) nonlinear parametric mixed models (typically a four-parameter logistic), where the collection includes all sensible random effects based on the assay design and experience with the assay system. Each of these models includes reference and all test samples.

- For each random effect full model, assess the similarity of each sample, typically using equivalence tests with bounds that have been selected to control the bias of potency due to nonsimilarity (based on unpublished work).

- For each random effect model, a (potentially partially) reduced model is fit based on the results of the similarity assessment.

- Choose among the (potentially partially) reduced models the random effect model to use to report similarity and potency results based on AIC, AICc, or BIC.

- Using the selected random effect model, for samples that pass similarity (have all parameters, joint parameters, or all measures with the similarity acceptance criteria) estimate and report log potency compared to reference standard.

5.4 Strategic Design

5.4.1 Design Goals

All experiment or assay designs are compromises among a diverse collection of goals. It is important that bioassays use designs that are practical in the laboratory (in many cases using grouped or serial dilutions and multichannel pipettes), provide protection against bias due to location and sequence effects, provide valid estimates of variation (to support inference), and be flexible enough to adapt to varying sample loads. It is desirable that manual and robotic versions of an assay be similar enough to share some initial or final steps, as well as share important statistical properties (most of the design structure). It is useful if the assay design is flexible enough to easily adapt to uses that require different levels of precision for similarity and potency results; some practical examples illustrate this issue. To qualify a new production facility or new reference lot it is usually important to establish that both curve shape and potency are closer to established values than for lot release. The range of potencies (and hence in-assay dilutions) needed for lot release may be wider for long-term stability studies than for lot release. It is also useful if the assay design can efficiently provide higher throughput when needed (perhaps by reducing the number of within-block replicates of some or all samples). For example, during late-stage clinical trials there are likely to be several clinical lots on stability while early commercial production lots are also being prepared for release; having an assay design that can efficiently handle multiple test samples in each assay can be particularly helpful.

5.4.2 Practical and Strategic Design Constraints

For many cell-based assays, compelling initial constraints are the volume requirements of the equipment and procedures that are familiar in the laboratory. For many labs these considerations lead to 24-well, 96-well, or 384-well cell culture plates, with many labs migrating to smaller volumes and higher density plates over time. There are often compelling reasons to use multichannel pipettes (minimize repetitive motions, avoid delays, etc.). These and other considerations often lead to designs with samples and dilutions assigned to plates rows (or columns) or parts of a row (or column) rather than assigning individual combinations of sample and dilution to arbitrary (or random) wells in any location on the plate(s).

For clarity, it is important to establish that a block in an assay is the collection of data from assay material that is set up close together in time by one analyst (or a small team of analysts working together). Further, an assay is the set of data used (together) to assess similarity of each test sample compared to standard. For each test sample that is similar to standard, the assay yields a potency estimate. Note that the reportable value for a sample (which is the value to be compared to a specification) may be based on combining log potency estimates from multiple bioassays.

Three examples of bioassays where blocks are convenient elements of the designs follow:

Example 1: A Strip-Unit Cell-Based Assay on Several (96-Well) Cell Culture Plates

This example is a cell-based assay that uses several plates, where each plate is a complete block. The edge wells of the plates are not used, samples are assigned to plate rows (with a separate randomization on each plate) and dilutions are assigned to columns (with a separate randomization on each plate); making the assay into a strip-unit design ([4,22], and Figure 5.3). Each sample is assigned to a single row on each plate and each dilution is assigned to a single column on each plate. To prepare samples for the assay, a deep-well setup plate can be used for preliminary dilutions, with one section (several adjacent columns) of the setup plate used for each assay plate. This works well if the assay uses two, three, four, five, or six cell culture plates and the preliminary dilution of samples (from the sample vial that is delivered to the lab, to the most concentrated column on the cell culture plate) is not too extreme to perform in a few dilution and mixing steps, each with a total volume near 1 milliliter. For an assay that uses three cell culture plates, a separate preliminary dilution is performed for each sample (using a freshly set pipette with a fresh tip) from the sample vial to the assigned row in columns 1, 5, and 9. The volumes used for each sample and diluent in columns 1, 5, and 9 are sample-specific; they may be intended to achieve the same protein concentration in each row. Subsequent dilutions on the deep-well setup plate are performed with six tips on a multichannel pipette to achieve a final concentration (in columns 4, 8, and 12) that are approximately four times the maximum target concentration on the cell culture plate dilution (using four times the target concentration allows for dilution onto the cell culture plate and dilution by later addition of cells in media). If the design uses two, four, five, or six cell culture plates, a different set of columns is used for the initial setup of samples on the deepwell setup plate, there are a different number of columns for preliminary dilution, and hence, different dilution steps are needed on the deepwell setup plate. Note that the bioassay design is blocked, with blocks represented by sections of the deepwell setup plate and the (associated) cell culture plate. The number of blocks could be fairly conveniently adjusted from two to six (and more with additional deepwell setup plates).

Example 2: A Blocked Cell-Based Assay on Several Six-Well Plates, or an Animal Bioassay that Has a Block Size of Six

This example captures two completely different bioassays with the same statistical design and analysis. A cell culture bioassay that requires large numbers of cells or large amounts of supernatant from each sample and dilution combination may use large-well plates that allow only three dilutions of each of two samples (standard and test) on each six-well culture plate. In this assay design each six-well plate will be treated as a block.

For an animal bioassay that uses relatively large animals or surgery as part of the assay, it may be practical to process only six animals each day even with a small team working together; the group of animals processed in a day constitutes a block in the assay.

Note that for both cases the block contains all combinations of two samples (standard and test) at each of three dilutions. In both of these assay designs, the within-block assignment of combinations of sample and dilution to well or animal is completely randomized and there is an independent preparation of each combination of sample and dilution for each block.

Example 3: An Animal Assay that Contains Three Test Samples, Each at Five Dilutions, with Thirty Animals for Each Combination of Sample and Dilution

In this assay the animals are housed in cages, with five animals per cage. All animals in a cage receive the same combination of sample and dilution. Note that it is important that there be an independent preparation of each combination of sample and dilution for each cage. While it is acceptable if these are independently prepared for each animal, doing so adds little value and requires appreciably more effort. In this design it is appropriate to consider the cages the experimental units for combinations of sample and dilution, animals are sampling units. Any analysis that treats the animals as experimental units when all animals in a cage receive the same combination of sample and dilution is incorrect; this would be a pseudo-replication error.

It may be discovered during the planning of this assay that the animal facility does not have the capacity to handle the required ninety cages with five animals in each cage all at the same time. The animal facility manager asks if the experiment could be divided into thirds, with two cages for each combination of sample and dilution performed in each of three sequential two-week time periods. The change that the animal facility manager requests would turn this into a blocked design, with three blocks. While that is a reasonable design, within-block replicates are rarely helpful (they are valuable only when they are very inexpensive compared to more blocks and the within-block variance among experimental units is large compared to the between-block variance). Better options would be to use six blocks, each containing fifteen cages (one cage from each combination of sample and dilution) or, if it is particularly convenient to have groups of near thirty cages at a time to consider designs with either more dilutions or more samples.

5.4.3 Other Bioassay Design Considerations

It is wise to make the assay large enough to reliably pass similarity of samples that are within the entire desired potency range of the assay; there is little benefit in making the assay larger than needed to reliably pass similarity. It is also strategically sensible to have the assay deliver a reported value based on a modest number of replicate assays.

A sometimes useful strategy for an assay that may be subject to certain types of location effects is to put specific dilutions (those not on the asymptotes or near the EC50 of reference) or specific samples (perhaps second replicates of reference or QC samples) in locations that may need to be removed (such as plate edges). With this approach in assays where it may be necessary to omit certain locations, the blocks (or assays) with more severe location effects can still be analyzed because these dilutions and samples are not essential.

Note that even if the intended analysis is a logit–log or probit–log analysis, there are well-accepted tools for doing mixed-model analyses of this type of data with block treated as a random effect.

5.4.4 Design Strategies during Bioassay Development

It is helpful if critical samples and dilutions are assigned to less variable locations. A sensible strategy is to put samples that are used primarily to monitor the performance of the assay are assigned to more variable locations (such as edges).

During the early development of a cell-based assays on 96-well culture plates it can be particularly effective to assign dilutions of a working standard to plate columns while assigning combinations of experimental factors to plate rows, with plates treated as blocks for factorial (or fractional factorial) designs. For example, combinations of cell number, pre-assay cell culture conditions, and media type (each at two levels) could be assigned to plate rows with all combinations appearing on each plate. Alternatively, some factors could have more levels, perhaps with four levels of cell number combined with two levels of media type; again with all combinations appearing on each plate. When there are more than eight combinations of levels of design factors that can be applied to plate rows, these factor combinations can still be assigned to rows, with a fraction of the full design (typically a fractional factorial) assigned to each plate (where the plate becomes a block in the development experiment). When there are more combinations of factors in the experiment than can be performed in a day (or a week), it is particularly valuable to treat what will become an assay (most likely the work performed by a single analyst in a day) as a block in the larger development or robustness experiment. This last idea is particularly helpful when a group of conditions (such as both levels of two factors, for a single combination of levels of other factors) all have good concentration response curves (large response ranges and small variation around the curves). Because the data in this group of conditions will not have come from a single day, early development data can demostrate that some combinations of conditions yield consistently (across day) good performance.

Some factors are not practical to apply to plate rows; for example, incubation time and plate washing are applied to an entire plate. For development experiments that involve factors applied to plates (or more generally, blocks), it is particularly helpful to have four, eight, or larger multiples of four (plates) blocks/assay; this supports good factorial and fractional factorial designs in blocks. For experiments that have different collections of development factors applied to each of several experimental units (for example, some factors applied to plate rows and other factors applied to plates), the development experiment is likely to be a fractional factorial in a split-unit. For these more complex designs it is helpful to look for either minimum aberration designs [11] or designs with maximal numbers of clear factor combinations [13].

Later in development it becomes important to include samples with a range of known potencies in each (or at least some) assays; at this stage it is often more practical to apply all development or robustness factors to within-assay blocks (perhaps plates) or assays rather than to within-plate rows.

It is important to emphasize that the strategic suggestion to use multiples of four blocks per assay is for development and validation (particularly for validation via robustness experiments). For production use of the assay the number of blocks per assay should be set to have enough in-assay replication to reliably pass the similarity bounds (that were chosen to help ensure that potency has appropriate properties). For production use of the assay, the number of replicate assays of each test sample (perhaps lot, or stability condition and time point from a lot) is chosen to yield acceptable precision for the (typically geometric) mean potency from the group of replicate assays used to produce a reportable value.

Because it is likely that a well-managed assay will, perhaps not initially, but over time (likely after changes based on experience), exhibit improved performance, it is valuable to have an assay design that can be adjusted without making drastic changes to the design or analysis. With a blocked assay design and analysis, it is fairly easy to to use either more or fewer within-assay blocks to change the expected width of the similarity confidence intervals. If the assay validation uses (say) four blocks per assay (for an assay that can reliably pass similarity for similar samples with three blocks per assay), the validation can support use of the assay with two, three, or four blocks per assay.

5.5 Other Ways to Be Strategic by Combining Design, Analysis, and Use of Bioassays

There may be a need to use a bioassay to make certain comparisons with particularly high (relative) precision. For example, it may be important to characterize the differences in curve parameters between a product (or potential product) and an international reference of a related, but nonidentical biological product. If it is important to make this, or other comparisons, using a bioassay that may not be fully developed or validated, it may be useful to perform a variation of the assay that uses many more blocks than the "in development" assay; this will yield appreciably more precision for similarity assessment.

When performing robustness testing it is appropriate to use both small fractions of factorial experiments (typically in blocks) and equivalence tests. The equivalence testing that is particularly relevant for use in robustness experiments on potency assays checks that any shifts in potency of samples with known potency stay inside appropriate equivalence bounds. It is useful to think of these bounds as another potential source of allowed bias in potency.

It is entirely sensible from a scientific and statistical viewpoint to perform a small number of assays on a lot that is intended for release and assess the potency estimate for the lot. If the estimated potency of the lot is near the center of the potency release range, it is reasonable to release the lot. If the estimated potency of the lot is well outside the potency release range, it is reasonable to fail the lot. If the potency of the lot is near either end of the potency release range, it is reasonable to perform additional assays; though the sampling scheme and testing rules must be well defined in advance. This thinking is central to sequential sampling, which is widely used in quality control. Sequential sampling strategies are cost-effective and sound; they are particularly appropriate for expensive low-precision bioassays, though time delays may be impractical.

5.6 Qualification/Validation Experiment Design and Analysis

The qualification experiment plan uses a slightly different version of the assay than what is shown in Figures 5.3 and 5.4; for the qualification experiment there are four plates per assay. If the assay qualification shows that the assay can reliably pass similarity for similar samples using three plates, the qualification experiment can be used to support a three plate version of the assay. The part of the qualification design that focuses on relative accuracy and precision of potency uses reference as test sample with samples added to the assay at shifted initial concentrations to create "test" samples with known $\log_2$ potencies of (for example): -0.6, -0.3, 0, 0.3, and 0.6 or potencies of 0.66, 0.81. 1, 1.23, and 1.52; note that these span a range wider than the product specifications for the protein product illustrated in Figure 5.1. Because the assay design contains six samples, these five test samples and reference standard can be included on each plate of each assay. Because two of the samples are at potency 1, (both reference standard and the "test" sample at potency 1 have known potency of 1), two different analyses are possible: One uses a single potency 1 sample as reference to assess similarity and report potency for each of the other five samples, another uses both potency 1 samples as within-assay replicates of reference standard and reports potency for each of the remaining four test samples; both analyses can be performed from the same laboratory data. The qualification experiment design uses three analysts, each of whom will perform a four-plate assay on each of three days; no two analysts perform an assay on the same day (this makes the qualification a nested design with day nested in analyst). While the experiment can be analyzed using variance components to partition variation in log potency at each target potency among days and analysts, and this partitioning is useful, ultimately the intermediate precision will be reported as variation among the nine assays. If the sample similarity failure rate is very low it is worthwhile to also reanalyze the experiment data using only three of the plates from each assay.

The qualification experiment data reported here is simulated data with known properties. The important properties are that the true potencies of each test sample is exactly on target, all test samples are actually similar to reference standard, and the residual standard deviation around the sample-specific, within-plate, concentration response curves is a constant 0.025, which represents 2.5% of the response range. Other simulation experiments demonstrate that (assuming a good design, a good analysis, and that all statistical assumptions are satisfied) the precision of measures of nonsimilarity and the precision of potency in cell-based bioassays with good design and good analysis is driven by the size of the residual standard deviation and the number of replicates in the assay.

The analysis of the qualification experiment includes no assay acceptance criteria; these must be set before a validation experiment. The sample acceptance criteria used for the qualification experiment require that the test sample have 90% confidence intervals for scaled shifts in range, no-dose asymptote, and the sum of range plus no-dose asymptote that are entirely within ±8% of long-term reference range, while scaled shifts in the shape or B parameter are entirely within ±40%. These equivalence test bounds are an educated guess selected to ensure that any bias in potency is less than 10% (but it is not yet known how much less than 10%).

5.6.1 Discussion of the Qualification Experiment Results

With the observed sample similarity failure rates it is not reasonable to use a three-plate version of the assay for production unless the similarity criteria are relaxed (which would likely allow more than acceptable bias in potency; Figure 5.5). Further, the similarity failures and the subtle U-shape in the precision profile plot demonstrate that the concentration range of the assay is either just barely wide enough (Figure 5.6), or not wide enough. For almost all assays, over time, the amount of variation in the shape of the reference standard curve tends to increase. To protect the assay from failures of assay and sample acceptance criteria, it is wise to use an appreciably wider concentration range in the assay than what is illustrated here.

Previous versions of the simulated qualification experiment that had ten-point dilution curves or had the log EC50 of the reference standard less well centered in the dilution range had much more pronounced U-shaped precision profiles (data not shown). These earlier versions had higher similarity failure rates, more relative bias of potency, and poorer precision of potency.

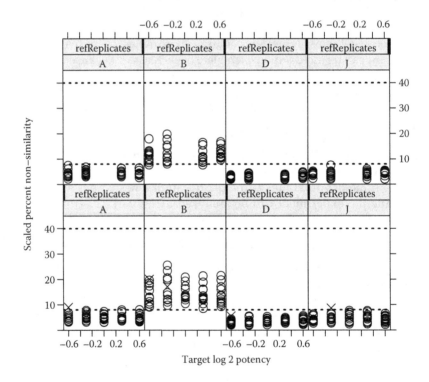

FIGURE 5.5
Nonsimilarity measures for each parameter and a combination of parameters. The lower row of panels is from analyses that used a single replicate of reference standard at potency one as reference and the other replicate of reference at potency one as a test sample; the upper row of panels used both replicates of reference at potency one as reference to assess similarity of all other test samples. Each column of panels corresponds to a measure of nonsimilarity with A = range, B = shape, D = no-dose asymptote, and J = range + no-dose asymptote. The horizontal dashed lines are at 40% and 8%, the similarity equivalence bounds. Each point represents one sample in one assay; circles are samples that passed all similarity criteria, Xs are samples that failed one or more similarity criteria. The points represent the absolute value of the most extreme endpoint (furthest from zero) of 90% confidence intervals for scaled shifts in measures of nonsimilarity.

It is clear that the bias and precision of potency estimates for the test samples improves when there are within-plate replicates of reference (Figures 5.6 and 5.7). Performing the qualification experiment in a way that allows analyses that use the same data in different ways is effective; it allows use of a single lab experiment qualification to support use of the assay with some flexibility in the assay format (Table 5.1).

The worst-case bias is reported as the most extreme 90% confidence interval of the target-specific potency estimates. The worst-case potency bias estimate is both simple and conservative; hence, it is an important first step. When there is no trend in target-specific potency bias it may be reasonable to pool bias estimates across the potency targets and produce a smaller potency bias estimate with a narrower confidence interval. The potency bias trend is reported as the 95% confidence interval on the worst-case change in potency that may occur across the potency range of the assay. This potency bias trend addresses linearity of potency in a way that is much more interpretable than R^2 or statements about the intercept or slope of a regression line relating observed log potency to target log potency. The potency bias trend can be combined with the worst case bias or added to the amount of degradation allowed during storage of the product. In combination, the total amount of bias from two or three sources can be thought of as "allowed bias from potency assay" as shown in Figures 5.1 and 5.2.

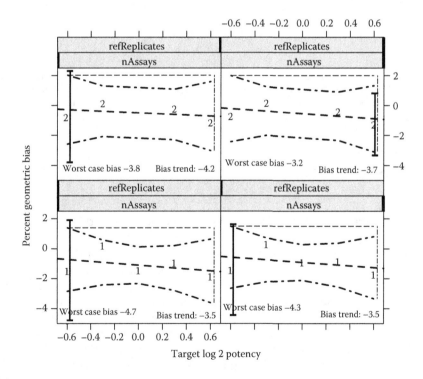

FIGURE 5.6

Percent geometric bias of potency vs. target $\log_2$ potency with one (lower panels, with plot symbol 1) or two (upper panels with plot symbol 2) within-block replicates of reference. The results shown are based on a qualification experiment with nine (left panels) or twelve (right panels) assays. The worst-case bias is shown in each panel; these represent the 90% confidence interval endpoints for bias that is furthest from zero. The bias trend is also shown on each panel, this represents the difference between the most extreme pair of 95% confidence intervals for a straight-line regression across the range of the assay.

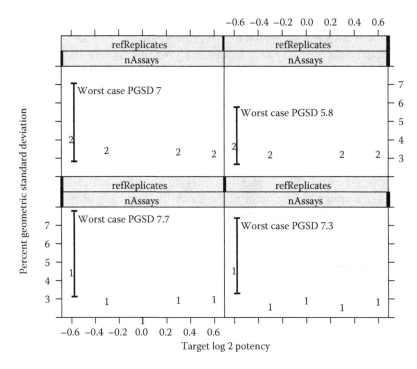

FIGURE 5.7
Percent geometric standard deviation of estimated potency vs. target $\log_2$ potency with one (lower panels, with symbol 1) or two (upper panels, with symbol 2) within-block replicates of reference. The estimates shown are based on nine (left panels) or 12 (right panels) assays. The worst-case percent geometric standard deviation (PGSD) is shown on each panel; this is the 90% confidence interval endpoint that is furthest from zero.

5.7 Summary

The analytic performance targets for bioassays must be informed by what is medically appropriate for the product and by what sample comparisons are to be made. For products with wide margins between safety and efficacy limits, it is reasonable to argue that the product specifications and other comparisons (such as similarity equivalence bounds as well as degradation limits) may be wider than for other products. Conversely, products with a narrow therapeutic window will require much more capable (low bias, high precision) bioassays. Further, there may be quite different bioassay performance requirements for different uses of an assay. For lot release of product from a stable process where there are multiple other analytic methods to support a conclusion that the process is producing the correct product, the precision requirements for similarity and potency, while demanding enough, may be not be as stringent as they will be when qualifying new reference material or demonstrating that a new production facility (or process) produces material that is comparable to an existing facility (or process). When a bioassay is used to qualify a new reference lot or qualify a new manufacturing facility or process, the precision and bias requirements for similarity or potency may be much more stringent.

It is important to keep clearly in mind during development, qualification, validation, routine use of, and monitoring of a bioassay that poor assay precision can be overcome with

TABLE 5.1

Expected Precision of Reported Values for Potency

nAssays	refReplicates	nAssaysInQual	sdRV	PGSDRV
1.00	1.00	9.00	0.11	7.72
2.00	1.00	9.00	0.08	5.40
3.00	1.00	9.00	0.06	4.38
4.00	1.00	9.00	0.05	3.79
6.00	1.00	9.00	0.04	3.08
8.00	1.00	9.00	0.04	2.66
1.00	2.00	9.00	0.10	7.01
2.00	2.00	9.00	0.07	4.91
3.00	2.00	9.00	0.06	3.99
4.00	2.00	9.00	0.05	3.44
6.00	2.00	9.00	0.04	2.80
8.00	2.00	9.00	0.03	2.42
1.00	1.00	12.00	0.10	7.34
2.00	1.00	12.00	0.07	5.14
3.00	1.00	12.00	0.06	4.17
4.00	1.00	12.00	0.05	3.61
6.00	1.00	12.00	0.04	2.93
8.00	1.00	12.00	0.04	2.54
1.00	2.00	12.00	0.08	5.75
2.00	2.00	12.00	0.06	4.03
3.00	2.00	12.00	0.05	3.28
4.00	2.00	12.00	0.04	2.83
6.00	2.00	12.00	0.03	2.31
8.00	2.00	12.00	0.03	2.00

Note: The expected standard deviation of reported values of log (base 2) potency (sdRV) and percent geometric standard deviation of reported values of potency (PGSDRV, which is %GCV of [21] for reported values) for various combinations of numbers of replicate assays of each sample (nAssays), with various numbers of reference replicates (refReplicates), and number of assays in the qualification experiment (nAssaysInQual). These are based on the worst-case PGSD values shown in Figure 5.7.

(admittedly expensive) replicates, while bias does not improve with additional replicates. Hence, the focus of development, validation, and monitoring should be on reducing bias of measures of nonsimilarity and bias of potency. Designs that protect bioassays against potential sources of bias such as location or sequence effects are important. Routine randomization and retrospective analyses are important tools.

The actual designs used for most industrial bioassays are more complex than "textbook" completely randomized designs. Analyses that ignore these important design features that produce blocked, split-unit, or strip-unit designs in bioassays are not only potential sources of bias (particularly in estimates of variation), they yield poor quality (low precision) estimates of similarity, making it difficult to pass equivalence tests with sensible bounds. Further, poor analyses yield meaningless estimates of the precision of estimated potency.

An essential part of the life-cycle management of a bioassay is periodic review of assay performance. This should include review of the frequency at which outliers are detected, what patterns can be found in where outliers appear, whether the transformation used is still appropriate, whether there have been any changes in the important sources of variation in the assay system, and whether the variation in the manufacturing system has changed, and if location or sequence effects have become important. Further elements for review include checks that the product specifications are still well supported, and whether it is appropriate to adjust the number of blocks (or replicates) in the assay or the number of replicate assays in reportable values.

References

1. Hirotogu Akaike. Information theory and an extension of the maximum likelihood principle. In B.N. Petrov and F. Caski, editors, *Proceeding of the Second International Symposium on Information Theory*. pp. 267–281, Academiai Kiado, Budapest, 1973.
2. Vic Barnett and Toby Lewis. *Outliers in Statistical Data*. Wiley Series in Probability and Mathematical Statistics. John Wiley & Sons, 3rd edition, 1994.
3. Douglas M. Bates and Donald G. Watts. *Nonlinear Regression Analysis and Its Applications*. Wiley, 1988.
4. G.E.P. Box and D.R. Cox. An analysis of transformations. *Journal of the Royal Statistical Society. Series B (Methodological)*, 26(2):211–252, 1964.
5. Kenneth P. Burnham and David R. Anderson. *Model Selection and Multimodel Inference*. Springer, 2nd edition, 2002.
6. J.D. Callahan and N.C. Sajjadi. Testing the null hypothesis for a specified difference – the right way to test for parallelism. *Bioprocessing Journal*, 2:71–78, 2003.
7. R.J. Carroll and D. Ruppert. *Transformation and Weighting in Regression*. Chapman & Hall, 1988.
8. Marie Davidian and David M. Giltinan. *Nonlinear Models for Repeated Measurement Data*. Number 62 in Monographs on Statistics and Applied Probability. Chapman & Hall, 1995.
9. NIST. Accessed from http://www.itl.nist.gov/div898/software/dataplot/refman1/auxillar/dixon.htm.
10. D.J. Finney. *Statistical Method in Biological Assay* 3rd Edition. Charles Griffen & Co. LTD, 1978.
11. Francis G. Giesbrecht and Marcia L. Gumpertz. *Planning, Construction and Statistical Analysis of Comparative Experiments*. Wiley, 2004.
12. W.W. Hauck, R.C. Capen, J.D. Callahan, J.E. DeMuth, H. Hsu, D. Lansky, N.C. Sajjadi, S.S. Seaver, R.R. Singer, and D. Weisman. Assessing Parallelism Prior to Determining Relative Potency. *PDA J Pharm Sci Tech*. 59:127–137, 2005.
13. Murat Kulahci, Jose G. Ramirez, and Randy Tobias. Split-plot fractional designs: Is minimum aberration enough? *Journal of Quality Technology*. 38(1):56–64, January 2006.
14. David Lansky. Strip-plot designs, mixed models, and comparison between linear and nonlinear models for microtitre plate bioassays. In A. F. Brown and A. Mire-Sluis editors, *The Design and Analysis of Potency Assays for Biotechnology Products*. Dev. Biol., Basel, Karger 107, 2002.
15. J.C. Pinheiro and D.M. Bates. *Mixed-Effects Models in S and S-Plus* Springer, 2000.
16. David A. Ratkowsky. *Handbook of Nonlinear Regression Models*. Marcel Dekker, 1989.
17. David A. Ratkowsky and Terry J. Reedy. Choosing near-linear parameters in the four-parameter logistic model for radioligand and related assays. *Biometrics*, 42:575–582, 1986.
18. Bernard Rosner. Percentage points for a generalized ESD many-outlier procedure. *Technometrics*, 25(2):165–172, 1983.
19. G.A.F. Seber and C.J. Wild. *Nonlinear Regression*. Wiley, 1989.

20. Charles Y. Tan. Sigmoid curves and a case for close to linear nonlinear models, 2009. Accessed from <http://www.mbswonline.com/upload/presentation Charles5-15-2009-14-32-2.pdf>.
21. Chapter <1030> Biological Assay Chapters – Overview and Glossary. *USP 40-NF 35*, US Pharmacopeial Convention, Rockville, MD 2017.
22. Chapter <1032> Design and Development of Biological Assays. *USP 40-NF 35*, US Pharmacopeial Convention, Rockville, MD 2017.
23. Chapter <1033> Biological Assay Validation. *USP 40-NF 35*, US Pharmacopeial Convention, Rockville, MD 2017.
24. Chapter <1034> Analysis of Biological Assays. *USP 40-NF 35*, US Pharmacopeial Convention, Rockville, MD 2017.
25. Chapter <111> Design and Analysis of Biological Assays. *USP 40-NF 35*, US Pharmacopeial Convention, Rockville, MD 2017.
26. W.N. Venables and B.D. Ripley. *Modern Applied Statistics with S*, 4th Edition. Springer, 2002.

6

Setting Specification

Harry Yang

CONTENTS

6.1 Regulatory Requirements

The safety, efficacy, and quality of a biological product is warranted through a set of effective control strategies, which include testing of raw materials, drug substance and product, in-process control, and manufacturing environment monitoring. Establishing specifications is at the heart of the overall control strategies and can be a formidable process. Various regulatory guidelines exist that are concerned with setting specifications for biological products. Of note is ICH Q6B, Test Procedures and Acceptance Criteria for Biotechnological/Biological Products (FDA 1999). Publication of ICH Q6B was intended to provide guidance on general principles for setting and justifying a uniform set of international specifications for biotechnological and biological products to support new marketing applications. In the document, specifications are defined as

> a list of tests, references to analytical procedures, and appropriate acceptance criteria, which are numerical limits, ranges, or other criteria for the tests described. It establishes the set of criteria to which a drug substance, drug product, or materials at other stages of its manufacture should conform to be considered acceptable for its intended use. "Conformance to specification" means that the drug substance and/or drug product, when tested according to the listed analytical procedures, will meet the acceptance criteria. Specifications are critical quality standards that are proposed and justified by the manufacturer and approved by regulatory authorities as conditions of approval.

Per this definition, a specification consists of three important components: (1) The quality attribute for which the specification is intended; (2) the analytical procedure used for measuring the quality attribute; and (3) acceptance criteria, used to make an acceptance or rejection decision of the batch of product. The acceptance criteria may be qualitative or quantitative. In the latter case, they are often expressed as numerical limit(s).

Traditionally, setting specifications was compliance-driven and largely based on a small number of commercial scale batches used for marketing approval. A subsequent batch would be tested to ensure it would meet the specification. As noted by Burdick et al. (2017), there are several drawbacks of the approach. First of all, the small data sets used for setting the specification lead to an under representation of all sources of variation. As a result, the probability of out-of-specification observations is greatly increased as more sources of variability are encountered. This may cause frequent root cause analysis and repeated testing. Secondly, application of statistical approaches may result in wide acceptance ranges due to one's inability to validate the assumption of data distribution. Overall, the traditional specification setting is an isolated exercise and neglects a vast amount of information regarding product safety, efficacy, and quality that can be gleaned from various sources.

In recent years, there has been a significant shift of regulatory expectations on assurance of product quality from the traditional "test to compliance" to a risk-based life cycle approach, as evidenced by the issuance of ICH Q8(R2) Pharmaceutical Development (ICH 2006), ICH Q9 Quality Risk Management (ICH 2007a), ICH Q10 Pharmaceutical Quality Systems (ICH 2007b), and ICH Q11 Concept Paper (ICH 2011). Within the new regulatory framework, specification is a part of an overall control strategy and development of specifications is a process driven by data obtained throughout the product life cycle. It includes several key elements: (1) Identification of critical quality attributes (CQAs), critical process parameters (CPPs), and input material attributes (MAs); (2) establishment of specifications from a holistic overall control strategy perspective; and (3) determination of acceptance criteria (EBE, 2013). Each of the above exercises requires enhanced understanding of process and product, use of statistical methods to estimate variability from various sources, and balanced risks between the consumer and producer.

6.2 Identification of Critical Quality Attributes

Identification of critical quality attributes (CQAs) begins with a risk assessment of all quality attributes (QAs) with regard to their potential impact on activity, PK/PD, safety, and immunogenicity with quality. Considerations are given to both severity and probability of occurrence. Figure 6.1 illustrates a scoring system for determining criticality of QAs.

	5	5	10	15	20	25
Severity	4	4	8	12	16	20
	3	3	6	9	12	15
	2	2	4	6	8	10
	1	1	2	3	4	5
	0	1	2	3	4	5

Occurrence

FIGURE 6.1
Risk-ranking based on severity and occurrence.

In this particular method, the total risk score is defined as the product of severity and occurrence. The highest risk, middle risk, and lowest risk corresponds to risk scores ≥ 15, 8 ≤ scores ≤12, and scores ≤7, respectively. There are other risk-based assessment tools, such as failure effect mode analysis (FEMA), that can also be used to determine the criticality of QAs (FDA, 2006). Risk-ranking is performed in order to justify the relative importance of individual quality attributes. After a score is assigned to each QA commensurate with its risk, the QA is classified into noncritical, key, or critical attributes corresponding to the lowest risk, middle risk, and highest risk, respectively.

Since changes in CQAs might have a significant impact on product safety and efficacy, it is critical to establish the relationships between CQAs and clinical performance and to use this knowledge to define acceptable ranges for CQAs. This knowledge provides a foundation for developing robust control strategies for the manufacturing process. However, it can be difficult to link a particular quality attribute to clinical performance (safety and efficacy).

In the literature, various models have been proposed to understand the relationships between CQAs and product safety and efficacy. For example, for process-related impurities, an impurity safety factor (ISF) is used to link to the toxicity of an impurity to the maximum acceptable level in the product through the following function (Schenerman et al. 2009):

$$\text{ISF} = \text{LD}_{50}/r \tag{6.1}$$

where LD_{50} is the amount of an impurity that results in lethality in 50% of animals tested, and r is the maximum amount of an impurity in the final product dose. The higher the ISF, the lower the safety risk caused by the impurity is. If a lower limit on the ISF is available (for example, from regulatory guidelines), it can be translated into a bound on the maximum amount of impurity in a final product dose.

Another example by Yang (2013) describes a method that provides a functional relationship between three correlated CQAs of a monoclonal antibody and a surrogate efficacy marker, namely, the area under the drug concentration curve (AUC). Such a linkage allows for the assessment of the impact of changes in these CQAs on the product efficacy, and also allows for the establishment of clinically relevant joint acceptance ranges for the CQAs. More examples of identifying CQAs can be found in Schenerman et al. (2009).

6.3 Selection of Critical Process Parameters and Input Material Attributes

After the CQAs are identified, a series of multivariate statistically designed experiments are carried out. The objectives of these experiments are to identify the previously mentioned

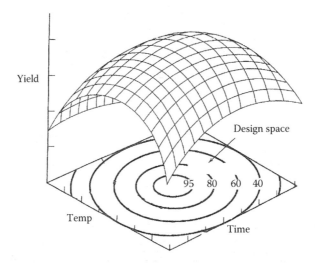

FIGURE 6.2
Design space.

process parameters (PPs) and input material attributes (MAs) that may impact the CQAs and establish relationships among between the CQAs and the PPs and MAs. Knowledge gleaned from these experimentations, coupled with historical data and manufacturing experience, can be used to develop a design space in which changes in PPs and MAs would have no major impact on the CQAs, thus rendering product quality assurance. The established design space is a key component of the overall control strategies. Figure 6.2 illustrates the concept of a design space. Suppose the two critical process parameters of a cell culture system are reaction times and temperature. An operation condition is deemed acceptable if it results in at least 60% of the maximum yield. The conditions within the circle labeled "60" is the design space as any combination of temperature and time gives rise to a yield no less than 60%.

6.4 Control Strategies

Per ICH Q11 (ICH 2012), a control strategy is

> a planned set of controls, derived from current product and process understanding, that assures process performance and product quality. The controls can include parameters and attributes related to drug substance and drug product materials and components, facility and equipment operating conditions, in-process controls, finished product specifications, and the associated methods and frequency of monitoring and control.

Once the CQAs, critical PPs, and MAs are identified, an overall control strategy can be developed to ensure each aspect of the manufacturing process is in a state of control. (See Figure 6.3.)

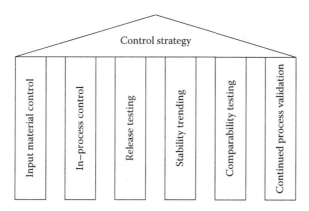

FIGURE 6.3
Overall control strategy.

6.4.1 Input Material Control

Input materials such as cell banks used for fermentation and excipients in the final product may have significant effects on a manufacturing process. The risk associated with the input materials may be mitigated through establishment of specifications either based on manufacturing experience or pharmacopoeial requirements, as well as acceptance sampling as described in Chapter 11, and qualification of new vendors.

6.4.2 In-Process Control

In-process control includes procedural control, control of process parameters, and in process testing.

6.4.2.1 Procedural Controls

Procedural controls are usually supported through the manufacturer's quality risk management system, and described in standard operating procedures (SOPs). These controls ensure manufacturing unit operations, equipment, and environment are operating within their expected ranges, resulting in consistent production of quality product.

6.4.2.2 Process Parameter Controls

Production robustness and consistency can be further assured when CPPs are controlled within the design space. Process analytical technology (PAT) can be used to control the manufacturing process through continued measurements of CPPs and input MAs that affect CQAs. Among the PAT tools are multivariate data analysis (MVDA) and multivariate statistical process control (MSPC), which are discussed in Chapter 9.

6.4.2.3 In-Process Testing

For a selected set of CQAs, in-process samples can be tested to verify that the process performs as expected. However for in-process testing, control criteria may be defined as either alert, action, or rejection, according to the internal quality system. It may also include defining of the adjustment of the subsequent operating units (EBE 2013).

6.4.3 Release Testing

For each drug substance or finished product lot, measurements of a set of CQAs are collected using analytical methods with associated acceptance criteria to ensure the lot is of the intended product quality to be released. The acceptance sampling plans discussed in Chapter 11 are typically used to aid the disposition of the lot while minimizing the chance of untoward rejection of a good lot and false acceptance of a bad lot. The lot may also be required to meet release limits, which are typically narrower than the specifications, to enhance the probability for the lot to meet the specification at the end of its shelf life.

6.4.4 Stability Trending

Some quality attributes such as impurity and potency may change over time. Stability testing can be carried out to ensure the product has its intended quality during its shelf life. Stability testing can also be performed to provide assurance of robustness of the manufacturing process after process changes (including site, scale, formulation, storage, shipping conditions, and/or delivery device).

6.4.5 Comparability Testing

For any postapproval changes, comparability testing is necessary to ensure the changes have no significant impact on the product quality. A specific testing plan is developed based on risk to product quality. The testing may include high-risk quality attributes QA with high-process capability (e.g., HCP) and some of the QAs with low criticality and moderate to high-process capability (e.g., DNA, methotrexate, and leached Protein A) (CMC Biotech Working Group 2009).

6.4.6 Continuous Process Verification

The control strategies described previously are often developed based on data collected from process development and quantification. As limited data from commercial production is used, it is likely that not all potential sources of variations in commercial manufacturing are incorporated. The continued process monitoring provides both a means to verify that the control strategy works as intended and opportunities to identify additional sources of variation and calibrate the overall control strategy as needed.

6.5 Considerations in Setting Acceptance Criteria

Establishment of acceptance criteria is a key component of setting specifications. This should be primarily driven by considerations concerning the product safety, efficacy, and quality. Relevant data include nonclinical and clinical experiences; historical knowledge of the product or similar products in the same class; analytical method variability; and manufacturing process capability, regulatory and pharmacopeial requirements.

Although clinical experience should take precedent over other sources of data, clinical data are often limited as usually clinical development only utilizes a few batches of the product. Therefore a robust strategy for setting acceptance criteria should allow the flexibility to set provisional limits for product release and update the limits based on data from post-marketing surveillance. This is consistent with the recent regulatory requirement of continued process validation and verification.

6.5.1 Frame of Reference

One common mistake in setting acceptance limits for a specification is that the frame of reference for intended use of the specification is not clearly defined (Burdick 2017). Here the "frame of reference" refers to the sampling population and parameter(s) of interest for statistical inference. Oftentimes, these limits are set based on measures of individual units from a product batch and used to assess conformance of the batch average, or vice versa. Since variability in individual measurements is larger than that of the average, acceptance limits can be either too wide or too narrow, thus inflating the consumer's or producer's risk. Consider an influenza vaccine for which a potency assay is performed as part of batch release test. Since the purpose of the test is to ensure that the potency of the batch is within the specification limits 6.5–7.5 $\log_{10}$ titer, the intent of the assay is to estimate the batch potency. For this assay, 12 samples from the batch are tested, giving rise to 12 readouts. The assay result is reported as the average of the 12 measurements and evaluated against the above acceptable limits. However, if an assay is intended to assess residual host cell DNA in the product, which may have unintended safety concerns, specification limits should be set for individual vials.

6.5.2 Sources of Variation

A manufacturing process is influenced by various sources of variation. When setting acceptable limits of a specification, it is important to use data encompassed of the full range of variability expected for the product and process (Burdick et al. 2017). This requires appropriate applications of experimental design and statistical analysis to estimate the variability and set specifications. In the following, we use two examples to illustrate how this can be accomplished.

> **Example 6.1: Setting Acceptance Range Based on Variance Component Analysis**
>
> Consider a situation in which a biopharmaceutical firm uses a large number of batches of raw materials from a vendor. To qualify an incoming batch, an assay is performed on a random sample of three determinations from the batch. The batch is accepted if the average of the three test results is within prespecified acceptable limits. Two sources of variation may impact the disposition of a batch: One is the assay variability, also referred to as *within batch variation*; the other is batch-to-batch variation, which is also called *between batch variation*. When setting the acceptable limits, one may test n_a samples from n_b randomly selected batches. The results of the test can be described by the following random effects model:
>
> $$X_i = \mu + A_i + \varepsilon_{ij} \tag{6.2}$$
>
> where A_i are random effects due to batch and assumed to be independent and following normal distribution $N(0, \sigma_a^2)$; ε_{ij} are measurement errors due to assay and are

independent and following a normal distribution $N(0, \sigma_e^2)$. A_i and ε_{ij} are also independent. The ANOVA table for this one-way random effect model is shown in Table 6.1.

The parameter μ is estimated as $\hat{\mu} = \overline{\overline{X}}$ using the least-square method or maximum likelihood. The variance components can be estimated as $\hat{\sigma}_a^2 = (MSA - MSE)/n_w$ and $\hat{\sigma}_e^2 = MSE$ by equating the mean squares with their corresponding expected mean squares. Accordingly, the total variance is estimated as $\hat{\sigma}^2 = \hat{\sigma}_a^2 + \hat{\sigma}_e^2 = MSA/n_w + (1 - 1/n_w)MSE$. These estimators are the same as those using the method of restricted maximum likelihood (REML) for balanced design. The REML gives unbiased estimations and is thus preferred to MLE.

For the previous example, suppose the following data in Table 6.2 were generated from an experiment in which three samples from each of five batches were tested. The data were fit to the mixed effects model in Equation 6.2, and the ANOVA table is given in Table 6.3.

TABLE 6.1

The Analysis of Variance (ANOVA) Table for One-Way Random Effect Model

Source of Variance	Degrees of Freedom	Sum of Square*	Mean Square	Expected Mean Square
Between-run	$n_a - 1$	$SSA = n_w \sum_{i=1}^{na} (\overline{X}_{i.} - \overline{\overline{X}})^2$	$MSA = \dfrac{SSA}{n_a - 1}$	$n_w \sigma_a^2 + \sigma_e^2$
Within-run	$n_a(n_w - 1)$	$SSE = \sum_i \sum_j (X_{ij} - \overline{X}_{i.})^2$	$MSE = \dfrac{SSE}{n_a(n_w - 1)}$	σ_e^2
Total	$n_a n_w - 1$	$SST = \sum_i \sum_j (X_{ij} - \overline{\overline{X}})^2$		

$^* \ \overline{\overline{X}} = \dfrac{1}{n_a n_w} \sum_i \sum_j X_{ij}; \ \overline{X}_{i.} = \dfrac{1}{n_w} \sum_{j=1}^{n_w} X_{ij}.$

TABLE 6.2

Results of Potency Assay from Testing Five Batches

Sample	Batch				
	1	2	3	4	5
1	101	106	102	99	96
2	99	104	100	97	93
3	100	104	102	98	97

TABLE 6.3

Summary of Analysis of Variance (ANOVA)

	ANOVA			
Source	df	SS	MS	EMS
Between-batch	4	147.74	36.94	$3\sigma_a^2 + \sigma_e^2$
Within-batch	10	17.99	1.80	σ_e^2
Total	14	165.73		

From Tables 6.2 and 6.3, we have

$$\bar{\bar{X}} = 99.97$$

$$\hat{\sigma}_e^2 = 1.80$$

$$\hat{\sigma}_a^2 = (36.94 - 1.80)/3 = 11.71.$$

The variability in the average of a random sample of three determinations from the batch is given by

$$\hat{\sigma} = \sqrt{\hat{\sigma}_a^2 + \frac{\hat{\sigma}_e^2}{3}} = \sqrt{11.71 + 1.80/3} = 3.51.$$

If the acceptance range is set as

$$\bar{\bar{X}} \pm 3\hat{\sigma},$$

it is calculated to be

$$99.97 \pm 3 \times 3.51 = (89.3, 110.4).$$

However, if one simply set the acceptance limits as

$$\bar{\bar{X}} \pm 3s,$$

where s is the sample deviation of the data in Table 6.2 and equal to 3.44, then as a consequence, the acceptance limits are estimated to be

$$99.97 \pm 3 \times 3.44 = (93.9, 105.8).$$

It is evident the latter method, which fails to correctly estimate the variability in the mean of three determinations, provides a narrow acceptance range.

Example 6.2: Use of Beta-Binomials to Capture Heterogeneity

This example concerns setting specifications for the integrity test of a manufacturing process that produces a product of monoclonal antibody. The finished product is a liquid form in vials. Since there are multiple fill lines used, a batch of product consists of vials from these fill lines. A sampling plan includes visual inspection of a fixed number of vials from the batch for defects such as foreign matters inside the vials, cracks on the vials, and insufficient sealing of the vials. The percent of defective vials is calculated and evaluated against the specification limit. The batch is accepted or rejected pending whether the percent of defectives from the sample inspection is below or above the acceptance limit. It is necessary to establish an acceptance limit for the percent of defectives.

In general, the number of defectives can be modeled through a binomial distribution. However, for this example, due to multiple fill lines in use, a hierarchical model that accounts for variation due to the fill lines and variation within the fill lines is more suitable for describing the data. Let Y be the total number of defectives in the sample $(X_1, \ldots, X_n)$ that follows binomial distribution $B(n, p)$, where p is the percent of defectives. Hence,

$$P[Y = y \mid p] = \binom{n}{y} p^y (1 - p)^{n-y}. \tag{6.3}$$

Assume that p is beta-distributed. That is,

$$\pi(p) = \frac{1}{B(\alpha, \beta)} p^{\alpha-1} (1 - p)^{\beta-1}, \ \alpha > 0, \ \beta > 0 \tag{6.4}$$

where $B(\alpha, \beta)$ is the normalization constant.

From Equation 6.3 and Equation 6.4, the marginal distribution of Y is the beta-binomial

$$P[Y = y] = \binom{n}{y} \frac{B(y + \alpha, n - y + \beta)}{B(\alpha, \beta)}. \tag{6.5}$$

Let $1 - \gamma$ be the confidence level of an upper control limit (UCL) and $(\hat{\alpha}, \hat{\beta})$ be the MLEs of the distribution parameters. The UCL can be chosen such that

$$\hat{UCL} = \min \left\{ m : \sum_{x=0}^{m} P[Y = y \mid \hat{\alpha}, \hat{\beta}] \geq 1 - \gamma \right\} / n, \tag{6.6}$$

Consider a situation in which 17 lots of vials of varying sizes were visually inspected. The results of inspection are presented in Table 6.4.

TABLE 6.4

Summary of Results of Visual Inspection of 17 Lots of Vials

Lot	Number of Vials Inspected	Defective Rate
1	210,370	0.07
2	300,430	0.02
3	147,110	0.04
4	566,308	0.06
5	489,441	0.07
6	186,799	0.04
7	670,281	0.05
8	667,680	0.04
9	170,940	0.03
10	472,440	0.05
11	167,700	0.05
12	671,330	0.05
13	671,597	0.04
14	221,993	0.03
15	673,060	0.04
16	665,140	0.06
17	668,200	0.02

TABLE 6.5

Upper Acceptance Limits for Various Lot Sizes

Batch Size	95% Upper Limit
10,000	0.0834
20,000	0.0834
30,000	0.0833
40,000	0.0833
50,000	0.0833
100,000	0.0833
150,000	0.0833
200,000	0.0833
500,000	0.0833
700,000	0.0833

By fitting the data to the model in Equation 6.5, the MLEs of the parameters (α, β) are $(\hat{\alpha}, \hat{\beta}) = (7.33, 127.27)$. From Equation 6.6, the 95% UCL for various lot sizes were determined and are presented in Table 6.5.

6.5.3 Impact of Correlation

Important assumptions of the mixed effects model (Equation 6.2) are that both the batch effects A_i and measurement errors are independently identically distributed according to two normal distributions and that A_i and ε_{ij} are also independent. There are situations in which these assumptions may be violated. For instance, in Example 6.2, if the five batches were produced using the same bulk drug substance, A_i are correlated; thus, no longer independent. Even if the specification is intended for individual measurement, direct use of $\bar{X} \pm ks$ as specification limits may not be appropriate, where $\bar{X} = \dfrac{1}{N}\sum_{i=1}^{N} X_i$ and $s = \sqrt{\dfrac{1}{N-1}\sum_{i=1}^{N}(X_i - \bar{X})^2}$ are sample means and the standard deviation (SD) is based on a sample X_i, $i = 1, ..., N$. This is due to the fact that when X_i are not independent, the sample SD may either under- or overestimate the population variability, causing wider or narrower acceptance limits (Yang et al., 2016). Assume $E[X_i] = \mu$, $Var[X_i] = \sigma^2$, and $cov[X_i, X_j] = \rho_{ij}\sigma^2$ for $i \neq j$. Yang et al. (2016) demonstrated

$$E[s] \leq \left[\sqrt{1 - \frac{1}{N(N-1)}\sum_{i \neq j} \rho_{ij}} \right] \sigma. \qquad (6.7)$$

Therefore the sample standard deviation s under- or overestimates the true standard deviation, quantified through $\dfrac{E[s] - \sigma}{\sigma}$, by at least a proportion of $\lambda = 1 - \sqrt{1 - \dfrac{1}{N(N-1)}\sum_{i \neq j} \rho_{ij}}$.

For $\rho_{ij} = \rho > 0$, $\lambda = 1 - \sqrt{1 - \rho}$. Table 6.6 provides a list of λ values for various values of correlation coefficient $\rho_{ij} = \rho \geq 0$, As seen from the table, with correlation coefficient being

TABLE 6.6

Lower Bound on Percent of Underestimation for Various Values
of Correlation Coefficient with $\rho_{ij} = \rho$

ρ	0	0.1	0.2	0.25	0.5	0.75	0.8
λ	0%	5%	11%	13%	29%	50%	55%

equal to 0.5, the sample standard deviation under-estimates the true reference product by at least 29%. The effect becomes more pronounced as ρ becomes larger. For example, the percent of underestimation reaches 55% when $\rho = 0.8$.

Yang et al. (2016) further illustrated the impact of correlation through analysis of two simulated data sets based on Equation 6.8,

$$X_{ij} = \mu + L_i + e_{ij} \tag{6.8}$$

and two variance-covariance matrices:

$$A = \begin{pmatrix} \sigma_L^2 + \sigma_e^2 & \sigma_L^2 & \sigma_L^2 & \sigma_L^2 \\ \sigma_L^2 & \sigma_L^2 + \sigma_e^2 & \sigma_L^2 & \sigma_L^2 \\ \sigma_L^2 & \sigma_L^2 & \sigma_L^2 + \sigma_e^2 & \sigma_L^2 \\ \sigma_L^2 & \sigma_L^2 & \sigma_L^2 & \sigma_L^2 + \sigma_e^2 \end{pmatrix} \tag{6.9}$$

$$B = \begin{pmatrix} \sigma_L^2 + \sigma_e^2 & \sigma_L^2 & 0 & 0 \\ \sigma_L^2 & \sigma_L^2 + \sigma_e^2 & 0 & 0 \\ 0 & 0 & \sigma_L^2 + \sigma_e^2 & \sigma_L^2 \\ 0 & 0 & \sigma_L^2 & \sigma_L^2 + \sigma_e^2 \end{pmatrix} \tag{6.10}$$

The former is referred to as a fully exchangeable correlation structure and the latter as a pair-wise exchangeable. The correlation between the two observations of the first data set is $\dfrac{\sigma_L^2 \left(\sigma_L^2 + \sigma_e^2 \right)}{\left(\sigma_L^2 + \sigma_e^2 \right)\left(\sigma_L^2 + \sigma_e^2 \right)} = \dfrac{\sigma_L^2}{\left(\sigma_L^2 + \sigma_e^2 \right)} = \rho$, a constant, whereas for the second data set the correlation between the two observations from batches 1 and 2 or 3 and 4 is ρ, and the correlation is 0 between other two observations from different batches.

Ten thousand Monte Carlo simulations were run for various values of the correlation ρ_R and with $N_R = 10$ and 16 to evaluate the distribution of s_R under fully exchangeable and pair-wise exchangeable correlation structures. Figure 6.4 shows a quartiles boxplot of s_R for selected values of ρ_R and N_R. Figure 6.5 shows the probability that $s_R < \sigma_R$ for a given value of ρ_R and N_R. From both Figures 6.4 and 6.5 it is clear that s_R typically underestimates σ_R, even when $\rho_R = 0$ and that the underestimation of σ_R by s_R worsens as ρ_R increases.

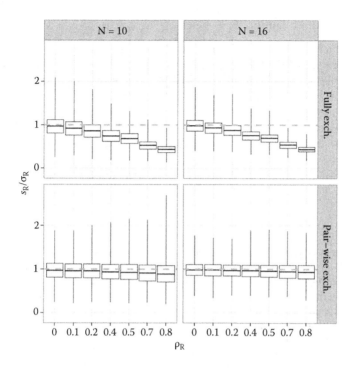

FIGURE 6.4
Quartiles boxplot of s_R/σ_R for selected values of ρ_R and N_R. (Adapted from Yang, H., Novick, S., and Burdick, R., *PDA J. of Pharm. Science and Technology.* 70(6), 1–13, 2016.)

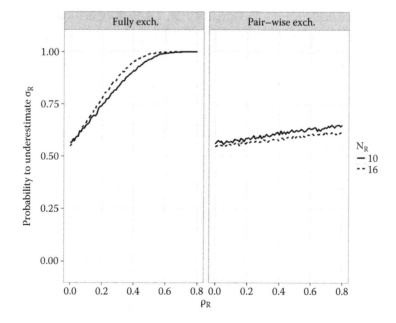

FIGURE 6.5
The probability that $s_R < \sigma_R$ for a given value of ρ_R and N_R. (Adapted from Yang, H., Novick, S., and Burdick, R., *PDA J. of Pharm. Science and Technology.* 70(6), 1–13, 2016.)

6.5.4 Clinical Relevance Limits

As noted by Burdick et al. (2017), clinically relevant specifications are most desirable as they are directly related to product safety and efficacy. In the published literature, there are several examples coping with how to link specification limits to clinical experience. Notable is the work by Capen et al. (2007) and Yang (2013). The former establishes potency specifications for antigen vaccines based on process capability data. The acceptable limits are shown to be appropriate through a clinical dose-ranging study. The latter uses a statistical model to establish the linkage between specifications of glycoforms to product PK parameters. The glycoform specifications were set so that a batch with glycoforms in spec would warrant a high probability for its PK characteristic to be within its acceptable range.

Example 6.3

We consider setting potency specification of a biological product of live virus. The product was successfully clinically demonstrated safe and efficacy when the number of the live viruses in the dose is in the range of $10^{6.5}$ and $10^{7.5}$. During the clinical development, an assay that directly counts number of viruses in a dose was used. Due to faster throughput, an indirect assay, called $TCID_{50}$, was planned to replace the direct assay. The assay measures the reciprocal of the dilution of viruses resulting in infection of 50% of host cells. The titer of the assay is estimated using the Karber method described in the following. It is of interest to set the specification of the $TCID_{50}$ assay.

KARBER METHOD

Let X_i be the i_{th} 1:10 dilution of the original undiluted test sample X_0. Define p_i to be the percentage of wells with positive CPE at the i_{th} dilution and X_f and X_l denote the first and last dilutions such that $p_f = 0$ at X_f, $p_l = 1$ at X_l. Using the Karber Method, the $\log_{10}$ $TCID_{50}$ titer of the original test sample X_0 is given by

$$\log_{10} TCID_{50} = k - \left(0.5 - \sum_{i=f}^{l} p_i \right). \tag{6.11}$$

Since for the $TCID_{50}$ assay, at each dilution level, there are eight wells tested for CPE, an estimate of p_i can be obtained as

$$\hat{p}_i = \text{total number of CPE positive wells}/8. \tag{6.12}$$

Combining Equations 6.11 and 6.12, the $\log_{10}$ $TCID_{50}$ titer estimate for X_0 can be estimated by

$$\log_{10} TCID_{50} = k - \left(0.5 - \sum_{i=f}^{l} \hat{p}_i \right). \tag{6.13}$$

An example is given in Figure 6.6.

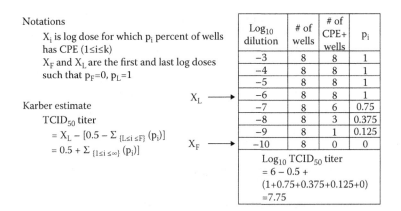

Notations

   X_i is log dose for which p_i percent of wells has CPE ($1 \le i \le k$)

   X_F and X_L are the first and last log doses such that $p_F = 0$, $p_L = 1$

Karber estimate

   $TCID_{50}$ titer

   $= X_L - [0.5 - \Sigma_{\{L \le i \le F\}} (p_i)]$

   $= 0.5 + \Sigma_{\{1 \le i \le \infty\}} (p_i)]$

Log$_{10}$ dilution	# of wells	# of CPE+ wells	p_i
−3	8	8	1
−4	8	8	1
−5	8	8	1
−6	8	8	1
−7	8	6	0.75
−8	8	3	0.375
−9	8	1	0.125
−10	8	0	0

$X_L \longrightarrow$ (−6 row)

$X_F \longrightarrow$ (−10 row)

Log$_{10}$ TCID$_{50}$ titer
= 6 − 0.5 +
(1+0.75+0.375+0.125+0)
=7.75

FIGURE 6.6
Calculation of viral titer based on the Karber method. Log$_{10}$ dilution = −3 means 1; 1000 dilution.

POISSON MODEL

Let Y be the number of infecting particles in a dilution X of THE original undiluted sample X_0, where 50% infectivity is expected. Assuming that y follows a Poisson distribution, Poisson(λ), with mean infecting particle λ.

$$0.5 = \text{Prob}[Y \ge 1] = 1 - e^{-\lambda}. \tag{6.14}$$

Solving Equation 6.14 for λ, we obtain

$$\lambda = \ln(2) = 0.69. \tag{6.15}$$

Let y_i be the number of infecting particles in X_i, the i_{th} 1:10 dilution of the original undiluted sample X_0 having a log$_{10}$ TCID$_{50}$ titer of $m + d$. Using (6.14) it can be inferred that y_i is also distributed according to a Poisson distribution, Poisson(λ_i), with expected value λ_i of Y_i being given by

$$\lambda_i = \frac{0.69 x 10^d}{10^{i-m}} = 0.69 x 10^{(m+d)-i}, \tag{6.16}$$

where $0 \le i \le n$.

Because of Equation 6.16, it can be readily proved that if $p_j = \text{Prob}[y_j \ge 1] = 1$, then $p_i = \text{Prob}[y_i \ge 1] = 1$ for $i < j$. Likewise, if $p_j = \text{Prob}[y_j \ge 1] = 0$, then $p_i = \text{Prob}[y_i \ge 1] = 0$ for $i > j$. These properties allows us to rewrite the Karber log$_{10}$ TCID$_{50}$ estimate in Equation 6.11 as

$$\log_{10} \text{TCID}_{50} = \left(\sum_{i=1}^{\infty} p_i \right) + 0.5 = \left(\sum_{i=1}^{\infty} \left(1 - e^{-0.69 x 10^{m+d-i}} \right) \right) + 0.5 \equiv K(m,d). \tag{6.17}$$

It can be readily shown that

$$k(m+1,d) = \left(1 - e^{-0.69 x 10^{m+d}} \right) + \left(\sum_{i=1}^{\infty} \left(1 - e^{-0.69 x 10^{m+d-i}} \right) \right) + 0.5 \approx k(m,d) + 1, \tag{6.18}$$

The relationship in Equation 6.18 implies that Karber $\log_{10}$ $TCID_{50}$ estimate of a sample, which has a theoretical $\log_{10}$ $TCID_{50}$ titer of *m + 1 + d* as would be obtained using the serial 1:10 dilutions described previously, is equal to the 1 plus Karber $\log_{10}$ $TCID_{50}$ estimate of a sample having a theoretical $\log_{10}$ $TCID_{50}$ titer of *m + d*.

RELATIONSHIP BETWEEN NUMBER OF VIRUSES AND $TCID_{50}$

Because there are 0.69 infecting particles in the dilution X of the original undiluted sample X_0, that results in 50% infectivity (refer to Equation 6.15), the total number of infecting particles in the X_0 is given by

$$10^{m+d} \times (0.69),\qquad(6.19)$$

which corresponds to a total number of viruses on a $\log_{10}$ scale of

$$\log_{10}[10^{m+d} \times (0.69)] = (m+d-0.16)\log_{10} FFU \equiv F(m,d).\qquad(6.20)$$

Comparing Equations 6.17 and 6.20, the difference between the Karber $\log_{10}$ $TCID_{50}$ estimate and the actual $\log_{10}$ number of viruses of the original test sample X_0 is given by

$$
\begin{aligned}
D(m,d) &= K(m,d) - F(m,d) \\
&= \left(\sum_{i=1}^{\infty} \left(1 - e^{-0.69 \times 10^{m+d-i}}\right) \right) + 0.5 - (m+d-0.16).
\end{aligned}
\qquad(6.21)
$$

From Equation 6.20, we obtain

$$F(m+1,d) = F(m,d) + 1.\qquad(6.22)$$

By Equations 6.18 and 6.22, it is evident that

$$
\begin{aligned}
D(m+1,d) &= K(m+1,d) - F(m+1,d) \\
&= [K(m,d)+1] - [F(m,d)+1] \\
&= K(m,d) - F(m,d) \\
&= D(m,d).
\end{aligned}
\qquad(6.23)
$$

Equation 6.23 implies

$$D(m,d) = D(0,d).\qquad(6.24)$$

In other words, the difference between the Karber $\log_{10}$ $TCID_{50}$ estimate and the actual $\log_{10}$ virus count of the original test sample X_0 is independent of *m*. Therefore, the theoretical relationship between $\log_{10}$ $TCID_{50}$ titer estimated using the Karber method and the number of infecting particles in a test sample has been established. It is shown that the two quantities differ by an amount, *D(0,d)*, which is only dependent on the fraction, *d*, of 1:10 dilution. Assuming *d* is uniformly distributed between 0 and 1, the expected mean titer difference between $\log_{10}$ $TCID_{50}$ assay titer and that of $\log_{10}$ virus count assay can be obtained as

$$D = \int_0^1 D(0,x)\,dx.\qquad(6.25)$$

TABLE 6.7

Log_{10} Titer Difference between $TCID_{50}$ and FFA Assay

True d	Estimated d		Difference between $TCID_{50}$ and FFU
	$TCID_{50}$ (Karber Method)	log_{10} FFU	
0	0.07	−0.16	0.23
0.1	0.17	−0.06	0.23
0.2	0.28	0.04	0.24
0.3	0.39	0.14	0.25
0.4	0.50	0.24	0.26
0.5	0.61	0.34	0.27
0.6	0.71	0.44	0.27
0.7	0.80	0.54	0.26
0.8	0.89	0.64	0.25
0.9	0.98	0.74	0.24

RESULTS

For any value of m, the theoretical difference $D(m,d)$ was calculated for d = 0, 0.1, ..., 0.9 and 1. The results are presented in Table 6.7. As seen from the table, the difference ranges from 0.23 to 0.27 with a minimum value of 0.23 and maximum of 0.27 achieved at d = 0 or 1, and 0.5, respectively. The sample average difference is about 0.25.

Based on the above analysis, the acceptable potency limits for the TCID50 assay may be obtained by calibrating the clinically acceptable range log_{10} 6.5 and log_{10} 7.5 by a factor of 0.25 log_{10} titer. This results in clinically justified specification limits of log_{10} 6.75 and log_{10} 7.75 for the $TCID_{50}$ assay.

6.5.5 Shelf Life

Most drug products degrade over time. Therefore, it is important to ensure that a drug product is safe and that its efficacy is within its shelf life. A biological product shelf life and storage condition can be established through a well-designed stability study. To capture broad manufacturing variability, the stability design should include multiple batches of the product. ICH Q1E (ICH 2003) suggests that at least three batches be used. It also states that regression analysis is considered an appropriate approach to evaluating the stability data for a quantitative attribute and establishes a retest period or shelf life. A typical model to describe stability data is given as

$$Y_{ij} = \alpha_i + \beta_i x_{ij} + \varepsilon_{ij} \tag{6.26}$$

where Y_{ij} are measured values of a stability attribute at times x_{ij}, $i = 1,...,n$; $j = 1,...,m$, α_i and β_i are intercept and slope of the ith batch, respectively, and ε_{ij} are measurement errors which are independently and identically distributed (*iid*) according to a normal distribution $N(0, \sigma^2)$.

In ICH Q1E, the batch effect characterized through α_i and β_i is considered as fixed. However, the batch effect also can be considered as random in Equation 6.26. The shelf life, defined as the time point at which the lower or upper one-sided 95% confidence interval of the predicted quality attribute value intercepts the lower or upper specification limit, can be determined either based on fixed or random effect assumptions. For the fixed-effect

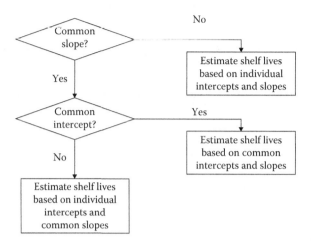

FIGURE 6.7
Flowchart for choosing models for shelf life estimation.

model, poolability tests are conducted according to the flowchart in Figure 6.7 to determine how data from different batches are used to estimate the shelf life. The tests are based on analysis of covariance (ANCOVA), using time as a covariate, to test the differences in slopes and intercepts of the regression lines among batches. As per ICH Q1E, each of these tests should be performed at a significance level of 0.25 to compensate for the expected low power of the design due to the relatively limited sample size in a typical formal stability study. The pooling tests should also be carried out in a proper order such that the slope terms are tested before the intercept terms.

Pending the outcomes of the poolability tests, the shelf life may be estimated using the model with individual slopes, common slope with individual intercepts, or common slope with common intercept. For the first case where the model with individual slopes is used, the pooled mean square error calculated from all batches should be used for estimating shelf lives of all batches. The shortest estimate is used for the shelf life of the product. Where a model of common slope and different intercepts is employed, pooled data should be used to estimate the common slope, individual intercepts, and their associated errors. Like the previous case, shelf lives of individual batches are estimated and the shortest is used as the product shelf life. For the common slope and intercept model, the shelf life is estimated based on the pooled data. Through use of an example, Chapter 7 describes in detail how the analysis for determining the shelf life is performed using the commercial software package JMP® (JMP 2007).

6.5.6 Release Limit

For quality attributes of a product that degrade over time, release limits are established to ensure a greater chance of compliance with specifications before the end of the product shelf life. The release limits are usually narrower than the specifications. Although not required by the FDA, EMA mandates that the limits be part of regulatory dossier. There are several sources of variation that may impact the determination of release limits. They include batch-to-batch variability, assay variation, and uncertainty with degradation rate estimate. Consider a situation in which the lower and upper potency specification limits are LSL and USL, respectively. While batches within this range are deemed to be good

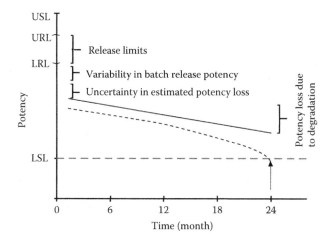

FIGURE 6.8
Release limit is established such that it takes into account the lower specification limit, total loss of potency over the shelf life of 24 months, maximum variability associated with the estimated potency at time zero, and degradation slope estimate.

for release, a batch with potency slightly above LSL at the time of release may not remain potent during the entire expiry period of 24 months, as shown in Figure 6.8. Furthermore, even if the test potency of the batch is 100%, the true potency of the batch might be lower because of assay variability. Additionally, the total potency loss over the shelf life is equal to degradation rate × shelf life. However, the degradation rate is usually unknown and estimated from data of stability studies. Therefore, there is an uncertainty associated with this estimate. To set appropriate lower and upper release limits (LRL and URL) this uncertainty also needs to be accounted for.

6.5.6.1 Fixed Effect Model

In the literature, several statistical methods have been proposed for determining release limits (Allen et al. 1991; Shao and Chow 1991; Wei 1998 and 2003). The most simplistic is the method by Allen et al. (1991), which is briefly described below.

For simplicity, we assume the quality attribute under consideration degrades over time. In such a case, the LRL and URL can be set as

$$\text{LRL} = \text{LSL} + b\text{T} + t_{1-\alpha,df}\sqrt{S_L^2 + \frac{S^2}{n}} \tag{6.27}$$

$$\text{URL} = \text{USL} - t_{1-\alpha,df}\sqrt{\frac{S^2}{n}} \tag{6.28}$$

where T is the shelf life, b is the average degradation rates, and bT represents the total loss due to degradation over the shelf life; $S_L = \text{SE}(b) \times T$ is the standard error associated with the total degradation loss bT; S is the assay variability estimated by the mean square error from fitting model 6.26; n is the number of samples tested at release; and $t_{1-\alpha,df}$ is the

$100(1 - \alpha)^{th}$ percentile of the central t-distribution with degrees of freedom (df) that can be estimated using the Satterthwaite approximation (Satterhwaite 1946):

$$df = \frac{\left(S_L^2 + \dfrac{S^2}{n}\right)^2}{\left(S_L^2\right)^2 /(n_b - 1) + \left(\dfrac{S^2}{n}\right)^2 /(n-1)}. \tag{6.29}$$

Since determination of the release limit requires estimates of degradation rate and various sources of variation, it relies on analysis of results from stability study of the product. As discussed in the previous section, the analysis follows a procedure shown in Figure 6.7. Basically, poolability tests of the batch slopes and intercepts are conducted. If the slopes are poolable, the combined data are used to estimate average slope and variability associated with both the slope and assay. If the slopes are not poolable, the worst slope from a single batch and assay variability estimated from the combined data is used for the release limit calculations.

Example 6.4

To demonstrate, consider a drug product with LSL= 90, shelf life T = 24 months, release test based on single determinations. A stability study was conducted using n_b = 3 batches. A poolablity test gave rise to a p-value of 0.31. Therefore, all three batches are poolable. Equation 6.26 was fit using the combined data, resulting in the parameter estimates, slope b = 0.15, Var(b) = 0.003, assay variability S = 0.025. The degrees of freedom df was calculated to be approximately equal to 2.3 and + 0.95, 2.3 = 2.676. Hence,

$$LRL = 90 + 0.5 \times 24 + 2.676 \times \sqrt{0.03 \times 24^2 + 0.95}$$
$$= 96.61.$$

RELEASE LIMIT BASED ON RANDOM EFFECTS MODEL

The method suggested by Allen et al. (1991) assumes that the batch effect is fixed. An alternate approach was proposed by Murphy and Weisman (1990), in which the batch effect is viewed as random. The poolability tests are not required. Instead the batches are considered poolable if the mean square error associated with the slopes in Equation 6.26 is less than or equal to total within-batch mean square error; otherwise, the batches are deemed to be not poolable. In the former case, data are fit to Equation 6.26 with batch being a fixed effect. The LRL is calculated using the related estimates from the model fitting. In the latter case, the stability components in Equation 6.26 are obtained from fitting Equation 6.26 with slopes being random effects. The standard error S_L associated with the total degradation loss is calculated to be

$$S_L = \sqrt{\left(\sigma_\beta^2 + S_T^2\right)T^2} \tag{6.30}$$

where σ_β^2 and S_T^2 are estimates of slope variance and batch to batch variance, respectively.

TABLE 6.8

Estimated from Analysis of Covariance

Parameter Estimates	Strain 1	Strain 2	Strain 3
Slope estimate (b)	0.023	0.021	0.019
Var(slope) $\left(\sigma_b^2\right)$	0.001796	0.001400	0.002168
Batch-to-batch variance $\left(S_T^2\right)$	0.000005	0.000007	0.000004
Random variance (S^2)	0.026000	0.016000	0.015000
DFL =No. of batches – 1	2	2	2
DFR = Total of Reps at 0 – No. of Batches	121	121	121
Degree of Freedom (df) for t	10.4	6.0	5.9

TABLE 6.9

Summary of Lower Release Limit Estimates

Input for LRL Calculations	Strain 1	Strain 2	Strain 3
LSL	6.5	6.5	6.5
Shelf Life (Weeks) (T)	20	20	20
b×T (Degradation Loss)	0.460	0.420	0.380
$T_{0.95,\,df}$	1.805	1.943	1.949
$S_L^2 = \left[\left(\sigma_b^2 + S_T^2\right)\times T^2\right]$	0.003	0.004	0.003
S^2/n	0.004	0.003	0.003
No. of Reps at Release (n)	6	6	6
Lower Release Limit	7.12	7.07	7.02

Example 6.5

In this example, we concern ourselves with setting release limits for a trivalent influenza vaccine. The shelf life of the product is 20 weeks in 2–8 C°. There batches of the product were placed on stability testing for over 24 weeks. The data were fit to a fixed effect model in Equation 6.26. Since the slope mean square error is greater than the within batch mean square error, it was decided to use the random slope stability model to derive the estimates needed for calculating LRL in Equation 6.27. The estimates were derived and are presented in Table 6.8.

Based on the estimates in Table 6.8, the release limits for all three strains were calculated and displayed in Table 6.9 along with the intermediate results.

6.6 Multivariate Specifications

As previously discussed, a specification consists of a list of tests. Since some of these tests may be correlated, the correlation structure of the quality attributes can have a significant impact on the probability of meeting the specification (Yang 2013; Peterson 2008). Yang et al. (2016) noted that for certain products, drug substance impurity and aggregation may produce a joint effect on immunogenicity. In other words, with less aggregation, a product with a high level of impurity may have more acceptable immunogenicity profile than those with a higher level of aggregate. Because the degree to which drug aggregate impacts the drug immunogenicity depends in part on impurity, understanding the relationship is critical to simultaneously set appropriate specification limits for both quality attributes. Establishing a joint specification for correlated quality attributes also has the advantage to control the overall Type I error, thus minimizing the chance of untoward rejection of product batches of good quality. A good example is provided by Yang (2013). Furthermore, since correlated tests may result in redundant information and incur unnecessary costs, it is of great benefit to identify a smaller set of "orthogonal" tests (Jenkins 1967).

6.7 Concluding Remarks

Setting specifications for drug substances and products used to heavily rely on process capability. It often resulted in much unnecessary testing. In addition, because there is no direct relationship between the specification and drug safety and efficacy, even if the product meets the specification, its quality remains uncertain to a certain extent. The QbD process development paradigm calls for adoption of a risk-based approach to the development of an overall control strategy. The strategy integrates input material controls, process parameter controls, in-process testing, release testing, characterization or comparability testing, and continued process monitoring to a manufacturing process to consistently deliver products that meet established quality specifications. It begins with determining criticality level of quality attributes and assessing capability of the process. The level of control for quality attributes and process parameters depends on the criticality of the attributes/parameters. As a result, the control strategy greatly reduces the number of tests throughout the production process. This chapter stresses the importance of using appropriate statistical design to gain understanding of various sources of variation. It also emphasizes the importance of ensuring that statistical methods used to establish specifications reflect the structure of the data.

References

Allen, P.V., Dukes, G.R., and Gerger, M.E. (1991). Determination of release limits: A general methodology. Pharmaceutical Research, 9(9), 1210–1213.

Burdick, R.K. et al. (2017). *Statistical Applications for Chemistry, Manufacturing, and Control (CMC) in the Pharmaceutical Industry*. Springer.

CMC Biotech Working Group. (2009). A-Mab: A Case Study in Bioprocess Development. Accessed on September 3, 2017, from www.casss.org/associations/9165/.../A-Mab_Case_Study _Version_2-1.pdf.

European Biopharmaceutical Enterprise (EBE). (2013). EBE Concept Paper: Considerations in setting specification. Accessed from http://www.ebe-biopharma.eu/documents/47/25/Considerations -in-Setting-Specifications.

Grimes, J.A., and Foust, L.B. (1994). Establishing release limits with a random slopes model. *Biopharmaceutical Proceedings*, pp. 498–502. Alexandri a, VA: American Statistical Association.

ICH. (1999a). CH Q6A. Specifications: Test Procedures and Acceptance Criteria for New Drug Substances and New Drug Products: Chemical Substances.

ICH. (1999b). ICH Q6B Specifications: Test Procedures and Acceptance Criteria for Biotechnological/ Biological Product. EMEA, September.

Jenkins, G.I. (1967). Multivariate methods applied to product testing and specifications. *Journal of the Royal Statistical Society Series D (The Statistician)*, 17(2), 141–155.

JMP®. (2007). *JMP User Guide, Release 7*. Cary, NC.

Manola, A. (2012) Assessing release limits and manufacturing risk from a Bayesian perspective. Mid-West Biopharamceutical Statistics Workshop, Muncie, ID.

Montgomery D.C. (1985). *Introduction to Statistical Quality Control*, 2nd ed. John Wiley & Sons: New York.

Murphy, J.R., and Weisman, D. (1990). Using random slopes for estimating shelf life. *Biopharmaceutical Proceedings*, 196–200. Alexandria, VA: American Statistical Association.

Owen, C.E.B. (2008). Parameter estimation for the beta distribution. Accessed from https://scholars archive.byu.edu/cgi/viewcontent.cgi?referer=https://www.google.com/&httpsredir=1&article =2613&context=etd.

Peterson, J.J. (2008). A Bayesian approach to the ICH Q8 definition of design space. *Journal of Biopharmaceutical Statistics*, 18: 959–975.

Satterthwaite, F.W. (1946). An approximate distribution of estimates of variance component. *Biometric Bulletin*, 2, 110–114.

Schenerman, M.A., Axley, M.J., Oliver, C.N., Ram, K., and Wasserman, G.F. (2009). Using a risk assessment process to determine criticality of product quality attributes, in *Quality by Design for Biopharmaceutical: Principles and Case Studies*, eds. Rathore, A.S. and Mhatre, R. Wiley.

Shao, J., and Chow, S.-C. (1991). Constructing release targets for drug products: A Bayesian decision theory approach. *Journal of Applied Statistics*, 40(3), 381–391.

Wei, G.C.G. (1988). Simple methods for determination of the release limits for drug products. *Journal of Biopharmaceutical Statistics*, 8(1), 103–114.

Wei, G.C.G. (2003). Release target, in *Encyclopedia of Biopharmaceutical Statistics*, ed. Chow, S.-C. Marcel Dekker, Inc.

Yang, H. (2013). Setting specifications of correlated quality attributes. *PDA Journal of Pharmaceutical Science and Technology*, 67, 533–543.

Yang, H. (2017). *Emerging Non-Clinical Biostatistics for Biopharmaceutical Development and Manufacturing*. Chapman & Hall/CRC.

Yang, H., Novick, S., and Burdick, R. (2016). On statistical approaches to demonstration of analytical similarity. *PDA Journal of Pharmaceutical Science and Technology*, 70(6), 1–13.

Yang, H., Zhang, J., Yu, B., and Zhao, W. (2016). *Statistical Methods for Immunogenicity Assessment*. Chapman & Hall/CRC.

7

Statistical Analysis of Stability Studies

Laura D. Pack

CONTENTS

7.1 Introduction

The stability program underpins all of the claims we make about the important ways a molecule changes over time. A comprehensive program includes compulsory studies required by regulatory agencies and studies to examine conditions of real-world use. Apart from studying new drug substances (DS) and drug products (DP), stability studies are routinely conducted on major process intermediates, reference standards, and critical laboratory reagents.

In any case, the principle of any stability study remains the same: Use reliable analytical methods to measure how a molecule changes over time under a specified storage condition or when subjected to a specific stressor. The information gained from a stability study informs us about the overall degradation profile, the degradation products formed under certain conditions, and how combinations of different conditions may affect overall product quality over time. Practical application of stability analysis leads to decisions about shelf life and product handling, and can inform decisions about potential container, formulation, or production changes.

Any commercially approved DP must have a labelled expiration date or shelf life (these terms are interchangeable). Per ICH Q1A, the shelf life is "the time period during which a drug product is expected to remain within the approved shelf life specification," provided that it is stored under the recommended storage conditions (RSC). Any DS must have an approved expiry or retest period, depending on the type of molecule. Further, a major process intermediate that is not immediately forward processed should be assigned an expiry or retest period. ICH Q1E defines an algorithm for setting the expiry/retest period for new DS and DP, and Q5C expands on these ideas for biological molecules. Q1E and Q5C also speak to study design for accelerated stability conditions (ASC).

Apart from determining shelf life, other stability studies are important to support conditions of real-world use. ICH Q1B defines requirements for demonstrating a molecule's photostability. Many molecules exhibit some degree of photosensitivity, so additional studies to establish allowable light exposure limits may be required. Additionally, a robust stability program includes studies that support any other storage or handling instructions communicated to prescribers or patients. Such claims may be included directly in the product label, or may be provided by the manufacturer upon request. Some examples of special stability studies include:

- Support for allowable excursions from RSC that may occur during shipping/handling, or at the clinic, pharmacy, or hospital.
- Support for allowable number of temperature cycles, especially for refrigerated or frozen products.
- Support for end-to-end stability where DS is held to its expiry/retest period and then filled into DP that is monitored through its expiry.

Not all of these special studies require statistical analysis, but analysis may be useful if predictions are desired based on a limited data set or if the claim is to be included in the product label.

ICH Q1E and Q5C guidance focuses on establishing an initial stability profile, but does not directly address postmarketing changes. Statistical analysis may not be required to extend commercial shelf life if three lots meet specifications at a time point prespecified in the annual stability protocol commitment (Huynh-Ba, 2009). Some jurisdictions have guidance that specifically addresses expiry extensions (e.g. Health Canada 2009, EMA 2012, TGA 2003), but most focus on requirements for applications and do not specifically address statistical analysis. However, the same statistical approaches employed in defining shelf life may be adapted to support extension.

Because the stability study focuses on how the molecule changes over time, stability studies can also be used to compare how two or more different groups change over time. Statistical analysis can be especially useful in comparability exercises, such as those that examine different container types, formulations, manufacturing sites, or process changes.

7.2 A Word about Study Design

The discussions in this chapter generally assume that available stability data follow the study designs called out in ICH Q1A, including specific storage conditions and time points tested. Since the general stability goal is to evaluate a molecule's behavior over time, most analysis focuses primarily on the estimation of the average slope of a regression line on the observed data. Points at the beginning and end of the time course have high leverage on the slope; in other words, these points have the potential to influence the slope estimate more so than do time points closer to the middle of the time course (Ott 2001). A typical stability study design results in observations that are more closely spaced at the beginning of a stability study, with testing typically at 0, 3, 6, 9, 12, 18, 24 months, and annually thereafter. As a stability lot ages, the results from the most recent time point (e.g., 24 months) have higher leverage than do some of the early time points (e.g., 6, 9 months).

When it is possible, replication of testing at a given time point can be statistically advantageous because it allows for more certainty in the slope estimate. Replication is more value added at the beginning and end of the time course because replicates can help to overcome potential influence from an unusual observation at a high leverage time point, especially at the later time points because degradation is expected (Chow 2007). Reasonably, only one result per time point is generated for product at RSC to avoid the potential for ambiguity that could arise from one result that is in specification and one that is out of specification (OOS), but replication may be possible in special studies not conducted at RSC or conducted on non-GMP lots. If replication cannot be built into the study design, additional closely spaced time points at the beginning and end of the study may help with more robust slope estimation. For example, an RSC study may include additional testing at 20 and 22 months for a product with a 24-month shelf life. As another example, a 3-month study at ASC may include additional testing at 0.25, 0.5, 2.5, and 2.75 months.

Bracketing is an approach that only studies low and high configurations of a product (e.g., strengths or fill volumes). In general, two strengths or fill volumes of the same formulation may be bracketed, but this type of stability program assumes two things: The low and high configurations have the same stability profiles, and any intermediate configurations fall along some continuum between the low and high configurations. Such assumptions should be verified using statistical analysis (as in Section 7.10.1) or minimally via qualitative evaluation by graphical comparison of results.

Matrixing can further reduce testing on stability by testing only a selected subset of the total number of possible samples for all factor combinations at a specified time point. The next time point studies a different subset of all possible samples. This chapter does not address study designs for matrixing; such designs are addressed in ICH Q1D and specific designs are proposed in Chow (2007). Matrixing studies are only appropriate for small molecules (per ICH Q5C), and assume a high level of product knowledge. When considering incorporating bracketing or matrixing into a stability program, one must consider the risk associated with not collecting data on the missing lots and time points, because once the stability study starts, time points that pass cannot be tested.

ICH Q1A also discusses selection of stability batches. The number of batches monitored on stability depends on the process validation life cycle strategy and regulatory requirements for intended registration jurisdictions. All lots manufactured during performance process qualification (PPQ) should be monitored on stability, unless a strong business justification exists for monitoring a subset of these lots. PPQ lots form the basis of knowledge of the product's stability profile, and this knowledge can prove especially valuable in post-commercialization comparability exercises. Additionally, it is valuable to collect stability information on pre-PPQ lots that are representative of the commercial process, such as clinical lots or other pilot-scale batches, because they can be used to set or extend expiry and can also augment the limited data set when a product is relatively new.

7.3 A Word about Source Data

The results of a statistical analysis are only as good as the quality of the data used to generate the analysis; this is sometimes known as the "garbage in, garbage out" principle. In other words, if data do not have enough significant figures, do not come from reliable analytical methods, or are unverified, the results of the statistical analysis may be unreliable.

Subsequent decisions made on an unreliable analysis may be inconsistent with the data even though the analysis seems to be data-driven. Reliable, high-quality data become even more important in stability analyses where we may make predictions about future behavior based on extrapolation of observed trends.

Burdick et al. (2017, Chapter 2) provide an excellent discussion of the appropriate number of significant digits for analysis. A basic rule is to provide two more digits than are present in the stability acceptance criterion (AC) or specification limit (Borman 2015). Because statistical analysis deals with quantifying uncertainty, some uncertainty in our measurements should be included so that the analysis can provide reliable results. Wheeler (2011) describes "chunky data," or data where information about measurement variation has been lost due to rounding; chunky data can make a predictable process appear unpredictable. Often, data sets with results rounded to specification precision have lost information about measurement variation.

Rounding intermediate calculations prior to statistical analysis tends to increase the difference between the estimate and the true value (Bluman 2014, Chapter 3), leading to biased estimates. A corollary principle taught in mathematics is to retain most decimal places from calculations until all operations are performed, and then round the final answer to the appropriate number of decimal places. In fact, the FDA Office of Regulatory Affairs (ORA) field manual specifies that an extra significant figure is retained during calculations used to generate reported results. Consider a statistical analysis as a set of calculations with numbers that should not be rounded until the final answer is obtained. Final analysis results can be formatted to the AC precision if desired.

Results from stability studies are most typically obtained from qualified or validated analytical methods. Consistent data generated with reliable measurement systems are of the utmost importance in stability analyses because results are gathered over such a long period. Special care should be taken when combining data from different analytical methods. Results generated under different versions of an analytical method could indicate an apparent stability trend when, in fact, the "trend" is an artifact of the differences in versions of the analytical method. Graphical evaluation of results generated under different analytical conditions can aid in decisions to combine data for stability analysis.

Unverified results may include incorrect values due to data entry errors or other assignable causes. Apparent outliers in a data set should be verified for accuracy before a statistical analysis is finalized. Once values are verified, extreme care should be taken before excluding outliers because they are presumably valid results from approved testing.

Stability data may follow a nonlinear degradation pattern (e.g., moisture content), or may not be normally distributed within a given time point (e.g., subvisible particulates). In most cases, it is much easier to transform data to linearity than to fit nonlinear models. This chapter focuses on analysis of linear data. Analysis should be performed on transformed data until conclusions are obtained, and then predicted values may be back-transformed for graphical purposes or for comparison to stability AC. Most often, it is easier to transform the measured value rather than transforming the predictor time, because the interpretation of a transformed response value is more straightforward than the interpretation of some function of time. However, the particular transformation chosen should be focused on the unmet model assumptions, and sometimes transforming the response does not completely resolve model fit issues.

Lastly, typically there are not the same number of observations for each stability lot because newly manufactured lots are constantly being placed on stability, and so are of differing ages. Most of the analysis techniques described in this chapter do not require every lot to have the same number of observations. Situations where it is undesirable to have unbalanced data are noted, as are implications that relate to analyzing lots with few observations.

7.4 Stability Models for Use in This Chapter

Note that all models described in this section are linear regression models, and assume that there are multiple lots in a data set. Some research questions may be addressed to the stability profile of a single lot, but it is generally best practice to analyze all available stability data together using a single statistical model and draw conclusions about individual lots after the model is fit.

Analyses suggested can be conducted in many different statistical software packages. Examples in this chapter are shown using JMP®, Version 13.0.

7.4.1 Fixed Lot Model

Purpose: The fixed lot model specified in Model 7.1 is the simplest stability model for more than one lot. It fits a separate intercept and slope to each lot in the stability data set. Model 7.1 can be reduced to fit a common slope with separate intercepts for each lot, or further reduced to fit a common slope and intercept to all lots. The fixed lot model is the model specified in ICH Q1E for establishing an initial shelf life.

Focus of inference: Only lots included in the analysis.

When to use: Use the fixed lot model regardless of the number of lots when we are interested in making inferences about *only the lots included in the data set*.

Generally, use the fixed lot model when data are available for up to three lots. This is a general guideline—Model 7.2 may be used when there are more than three lots, as discussed in Stroup & Quinlan (2016).

Benefits of fitting this model: Simple, expressly detailed in ICH Q1E.

Disadvantages of fitting this model:

1. The conclusions from this model apply only to the lots included in the data set, and are not necessarily applicable to future batches. This may be a disadvantage if we want our conclusions to apply to all future batches.

2. Fitted regression lines do not consider the way other lots in the data set behave.

3. The model may result in artificially steep slopes due to highly influential observations at the beginning or end of the time course for a particular lot, especially for lots with few data points.

Model specification:

$$Y_{ij} = \beta_0 + \beta_1 Lot_i + \beta_2 Time_j + \beta_3 (Lot^*Time)_{ij} + E_{ij} \qquad (7.1)$$

$$i = 1, \ldots, n; j = 1, \ldots, T_i$$

Where

    Y_{ij} is the observed value for lot i at time point j

    β_0 is the average y-intercept across all lots

    β_1 is the adjustment to the average intercept for the ith lot

    β_2 is the average slope across all lots

    β_3 is the slope for the ith lot

    $Time_j$ is the jth time point

    E_{ij} is a normal random error term created by model misspecification and measurement error; E_{ij} is assumed $\sim N(0,\ \sigma_E^2)$

    n is the number of lots

    T is the number of responses obtained for lot i

7.4.1.1 Statistical Assumptions for the Fixed Lot Model

1. The overall degradation pattern is linear.

2. The response is normally distributed at a given time point (i.e., E_{ij} are normally distributed).

3. The residual variability of the response within a lot is equal for each data point and across lots (i.e., E_{ij} have the same variance); this assumption is called *homogeneity of variance* for lots.

4. The responses for each lot at each time point are independent (i.e., E_{ij} for one result is not correlated with the E_{ij} for another result). Sometimes, stability data violate this assumption because multiple samples are tested together in the same assay.

7.4.1.2 Fitting the Fixed Lot Model in JMP®

Figure 7.1 shows the JMP window specifying the fixed lot model in the **Fit Model** platform. To create this model:

1. From an open JMP data table, navigate to **Analyze → Fit Model**.

2. Add the responses from **Select Columns**:

    a. Select the response variable and click **Y**.

    b. Select Lot and Time and click **Add** in **Construct Model Effects**.

    c. Select Lot and Time, then click **Cross** to add the Lot*Time term.

    Note that to make predictions for extrapolated time points, the data table should contain a row that has no Y value at the intended time point of prediction for each lot *before the model is fit*.

3. Click the drop-down arrow by **Model Specification**. Uncheck **Center Polynomials** because 0 represents a meaningful value of the predictor, Time. By default, JMP centers polynomials, but leaving this option checked will lead to misalignment in parameter estimates compared to other statistical software (e.g., SAS). In other words, Time should not be a "coded" variable.

4. If appropriate, adjust the confidence level for the analysis.

    a. The default alpha level for calculated confidence intervals on the mean is $\alpha = 0.05$ (i.e., 95% confidence). An overall $\alpha = 0.05$ is used for a two-sided 95% confidence

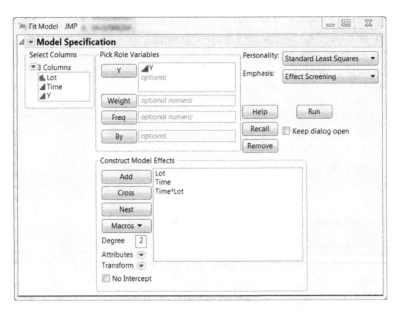

FIGURE 7.1
JMP dialogue used to fit fixed lot model.

interval (CI) on the regression line, which is the case when the stability specification has both a lower and an upper limit.

b. For a one-sided specification, use the appropriate one-sided 95% confidence bound (CB) on the mean, so the overall confidence level for the regression is 90% (i.e., $\alpha = 0.1$). Do this using the drop-down menu Model Specification → Set Alpha Level, and enter 0.1, as shown in Figure 7.2.

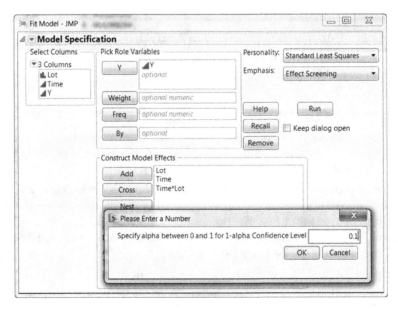

FIGURE 7.2
Changing the confidence level in the JMP fit model dialogue.

5. Select **Personality**: "Least Squares" and **Emphasis**: "Effect Screening" to automatically generate key output for model interpretation.

6. **Run** the analysis.

7.4.1.3 Obtaining Output from the Fixed Lot Model Fit in JMP®

This section provides details on how to obtain JMP output for the fixed lot model. Information about interpretation of results is discussed in sections pertaining to specific research questions.

1. Figure 7.3 shows an example of key statistical output obtained for the fixed lot model from the JMP **Fit Model** platform.

    a. **Effects Tests** are used to determine the statistical significance of model terms, and **Parameter Estimates** are used to estimate values at given settings of model parameters.

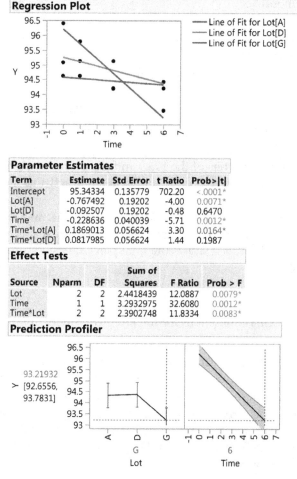

FIGURE 7.3
Key statistical output for the fixed lot model.

b. The **Prediction Profiler** is an interactive tool that can be used to determine predicted means for any combination of lot and time point. The predicted value is shown on the Y-axis. The predicted value represents both the predicted value of an individual response as well as the mean for all responses for the given lot and time values. The confidence interval on the average of all responses shown in brackets.

The example in Figure 7.3 shows the predicted value at six months for Lot G: 93.22% with lower one-sided 95% CB on the mean = 92.66%.

2. Figure 7.4 shows screenshots of the JMP windows used to build a plot of the regression that is aligned with the example plots provided in ICH Q1E. To make the plots in Figure 7.4:

a. Save columns from the **Fit Model** Output window: using the drop-down arrow by **Response**, select **Save Columns**, and save **Predicted Values** and **Mean Confidence Interval** to save these values to the data table.

b. Select rows for the lot of interest if data from only one lot should be plotted. Figure 7.4 plots the regression line for Lot G, the lot with the lowest predicted value at 12 months.

c. Use the graph builder to construct a scatter plot of Y, Y Pred, and the appropriate confidence bound(s) vs. Time, with points connected by the smoother. Follow these steps to refine the plot:

   i. Right click anywhere in the plot area, select **Smoother**, **Y**, and select only **Predicted Y** and **Lower 90% Mean Y**.

   ii. Right-click anywhere in the plot area, select **Points**, **Y**, and select only **Y**.

   iii. Right-click in the legend area and select **Legend Settings** to make sure all variables show on the plot.

   iv. Change the properties of the lines and the points by right clicking on the individual legend entries either in the **Legend Settings** menu or directly in the legend.

   v. Add a horizontal reference line for the stability AC and a vertical reference line at the time point of proposed expiry, and adjust axis ranges as desired. The plot in Figure 7.4f shows the final plot suggested for an expiry evaluation in ICH Q1E.

7.4.1.4 *Verifying Statistical Assumptions for the Fixed Lot Model in JMP®*

1. A scatter plot of the data can be used to decide whether the data follow a sufficiently linear degradation pattern, as shown in the example **Regression Plot** from Figure 7.3. The data in Figure 7.3 appear approximately linear for each lot.

2. Model residuals should be examined to validate assumptions about distribution and correlation of the error term. With a limited data set, only severe departures from the guidelines below are cause for concern. The data and all diagnostic plots should be taken together with scientific knowledge to decide whether model assumptions are reasonable.

a. Figure 7.5 shows example diagnostic plots generated with **Emphasis**: "Effect Screening" in the Fit Model dialogue; these plots can also be accessed from

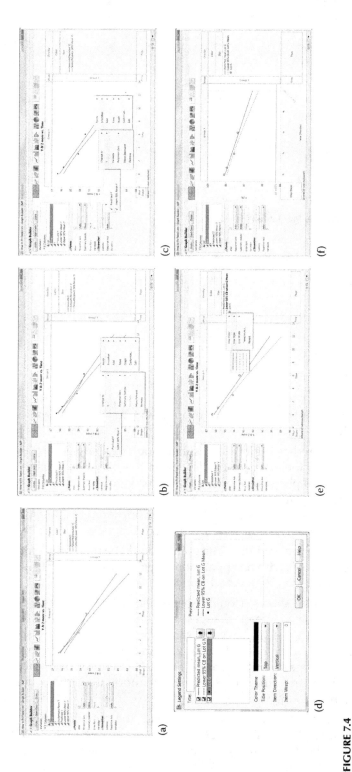

FIGURE 7.4

Creating a plot of predicted values and confidence bounds in JMP. (a) Initial plot. (b) Change points. (c) Change smoother. (d) Change legend. (e) Adjust markers. (f) Final plot per ICH Q1E.

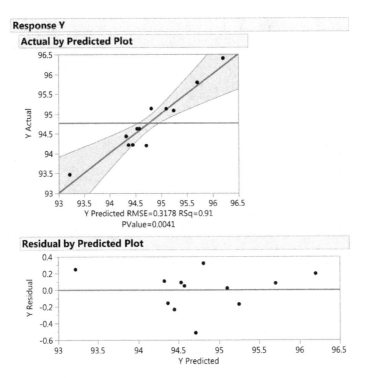

FIGURE 7.5
Example diagnostic plots for fixed lot model.

the Fit Model output using the drop-down arrow by **Response → Row Diagnostics**.

- Actual by Predicted Plot: The points should fall approximately along the straight line; the example plot supports that the assumption of linearity is met. If this plot shows points that look S-shaped or have severe curvature, the data may not be linearly related to time. Attempt to transform the response to achieve linearity using an appropriate transformation (Box 1964; Kutner 2005), or fit a nonlinear model.

- Residual by Predicted Plot: The points should be randomly scattered about a center line of 0, with no apparent pattern; the example plot shows that the homogeneity of variance assumption is met.

  - If this plot shows a bugle shape, then the variance is changing as the predicted mean changes, and the assumption of homogeneity of variance (i.e., E_{ij} have the same variance) is violated, so the model predictions are not valid. To address this, try transforming the data using a logarithmic, square root, or other appropriate transformation. Freeman and Tukey (1950) provides information on variance stabilizing transformations.

  - If this plot shows any type of trend, the model may be missing an important term. To address this, ensure that there are no differences in results due to lurking variables, such as method changes or different containers.

b. Figure 7.6 shows an example of a normal quantile (Q–Q) plot of Studentized residuals; the example plot shows that the assumed normal distribution is adequate.

All values should fall approximately along the straight line. Any curvature in this plot indicates that the data may not follow the assumed distribution (e.g., normal). Extreme observations may be apparent in the Q–Q plot as points that don't fall along the otherwise approximately straight line.

Figure 7.7 shows how to generate the Q–Q plot for the Studentized residuals. First, save the Studentized residuals from the model: Using the drop-down

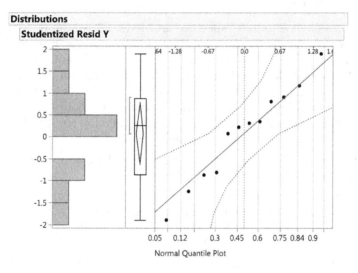

FIGURE 7.6
Example normal quantile plot of Studentized residuals from fixed lot model.

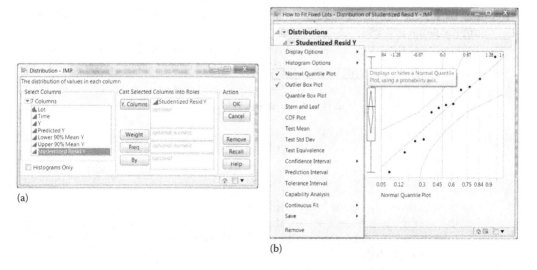

FIGURE 7.7
JMP dialogues to create normal quantile plot of Studentized residuals from model. (a) Creating distribution of studentized residuals. (b) Creating the Q–Q plot of studentized residuals.

arrow by **Response**, select **Save Columns**, and select **Studentized Residuals** to save these values to the data table. Next, create the Q–Q plot using **Analyze → Distribution**. Select "Studentized Resid" as **Y**, then **OK**. From the drop-down arrow by **Studentized Resid**, select **Normal Quantile Plot**.

3. Any of the plots in Figures 7.3, 7.5, and 7.6 can be used to visualize potential outliers in the data set; the example plots do not show any apparent outliers. Verify the validity and accuracy of any unusual results before excluding them, and only exclude values with scientific justification, especially if they are for commercial lots.

7.4.2 Random Lot Model

Purpose: The random lot model specified in Model 7.2 is a more computationally complex stability model than the fixed lot model, and is adapted from ICH Q1E. It considers lots as a random outcome of a consistent manufacturing process, as opposed to the fixed lots model that considers the trend for each lot in isolation. The random lot model allows the intercept to vary from lot to lot, and allows the slope to vary from lot to lot, depending on the sources of random variability in the data. Model 7.2 can be reduced to remove random intercept and slope variance components based on various model fitting strategies.

Focus of inference: Lots included in the analysis and all future lots manufactured under the same process.

When to use: Data are available for multiple lots and a relatively large data set (e.g., more than 15–20 total data points) and we want to extend our conclusions to the population of all current and future lots. There is no definitive guidance on the exact number of lots required to fit the random lot model instead of the fixed lot model. Stroup & Quinlan (2016) have shown that the random lot model performs quite well with six lots, and can make reasonable predictions with three lots. However, predictions based on three lots are likely to result in artificially short expiry periods when the random lots model is used to establish or extend expiry.

Benefits of fitting this model: Conclusions apply to all future lots manufactured using the same process.

Disadvantages of fitting this model: May require more data than the fixed lot model

Model specification:

$$Y_{ij} = \beta_0 + L_i + (\beta_1 + B_i)\text{Time}_j + E_{ij} \tag{7.2}$$

$$i = 1,\ldots,n; j = 1,\ldots,T_i$$

Where
  Y_{ij} is the observed value for lot i at time point j
  β_0 is the average y-intercept across all lots
  L_i is a random variable that allows the y-intercept to vary from lot to lot; L_i is assumed $\sim N(0,\ \sigma_L^2)$
  β_1 is the average slope across all lots
  B_i is a random variable that allows the slope to vary from lot to lot; B_i is assumed $\sim N(0,\ \sigma_B^2)$

E_{ij} is a normal random error term created by model misspecification and measurement error; E_{ij} is assumed $\sim N(0, \sigma_E^2)$

n   is the number of lots

T   is the number of responses obtained for lot i

7.4.2.1 Statistical Assumptions for the Random Lot Model

All assumptions are the same as those for the fixed lot model. Additionally, assume that

- Lots are random outcomes of a consistent manufacturing process.
- The random effects Lot and Lot*Time are independent. In other words, L_i and B_i are not correlated with each other.
- Observations for one lot are correlated with each other more strongly than are observations across lots.

7.4.2.2 Fitting the Random Lot Model in JMP®

Figure 7.8 shows the JMP window specifying the random lot model in the **Fit Model** platform. To create this model:

1. From an open JMP data table, navigate to **Analyze → Fit Model**.
2. Add the responses from **Select Columns**:
   a. Select the response variable and click **Y**.
   b. Select Lot and Time and click **Add** in **Construct Model Effects**.
   c. Select Lot and Time, then click **Cross** to add the Lot*Time term.
3. Designate the appropriate terms as random effects by selecting Lot and Lot*Time, click the drop-down arrow by **Attributes**, and select **Random Effect**.

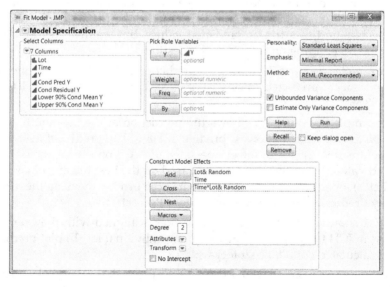

FIGURE 7.8
JMP model dialogue used to fit random lot model.

4. Click the drop-down arrow by **Model Specification**. Uncheck **Center Polynomials** because 0 represents a meaningful value of the predictor, Time.

5. If appropriate, adjust the confidence level for the analysis.

6. By default, the **Unbounded Variance Components** box is checked; this option allows variance estimates to be negative. Although variances are always positive, negative estimates can occur when there are few levels corresponding to the variance component (e.g. small number of lots). Leave this box checked because the focus of inference is on fixed effects, and constraining variance estimates to be positive may lead to bias in fixed effects tests (JMP 2017). If a situation arises where we are *only interested in the variance component estimates*, one can choose to uncheck this box.

7. **Run** the analysis.

7.4.2.3 Obtaining Output from the Random Lot Model Fit in JMP®

The output from the random lot model looks very similar to that for the fixed lot model. However, there are some important differences, especially when it comes to making conclusions about similarity of lots and predictions about individual lots.

1. Figure 7.9 shows an example of key statistical output obtained for the random lot model from the JMP **Fit Model** platform. **Fixed Effects Tests** are used to determine the statistical significance of model terms (i.e., Time), and **REML Variance Component Estimates** are used to examine the contribution to the total variance made by the random Lot and Lot*Time model terms. **Parameter Estimates** are used to estimate the overall average at a given time point and the overall average slope.

2. Figures 7.9 and 7.10 show examples of the JMP **Prediction Profiler** that can be used to obtain predictions from the random lots model.

   Difference between fixed and random lots model: Predictions can be generated for the overall mean or for individual lots at certain time points. Because lots are considered random outcomes of a consistent process, their individual slopes are not explicitly required to estimate predicted values, but we may desire to examine specific lots, depending on the research question.

   The example in Figure 7.9 shows the prediction at the six-month time point for the overall mean: predicted mean = 93.96% and lower one-sided 95% CB on the mean = 93.56%.

   The example in Figure 7.10 shows the prediction at the six-month time point for Lot N, the lot with the lowest predicted value. The predicted mean of Lot N at six months = 93.61% with lower one-sided 95% CB on the mean = 93.31%. The predicted values for individual lots are based on the best linear unbiased predictors (BLUPs) for each lot, and can be shown in the profiler by using the drop-down arrow by **Prediction Profiler → Conditional Predictions**.

3. Figure 7.11 shows a plot of the regression that is aligned with the example plots provided in ICH Q1E using the BLUP for an individual lot. To plot predicted values and calculated confidence intervals:

   a. Save columns from the **Fit Model** Output window. Using the drop-down arrow by **Response**, select **Save Columns**, and save **Conditional Pred Values** and **Conditional Mean CI** to save these values to the data table.

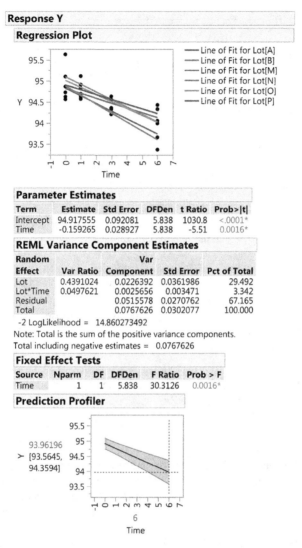

FIGURE 7.9
Key statistical output for the random model.

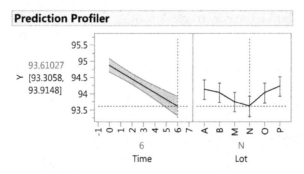

FIGURE 7.10
Example prediction profiler for individual lots from random lot model.

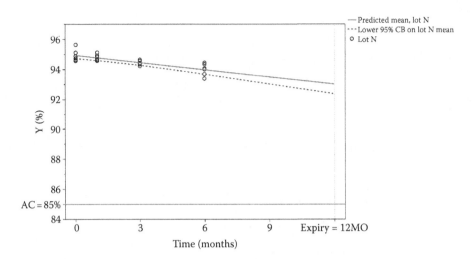

FIGURE 7.11
Example plot of conditional predicted values and confidence bound from random lot model.

b. Select rows for the lot of interest if data from only one lot should be plotted. Figure 7.11 plots the regression line for Lot N, the lot with the lowest predicted value at 12 months.

c. Use the graph builder to construct a scatter plot of Y, Cond Pred Y, and the appropriate confidence bound(s) vs. Time, with points connected by the smoother as detailed in Figure 7.4.

7.4.2.4 Verifying Statistical Assumptions for the Random Lot Model in JMP®

The random lot model assumptions are the same as those of the fixed lot model; therefore, the same types of plots are used to verify model assumptions. However, when random variance components are present in the model, the *conditional predictions and residuals* must be examined. Comparing the unconditional residuals (i.e., those shown in the default model output) to the conditional residuals can show how fitting the Lot and Lot*Time terms as random effects improve the model fit. However, only the conditional residuals need be used to verify model assumptions.

To create plots of the conditional residuals: use the drop-down arrow by **Response →** **Save Columns**, and save **Conditional Pred Values** and **Conditional Residuals** to the data table. Use the graph builder to construct plots of Actual Values vs. Conditional Predicted Values and of Conditional Residuals vs. Conditional Predicted Values. Create the Q–Q plot by evaluating the distribution of the conditional residuals.

Figure 7.12 shows the plots of conditional residuals used to verify assumptions of linearity and homogeneity of variance. Figure 7.13 shows the Q–Q plot for the conditional residuals. The example plots show that the model assumptions are met.

7.4.3 Qualitative Predictor model

Purpose: The qualitative predictor model specified in Model 7.3 is used to compare stability data from two or more groups that differ based on a qualitative variable, X, such as container type, formulation, manufacturing site, or pre/post

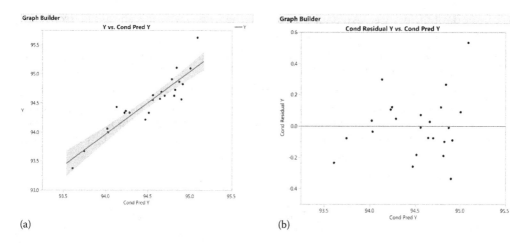

FIGURE 7.12
Example diagnostic plots for the random lot model. (a) Actual vs. conditional predicted values. (b) Conditional residuals vs. conditional predicted values.

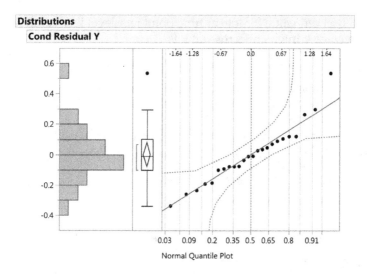

FIGURE 7.13
Example normal quantile plot of conditional residuals from random lot model.

manufacturing change. For example, if X is container type, then we might compare x_1 = vial versus x_2 = syringe. This model considers lots as a random outcome of a consistent manufacturing process, and does not compare the trends for individual lots. Instead, it compares the trend for each level of X, considering X as a fixed variable where each group may have a unique slope and intercept.

Focus of inference: The lots included in the analysis and all future lots manufactured under the same processes.

When to use: Data are available for multiple time points on multiple lots for each level of X. There should be at least two lots for each level of X, with at least four to five time points on each lot to ensure that sample sizes are large enough to detect important differences. All data grouped as the same level of X should be from the same or comparable manufacturing processes.

Benefits of fitting this model: Conclusions apply to all future lots manufactured under the same conditions as those in the data set.

Disadvantages of fitting this model: Requires multiple measurements on multiple lots for each level of X, so may not be useful if only one lot of one configuration has been studied. If limited time exists to generate stability data for profile comparison, additional intermediate time points should be tested (e.g., 0, 0.25, 0.5, 2.5, 2.75, and 3 months).

Model specification (shown when X is indicator variable):

$$Y_{ijk} = \beta_0 + L_{i(k)} + \beta_1 Time_j + \beta_2 X_k + \beta_3 (X^*Time)_{jk} + E_{ijk} \qquad (7.3)$$

$$i = 1, \ldots, n; j = 1, \ldots, T_i, \ k = 1, \ldots, m - 1$$

Where

Y_{ijk} is the observed value for lot i at time point j for level k of variable X
β_0 is the average y-intercept across all lots
L_i is a random variable that allows the y-intercept to vary from lot to lot; L_i is assumed $\sim N(0, \sigma_L^2)$; nested in X
β_1 is the average slope across all lots
β_2 is the adjustment to the average intercept for the kth level of X
β_3 is the slope for the kth level of X
E_{ijk} is a normal random error term created by model misspecification and measurement error; E_{ijk} is assumed $\sim N(0, \sigma_E^2)$
n is the number of lots
m is the number of levels of X
T is the number of responses obtained for lot i

7.4.3.1 Statistical Assumptions for the Qualitative Predictor Model

1. All assumptions are the same as those for the random lot model, including that all lots are random outcomes of a consistent manufacturing process.
2. All levels of X have the same variance (i.e., homogeneity of variance).
3. All lots within a level of X are expected to degrade in the same way, apart from random process variation.

7.4.3.2 Fitting the Qualitative Predictor Model in JMP®

Figure 7.14 shows the JMP window specifying the qualitative predictor model in the **Fit Model** platform. To create this model:

1. From an open JMP data table, navigate to **Analyze → Fit Model**.
2. Add the responses from **Select Columns**:
   a. Select the response variable and click **Y**.

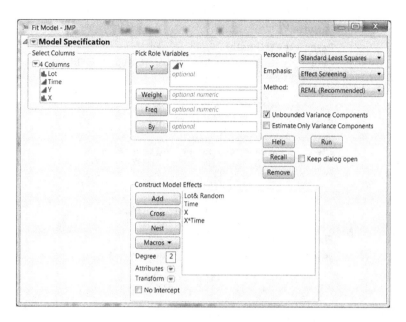

FIGURE 7.14
JMP model dialogue used to fit the qualitative predictor model.

   b. Select Lot, Time, and X and click **Add** in **Construct Model Effects**. X should have a red histogram icon next to it in the **Select Columns** box to indicate that it is a qualitative variable.
   c. Select X and Time, then click **Cross** to add the X*Time term.

3. Designate Lot as a random effect by selecting Lot, click the drop-down arrow by **Attributes**, and select **Random Effect**.

4. Click the drop-down arrow by **Model Specification**. Uncheck **Center Polynomials** because 0 represents a meaningful value of the predictor, Time.

5. If appropriate, adjust the confidence level for the analysis.

6. By default, the **Unbounded Variance Components** box is checked. Leave this box checked because the focus of inference is on fixed effects, and unchecking it could lead to bias in tests for fixed effects (JMP 2017).

7. **Run** the analysis.

7.4.3.3 Obtaining Output from the Qualitative Predictor Model Fit in JMP®

The output from the qualitative predictor model looks similar to output from the random lots model except that it contains additional information about the qualitative variable X. The focus of inference is now on X instead of the trend of just one group.

1. Figure 7.15 shows an example of key statistical output obtained for the qualitative predictor model from the JMP **Fit Model** platform.
   a. **Fixed Effects Tests** are used to determine the statistical significance of model terms (i.e., Time, X, and X*Time), and **REML Variance Component Estimates** are used to examine the contribution to the total variance made by the random Lot term.

Response Y

Parameter Estimates

Term	Estimate	Std Error	DFDen	t Ratio	Prob>|t|
Intercept	95.036472	0.1183	13.55	803.35	<.0001*
Time	-0.197684	0.028474	22	-6.94	<.0001*
X[X1]	0.0218921	0.1183	13.55	0.19	0.8559
X[X1]*Time	0.0225836	0.028474	22	0.79	0.4362

REML Variance Component Estimates

Random Effect	Var Ratio	Var Component	Std Error	Pct of Total
Lot	0.2743163	0.0350302	0.039837	21.527
Residual		0.1277001	0.038503	78.473
Total		0.1627303	0.0482518	100.000

-2 LogLikelihood = 43.328704643

Note: Total is the sum of the positive variance components.
Total including negative estimates = 0.1627303

Fixed Effect Tests

Source	Nparm	DF	DFDen	F Ratio	Prob > F
Time	1	1	22	48.1984	<.0001*
X	1	1	13.55	0.0342	0.8559
X*Time	1	1	22	0.6290	0.4362

FIGURE 7.15
Key statistical output for the qualitative predictor model.

    b. Model predictions are obtained from the **Parameter Estimates** table. The value for "Intercept" is the average for all levels of X at time 0, and the value for "Time" is the average slope for all levels of X.

2. Figures 7.16 and 7.17 show examples of the JMP **Prediction Profiler** that can be used to obtain predictions from the qualitative predictor model for different levels of X.

    The example in Figure 7.16 shows the prediction at the six-month time point for the overall mean of group X2: Predicted mean = 93.69% with lower bound from a two-sided 95% CI on the mean = 93.32%.

    The example in Figure 7.17 shows the prediction at the six-month time point for Lot N: 93.62% with lower one-sided 95% CB on the mean = 93.25%. The predicted values for individual lots are based on the BLUPs for each lot, and are obtained by selecting **Conditional Predictions** from the drop-down arrow by **Prediction Profiler**. Note that the X setting in the profiler must match the lot's level of X in

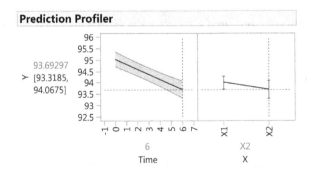

FIGURE 7.16
Example prediction profiler for mean of X2 from the qualitative predictor model.

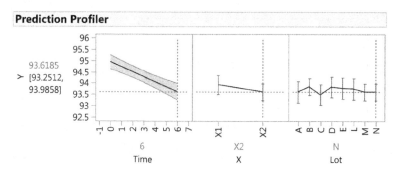

FIGURE 7.17
Example prediction profiler for individual lots from the qualitative predictor model.

order to obtain accurate predictions for that lot (i.e., X must be set at X2 when predicting for Lot N because Lot N is from group X2).

3. Figure 7.18 shows a scatter plot of the data with the estimated regression lines for each level of X. Symbols and lines are differentiated by level of X because we are primarily interested in comparing the profiles of the two groups.

To plot predicted values and calculated regression lines by level of X:

a. Save the **Predicted Values** column from the **Fit Model** Output window.

b. Use the graph builder to construct a scatter plot of Y and Predicted Y vs. Time. To plot symbols and regression lines for each level of X, select X as the **Overlay** variable. The plot can be further refined as shown in Figure 7.4.

4. Figure 7.19 shows an alternate plot that may prove useful for some applications of the qualitative predictor model. In this plot, each level of X has the same color; however, each lot has a different symbol and the regression line for each lot is shown.

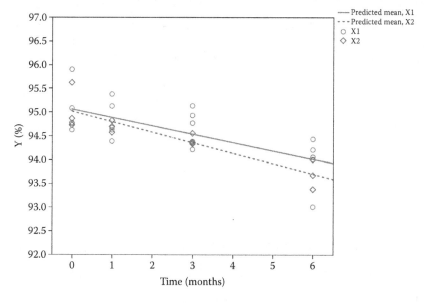

FIGURE 7.18
Example plot of average predicted values by level of X from the qualitative predictor model.

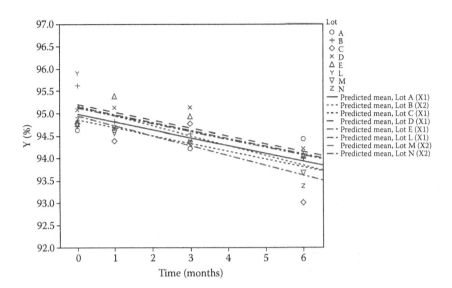

FIGURE 7.19
Example plot of conditional predicted values by lot from the qualitative predictor model.

To plot the predicted values and calculated regression lines by lot, save and plot the **Conditional Pred Values**, select Lot as the **Overlay** variable, and **Color** by X. Further refine the plot as shown in Figure 7.4.

7.4.3.4 Verifying Statistical Assumptions in JMP®

As with the random lot model, the conditional predictions and conditional residuals must be examined because the qualitative predictor model fits Lot as a random term. It may be useful to color the residuals by level of X to visualize potential differences in variability between the groups.

Figure 7.20 shows the plots of conditional residuals used to verify assumptions of linearity and homogeneity of variance. Figure 7.21 shows the Q–Q plot for the conditional residuals. The diagnostic plots show that model assumptions are reasonable.

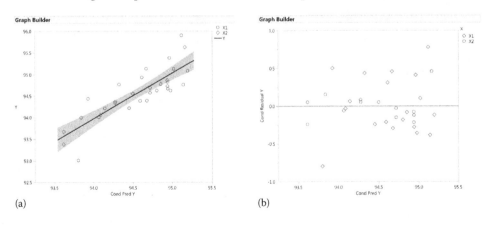

FIGURE 7.20
Example diagnostic plots for the qualitative predictor model. (a) Actual vs. conditional predicted values. (b) Conditional residuals vs. conditional predicted values.

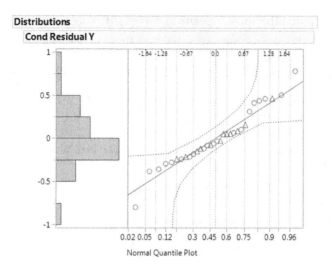

FIGURE 7.21
Example normal quantile plot of conditional residuals from qualitative predictor model.

7.5 Outline

The type of statistical analysis and subsequent interpretation of results depends on the particular research question of interest. The same statistical model may be used to answer different research questions, depending on the way analysis results are presented. If we ever struggle with the practical implications of our findings, it is instructive to return to the research question we are trying to answer. It may be that our analysis did not answer the intended research question, and that a different analysis should be applied.

The following sections relate the stability models from Section 7.4 to specific research questions that may arise as a stability program develops.

7.6 Is there a trend on stability?

    7.6.1 Can a particular CQA be considered "stability indicating"?

    7.6.2 Is the change over time statistically significant?

    7.6.3 Is the change over time practically significant?

    7.6.4 Is an individual result "in trend"?

    7.6.5 Is a stability lot in trend?

    7.6.6 How can I establish a stability trending program?

    7.6.7 How can I perform an annual "trend analysis" as required for commercially approved products?

7.7 How is the stability profile related to the expiry/retest period?

    7.7.1 What is the appropriate expiry or retest period for my product?

    7.7.2 Will an individual lot meet its intended expiry period?

    7.7.3 Can I extend the expiry period?

    7.7.4 How can I model behavior for end-to-end stability for multiple product stages?

7.8 How does the stability profile relate to the specification limit?

    7.8.1 What is the appropriate specification limit to achieve a desired expiry or retest period?

    7.8.2 Is it appropriate to have a tighter specification limit at lot release?

    7.8.3 Does changing the specification limit impact the expiry?

    7.8.4 What is the probability of an individual OOS result on stability?

7.9 How much exposure to a particular condition can be allowed without impacting the shelf life?

    7.9.1 What is an appropriate limit for exposure to temperatures above recommended storage?

    7.9.2 How much light exposure is acceptable?

    7.9.3 Does temperature cycling impact my product?

7.10 Do two (or more) different permutations of my molecule change the same way over time?

    7.10.1 Can I apply a bracketing approach to several different configurations of the same product formulation?

    7.10.2 Is one formulation, container, or configuration more stable at a given temperature?

    7.10.3 Is the stability profile the same after a manufacturing or process change?

7.6 Is There a Trend on Stability?

Trend is a broad term that simply means some type of noticeable pattern in data. Sometimes, there can be an obvious trend in a graph, and little more than a picture is needed to establish the pattern. Other times, we want to use statistics to objectively characterize any stability trends. There are several possible interpretations of the question, "Is there a trend on stability?" We may speak of a change over time, whether a result is expected based on other data, or a summary of the general conclusions from the overall stability program.

The question of "trend over time" is perhaps the most fundamental question answered by an analysis. A stability program is typically focused on monitoring only those CQAs that are expected to change over time, or those that, if they did change over time, may affect patient safety or product efficacy. In addition to interest in the presence of a trend, demonstrating its absence may allow monitoring on stability only a subset of the CQAs measured at lot release.

We could also speak of whether a specific result is "in trend." Apparent out of trend stability results can be investigated in a timely fashion. A stability trending program is analogous to trending of lot release data, and provides information about the degree of process consistency.

A summary of the overall stability trend may incorporate evaluation of trend over time, summarize out of trend results, examine how lots trend as a group, and compare trends to established specifications. An overall stability trend summary can provide evidence of manufacturing consistency over the product life cycle.

7.6.1 Can a Particular CQA Be Considered "Stability Indicating"?

The stability indicating properties of an analytical method are typically confirmed during method validation, inferring that the method is capable of detecting degradation if it is present. CQAs monitored on stability are typically those that are shown to be "stability indicating," meaning that there is a measurable change over time. However, the measured CQA may only show appreciable change at ASC, so monitoring it on stability may provide value to confirm that no change occurs at RSC. Evaluating whether a CQA is stability indicating may be undertaken either to demonstrate the CQA is changing over time or to provide evidence that there is no change over time.

In many instances, graphical evidence is sufficient to support a claim that a particular CQA is stability indicating. In fact, the very first thing to do in any stability analysis is to *plot the data*. Much can be learned from a simple scatter plot of data vs. time, with lots denoted by different symbols. Figure 7.22 shows several example scatter plots based on the data given in Table 7.1: In Figure 7.22(a), there is a clear trend over time, and in Figure 7.22(b), there is no apparent trend. However, as shown in Figure 7.22(c), there may be instances where it is difficult to make an objective claim about the trend over time; in these cases, leaving interpretation up to the reader may lead to differing opinions, and statistical analysis can help to make a more objective statement about the presence or absence of a trend.

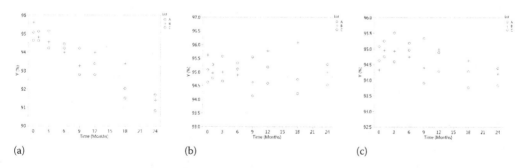

(a) (b) (c)

FIGURE 7.22
Scatter plots of example stability trends. (a) Clear trend over time. (b) No trend over time. (c) Potential trend over time.

TABLE 7.1

Data Used for Figure 7.22 Example

Lot	Time	Clear Trend Over Time (7.22a)	No Trend Over Time (7.22b)	Potential Trend Over Time (7.22c)
A	0	94.622	94.622	94.622
A	1	94.622	94.772	94.747
A	3	94.213	94.663	94.588
A	6	94.430	95.330	95.180
A	9	92.773	94.123	93.898
A	12	93.382	95.182	94.882
A	18	91.506	94.206	93.756
A	24	90.825	94.525	93.825
A	36	89.576	94.976	94.076
A	48	87.596	94.796	93.596
B	0	95.622	95.622	94.322
B	1	94.821	94.971	94.946
B	3	94.551	95.001	94.926
B	6	93.995	94.895	94.745
B	9	93.271	94.621	94.396
B	12	93.977	95.777	94.977
B	18	93.381	96.081	94.631
B	24	91.395	94.995	94.195
B	36	89.997	95.397	94.497
B	48	87.936	95.136	93.936
C	0	95.077	95.077	95.077
C	1	95.122	95.272	95.247
C	3	95.128	95.578	95.503
C	6	94.208	95.108	94.958
C	9	94.204	95.554	95.329
C	12	92.781	94.581	94.281
C	18	92.021	94.721	94.271
C	24	91.684	95.284	94.384
C	36	89.121	94.521	93.621
C	48	87.680	94.880	93.680

7.6.2 Is the Change over Time Statistically Significant?

Asking whether a change over time is statistically significant implies that we are conducting a statistical hypothesis test. Specifically, we are testing whether the slope of the regression line is different from 0 where H_0: $\beta = 0$ vs. H_A: $\beta \neq 0$, and β is the slope. The hypothesis test is conducted by fitting a regression model to the stability data and then examining the p-value for the Time term, which is derived from a t-test on the slope parameter. The p-value for Time is compared to a stated significance level, typically $\alpha = 0.05$. A p-value < 0.05 for Time is taken as evidence that there is a statistically significant trend over time at the 95% confidence level. Note that a p-value greater than 0.05 does not prove that there is no trend over time; rather, we can only state that there is not enough evidence to demonstrate that there is a trend over time.

Model 7.1 or Model 7.2 can be used to conduct a statistical test for change over time. As noted earlier, the focus of inference determines the more appropriate model.

- Fit Model 7.1—the fixed lot model—if we are only interested in making statements about the particular lots in the data set. The fixed lot model examines each lot individually, so t-tests are provided for not only the Time term, but also the Lot*Time term. Since there are two Time-related terms in the model, there are four potential conclusions relating to the significance of the trend over time, depending on the p-values for the Time and Lot*Time terms.

- Fit Model 7.2—the random lot model—if we are interested in making statements about all of the lots that have been or will be manufactured. Fitting the random lot model provides a model with only one fixed term, Time, so there are two potential conclusions relating to the significance of the trend over time.

Table 7.2 outlines the possible conclusions of the hypothesis test of the stability trend, depending on whether Model 7.1 or Model 7.2 is fit to the data.

Many articles speak to the pitfalls of using the p-value as a measure of evidence. Often, we are less likely to observe a significant p-value with smaller data sets, and more likely to observe a significant p-value with larger data sets or measurements that are more precise (Wasserstein and Lazar 2016). In the case of a stability analysis, using a p-value alone may lead to erroneous conclusions or conclusions that could change with the addition of each new data point. Therefore, in addition to reporting any p-values, it is best practice to provide a scatter plot of the data and report the CI on the slope, which affords some statement

TABLE 7.2

Possible Conclusions for Hypothesis Test of Statistically Significant Trend over Time

Model Fit to Data	p-value for Time Term	p-value for Lot*Time Term	Conclusion
Model 7.1	$p \geq 0.05$	$p \geq 0.05$	There is no evidence that there is an overall trend over time. There is no evidence that the slope of any one lot differs from the slope of the other lots.
	$p \geq 0.05$	$p < 0.05$	There is no evidence that there is an overall trend over time. There is evidence that the slope of at least one lot differs from the slope of the other lots.
	$p < 0.05$	$p \geq 0.05$	The average trend over time is statistically significant at the stated confidence level (95% for $p = 0.05$). There is no evidence that the slope of any one lot differs from the slope of the other lots.
	$p < 0.05$	$p < 0.05$	The average trend over time is statistically significant at the stated confidence level (95% for $p = 0.05$). There is evidence that the slope of at least one lot differs from the slope of the other lots.
Model 7.2	$p \geq 0.05$	N/A	There is no evidence that there is an overall trend over time.
	$p < 0.05$	N/A	The average trend over time is statistically significant at the stated confidence level (95% for $p = 0.05$).

Note: N/A: Lot*Time is not a fixed effect in Model 7.2, so it does not contribute to the conclusion about trend over time.

about the range of possible slopes. Note that if the CI on the slope contains 0, then there is no statistical evidence that the slope differs from 0.

The example output in Figure 7.23 shows the results of two different examinations for the presence of a statistically significant trend over time using the same data set; the data are those for a "clear trend over time" from Table 7.1. Since the trend over time is obvious, a scatter plot of the data with estimated regression line shown in Figure 7.24 is sufficient to demonstrate the presence of a trend. The statistical output is useful for making quantitative statements about the trend.

Figure 7.23(a) shows the results from Model 7.1—the fixed lot model.

- The p-value for Time is <0.0001, so the trend over time is statistically significant (at any stated confidence level).

- The p-value for Lot*Time is 0.5310, so there is no evidence that the slopes differ by lot.

- The p-value for Lot is 0.4437, so there no evidence that the intercepts differ by lot.

- The parameter estimate for Time gives the average slope for all lots. The average slope is −0.155445%/month. The range of possible slopes is given by the two-sided 95% CI on the slope = (−0.18, −0.13)%/month.

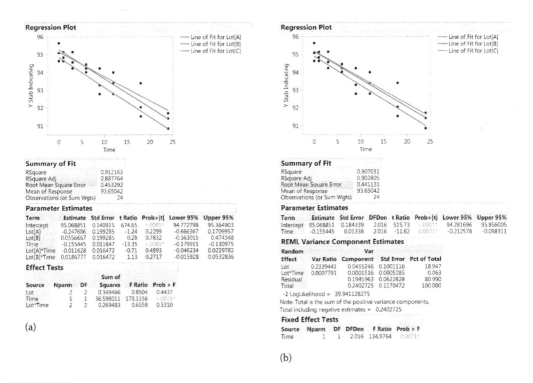

(a)

(b)

FIGURE 7.23
Example output for models evaluating statistical significance of trend over time. (a) Fixed lot model. (b) Random lot model.

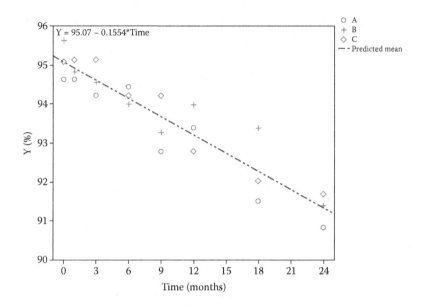

FIGURE 7.24
Scatterplot of data and regression line from Figure 7.23 example.

Figure 7.23(b) shows the results from Model 7.2—the random lot model.

- The *p*-value for Time is 0.0071; therefore, the trend over time is statistically significant at the 95% confidence level.
- The percent of total variance due to Lot is about 19% and the percentage due to Lot*Time is essentially 0%. Therefore, there is considerable lot-to-lot variability at the time of manufacture, but there is not measurable variability in the slopes of the lots.
- The parameter estimate for Time gives the average slope for all lots. The average slope is −0.155445%/month. The range of possible slopes is given by the two-sided 95% CI on the slope = (−0.21, −0.10)%/month.

Note that the slope estimate for Model 7.2 is the same as that for Model 7.1 in this example because the data are balanced (i.e., every lot has the same number of observations at each time point). In general, the slope estimates will differ for Model 7.1 and Model 7.2 when the data are unbalanced. The CI on the slope is wider for the random lot model because lot-to-lot variation is considered as part of the total variance used to calculate the CI.

When initially assessing the presence of a trend over time, the number of lots available for examination may be limited. We may wish to assess the trend for the first stability lot at the outset of a clinical program, to examine the behavior of a reference standard lot or other critical reagent lot, or because we have conducted a special stability study of some kind on only one lot.

If there is only one lot available in the data set, or if there is no evidence that the lots differ in slope or intercept, Model 7.1 reduces to Model 7.4:

$$Y_i = \beta_0 + \beta_1 \text{Time}_i + E_i \tag{7.4}$$

$$i = 1, \ldots, T$$

Where
  Y_i is the observed value at time point i
  β_0 is the average y-intercept
  β_1 is the average slope
Time$_i$ is the ith time point
  E_i is a normal random error term created by model misspecification and measurement error; E_j is assumed $\sim N(0, \sigma_E^2)$
  T   is the number of time points

The statistical output obtained from fitting Model 7.4 is similar to that from Model 7.1, but lacks a p-value for Lot*Time. The interpretation of the p-value for Time remains the same as described in Table 7.2. However, with only one lot, the conclusions drawn from this analysis apply only to this lot. One must be careful not to extend the conclusions to all future lots until further data on more lots are obtained.

When fitting a model to only one lot, including data for more time points is better, because data at the beginning and end of the time course are highly influential to the slope of the regression line. Further, having more time points towards the ends of the regression line will make for a better slope estimate. For example, a study with time points at 0, 0.25, 0.5, 3, 5.5, 5.75, and 6 months will be less prone to influence from extreme observations than a study with time points at 0, 1, 2, 3, and 6 months. Although it only takes two points to estimate a straight line, having four or five data points will result in a more robust estimate of the slope.

7.6.3 Is the Change over Time Practically Significant?

A statement on the statistical significance of the Time effect using a p-value is weak evidence of the absence or presence of a trend because it does not quantify the potential change. A CI on the slope parameter quantifies the magnitude of the estimated change and provides the range of possible slope values, which also gives some measure of the uncertainty associated with the slope estimate. The p-value and CI on the slope parameter are sufficient evidence to demonstrate that a trend *is* present. However, to demonstrate that a trend is *not* present, our analysis findings must be presented in a different way. A statistically significant trend may not be practically significant because it may not be of a magnitude that is consequential when considered in conjunction with the precision of the analytical method, the expiry period, the stability AC, or other scientific considerations.

In order to demonstrate that there is no trend over time, we can conduct two one-sided t-tests (TOST) of the hypotheses: H_0: $|\beta| \geq EL$ vs. H_A: $|\beta| < EL$ where EL represents the equivalence limit. A subject matter expert selects the EL value; the EL is a slope value that represents no practically important change over time. TOST is commonly known as an equivalence test, and it aims to prove that the possible values are less than a practically meaningful value, and that the slope is thus practically equivalent to 0. In this construct,

β can be either the slope parameter or the total change over a given time period (i.e., $\beta \times$ Time point) because either measure is a way to quantify the potential trend.

The equivalence test is conducted as a three-step process:

- First, define the amount of change that is *not* practically important, known as the equivalence limit (EL). The EL is defined as a positive quantity. The entire range −EL to +EL defines the range of possible β values that are considered not practically important, and therefore can be considered practically equal to 0. It is ideal to choose EL based on scientific or regulatory rationale.

- To quantify the amount of change over time, fit a regression to the data using either Model 7.1, Model 7.2, or Model 7.4. Calculate β and a two-sided CI on β (i.e., two one-sided confidence bounds on β). In practice, two one-sided 95% confidence bounds may be calculated, which together result in a 90% CI. Although the CI is calculated with 90% confidence, the significance level of the test is 0.05, as demonstrated by Berger and Hsu (1996).

- To conduct the equivalence test, compare the CI on β to the range from −EL to EL. If the CI on β falls entirely within ±EL, then the observed change over time has been shown to be less than the change that is considered practically equal, or equivalent, to 0; this result can be taken as evidence that there is no practically significant trend in a CQA over time. If the CI does not fall entirely within the interval from −EL to EL, then there is not sufficient evidence to claim that the slope is not practically significant. In such cases, scientific rationale should be used to determine if the observed change over time is meaningful.

In practice, defining the EL may be difficult, because an acceptable value of the allowable change may be difficult to discern. When defining the EL, remember that it must be scientifically defensible because the overall conclusion of the equivalence test depends on the stated practically important value for the slope. A practically important slope may take into consideration things such as the analytical method precision, the amount of change that impacts the ability to meet specifications, or the amount of change the may affect other product characteristics.

One way to objectively define an EL is to consider the analytical method's intermediate precision (IP), which can be taken from method validation or assay trending data. One may choose to define the EL as a multiple of the IP. For example, for a method with an IP standard deviation of 0.5%, define any change that exceeds 2*IP as a practically important change. If evaluating the total change over time, then the EL is 2*0.5% = 1%, and an observed a change of more than 1% over the studied time period is practically significant. If evaluating the slope, allowing a shift of no more than 2*IP (or 1%) over 24 months would result in an EL of ± (1%/24months) = ± 0.042%/month. If the slope exceeds 0.042%/month in absolute value, then the slope exceeds two times the change expected based on the method variability, and may be considered a practically significant change. When defining the slope EL based on the method's IP, the acceptable slope differs as the observed study duration differs because the IP is constant.

Figure 7.25 shows example output from an analysis for practically significant change over time for the data sets provided in Table 7.1 and plotted in Figure 7.22: 7.25(a) shows data with an obvious trend, 7.25(b) shows data with no obvious trend, and 7.25c shows data where a trend may be present. Model 7.2 is used to fit the regression because we assume that every lot is degrading at the same rate, and any differences are due to random process

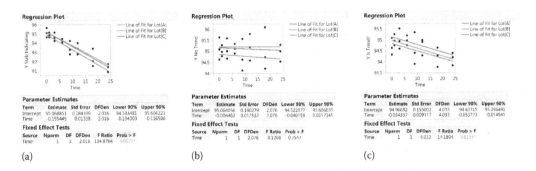

FIGURE 7.25

Example analysis examining practically significant change over time. (a) Practically significant change over time. (b) No practically significant change over time. (c) Potential practically significant change over time.

and method variation. Using the example EL of 0.042%/month for the slope parameter, the results of the evaluation are stated as follows:

- Figure 7.25(a): The 90% CI for the slope parameter is (−0.194, −0.117)%/month. The slope is practically significant because the 90% CI falls entirely outside of the EL interval from −0.042 to 0.042%/month.

- Figure 7.25(b): The 90% CI for the slope parameter is (−0.040, −0.031)%/month. The slope is not practically significant because the 90% CI on the slope falls entirely inside of the EL interval.

- Figure 7.25(c): The 90% CI for the slope parameter is (−0.054, −0.015)%/month. The slope is not equivalent to 0, and may be practically significant because the 90% CI on the slope falls partially outside of the EL interval. Scientific justification is required to make a definitive statement about the practical importance of the change over time.

Note that Figure 7.25 also shows the p-values for Time because the same model can be used to test for either practical significance or statistical significance. In general, it is best practice to state only one conclusion in case the conclusion about statistical significance conflicts with the conclusion about practical significance. Specifically, a change might be statistically significant but not practically significant, so including the p-value may complicate the explanation of the overall conclusion that the trend is unimportant. For example, notice that in Figure 7.25(c), the equivalence test is inconclusive, but the p-value for Time is less than 0.05. Although it may be tempting to use the p-value to make a definitive statement about the slope after the equivalence test is conducted, the more appropriate course of action is to state the equivalence conclusion and use scientific rationale to justify the importance of the potential slope.

7.6.4 Is an Individual Result in Trend?

We often ask the question of whether an individual result is "in trend" because it appears unusual compared to our current knowledge. It is important to examine unusual results in real time so that their validity can be investigated as soon as they are observed; otherwise, a suspect result may make it into the historical stability data set and could influence stability conclusions about expiry, specifications, and future expected trends. A timely examination of an out-of-trend (OOT) result may lead to discovery of lab errors, previously unknown impact from method changes, or some type of impact from a process change. An apparent OOT result could also be due to random method and/or process variation and thus be perfectly acceptable.

In order to determine if a particular result is in trend, one must define what values can reasonably be expected based on the stability data observed to date. The way to approach this question will depend on the extent of knowledge about the stability profile. At the outset of a stability program, when little data are available, the best tool may be a simple scatter plot of the data. Although a plot of the data is a qualitative way to detect unusual observations, it provides a visual representation that allows discussion of whether a result is odd enough that it bears closer examination.

As knowledge grows, statistical analysis can be incorporated. Before using statistical analysis for trending, it is important to have a good idea of the expected stability profile. Statistical intervals are used to define a region of expected results based on information already obtained. Clearly, the robustness of the limits will rely upon having studied a sufficient number of lots for a reasonable amount of time.

To determine if a particular result is in trend, an interval that applies to individual results is employed. Such an interval will take the form of the predicted mean at a given time point ± some multiple of the population standard deviation, also represented as $\overline{x_T} \pm k \times s$. There are many ways to determine the multiplier, k, depending on the interval's purpose and the available amount of information. At its simplest, a statistical interval on individual results may use $k = 3$, similar to a control chart: We expect 99.73% of observations to fall within ±3 standard deviations of the mean, based on normal probability assumptions. With very little information, one could choose to use this kind of basic interval at each time point. However, an estimate of the true standard deviation based on a small sample size has little certainty, and so the interval may not be very precise.

A tolerance interval (TI) is a better way to check that a new stability result is within expectations because this interval to applies to *all future results* generated under current process conditions. A TI describes the region expected to contain a certain proportion of future results (p, also known as coverage) with a specified level of confidence $(1 - \alpha)$%. For example, a 95% confidence, 99% coverage TI is expected to contain *at least* 99% of future observations with 95% confidence, denoted as a 95/99 TI. Although p and α can theoretically take any values, a 95/99 TI is commonly used in industry because it generally provides intervals of a practical width when calculated using a reasonably sized data set.

Bear in mind a few important properties of TIs:

- TIs depend heavily on the assumption of normality because they are symmetric about the estimated mean. Specifically, the observations at each time point should be normally distributed about the fitted regression line; this assumption should be verified as described in Section 7.4 before proceeding with TI calculations. If this is not a valid assumption, then data should be transformed prior to calculations described below, or nonparametric intervals can be calculated as described in Section 5 of Hahn et al. (2017).

- A TI can be either one-sided or two-sided. A two-sided TI is recommended since interest is generally in whether a result is unusual in either the positive or the negative direction. If a one-sided TI is desired, the appropriate bound of the two-sided interval may be used, or exact calculations for one-sided bounds may be found in Burdick et al. (2017).

- The TI will become narrower as more data are collected because k is a function of sample size.
- Interval width is adjusted by changing p and α, but the best practice is to be consistent in the choice across CQAs within one analysis.
  - The width of the TI is impacted more by changing p than α.
  - Changing p implies coverage of either a greater or lesser proportion of the total distribution of data.
  - A more conservative TI (i.e., narrower width) will have a smaller p value and/ or a smaller α value.
- The value for p is related to the expected excursion rate: The TI is expected to contain $p\%$ of future observations, so it is expected to not contain $(1 - p)\%$ of future observations. Therefore, for a TI with 99% coverage, about 1% of future observations are expected to fall outside of the TI due to random chance.

Before calculating a TI for individual stability results, we must assume that all lots are degrading approximately the same way over time. Without this assumption, the OOT status of a result would depend on the slope of the individual lot. Since we assume that the manufacturing process is consistent and validated, it should be reasonable to assume consistent degradation among lots. The slopes of each lot can be monitored separately as described in Section 7.6.5.

The calculation of a TI depends on the sources of variation present in the data set: Is most of the variation due to method error and other unexplained sources, or is a large portion due to lot-to-lot variation at the time of manufacture? If lot-to-lot variation is present, then a TI that does not properly account for this variation may be too narrow.

To examine the sources of variation in the data, begin by fitting a reduced version of Model 7.2 that considers only the random Lot term, and exclude the random Lot*Time term (because a common slope among lots is assumed):

$$Y_{ij} = \beta_0 + L_i + \beta_1 Time_j + E_{ij} \tag{7.5}$$

$$i = 1, \ldots, n; j = 1, \ldots, T_i$$

Where
- Y_{ij} is the observed value for lot i at time point j
- β_0 is the average y-intercept across all lots
- β_1 is the average slope across all lots
- L_i is a random variable that allows the y-intercept to vary from lot to lot; L_i is assumed $\sim N(0, \sigma_L^2)$
- E_{ij} is a normal random error term created by model misspecification and measurement error; E_{ij} is assumed $\sim N(0, \sigma_E^2)$
- n is the number of lots
- T is the number of responses obtained for lot i

If σ_L^2 from Model 7.5 is 0, then it reduces to Model 7.4, where the only variation in the data set is attributed to method error and other unexplained sources of variation. In general, if σ_L^2 from Model 7.5 is less than 5% of the total variance, Model 7.4 can be considered adequate. However, if σ_L^2 is greater than about 5% of the total variance, then it should be considered in the TI calculations.

An approximate two-sided TI is of the form:

$$TI = \bar{x}_T \pm k_2 \sqrt{\sigma^2} \tag{7.6}$$

Where

$\bar{x}_T$ is the predicted value of the regression line at time point T
$\sqrt{\sigma^2}$ is the square root of the estimated total variance from Model 7.4 or Model 7.5
N is the total number of observations in the data set
k_2 is the multiplier, and is based on N, p, α, and the variance components in the data

The values of k_2 and $\sqrt{\sigma^2}$ depend on whether Model 7.4 or Model 7.5 is fit to the data. When Model 7.4 is adequate, $\sqrt{\sigma^2} = \sqrt{\sigma_E^2}$, or the square root of the estimated residual variance from the regression (i.e., RMSE). Equation 7.7 is used to calculate $k_{2,\text{Fixed}}$ for the TI as recommended by NIST in the Engineering Statistics Handbook (2012), with an adjustment for unequal number of observations per lot as provided in Chapter 2 of Burdick et al. (2017).

$$k_{2,\,\text{Fixed}} = \sqrt{\frac{\left(1 + \dfrac{1}{n_H}\right) Z^2_{(1+p)/2} \times df_{\text{error}}}{\chi^2_{df_{\text{error}},\alpha}}} \tag{7.7}$$

Where

n_H is the harmonic mean of the observations per lot

$n_H = \dfrac{L}{\displaystyle\sum_{i=1}^{L} \dfrac{1}{n_i}}$ for L = number of lots

$Z^2_{(1+p)/2}$ is the critical value of the standard normal distribution with cumulative probability $(1 + p)/2$

df_{error} is the error degrees of freedom after estimation of the regression

$\chi^2_{df_{\text{error}},\alpha}$ is the critical value of the chi-squared distribution with degrees of freedom df_{error} and area α to the left

When Model 7.5 is required, the TI from Equation 7.6 uses $\sqrt{\sigma^2} = \sqrt{\sigma_L^2 + \sigma_E^2}$. The calculation of k_2 is computationally intensive, and will not be described here; details on these calculations can be found in Hoffman and Kringle (2005).

JMP cannot directly calculate a TI that accounts for a trend over time; it also does not adjust for data sets containing lots with studies of differing lengths (i.e., "unbalanced" data sets where not all lots have the same time points). However, the TI calculations can be done in JMP with the aid of the regression model output and Equation 7.7 for $k_{2,\text{Fixed}}$.

The data in Table 7.3 are used in an example 95/99 TI calculation.

The 95/99 TI is calculated using the following steps:

- Fit Model 7.5 to ensure random Lot variance is less than about 5% of the total. Figure 7.26(a) shows that the variance due to Lot is 2.851%, so re-fit the data with Model 7.4 as shown in Figure 7.26(b).

TABLE 7.3

Data for Example TI Calculation

Time (Months)	Lot A	Lot B	Lot C	Lot D	Lot E	Lot F	Lot G
0	95.572	96.010	94.784	93.842	95.270	94.714	94.618
1	94.245	95.240	94.558	94.575	95.264	95.217	94.772
3	94.035	94.964	95.267	94.409	95.068	94.193	94.812
6	94.883	93.723	93.508	93.833	93.691	94.169	94.374
9	93.944	94.455	93.514	94.139	93.028	94.112	93.706
12	94.031	93.305	93.123	93.052	93.031	93.562	93.272
18	92.074	92.400	92.530	92.787	91.986		
24	91.359	92.148	91.631	91.047			
36	90.311	90.035	90.565				

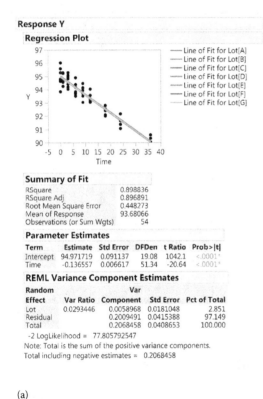

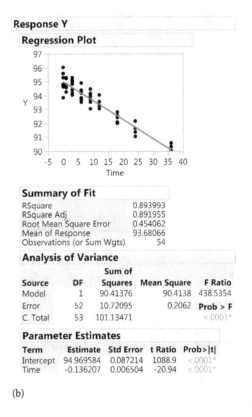

FIGURE 7.26

Example model fit for tolerance interval calculations. (a) Model (5). (b) Model (4).

- Obtain the predicted values from the model by saving the **Predicted Y** values to the data table. These values are $\bar{x}_T$ for each time point. Note that each lot will have the same $\bar{x}_T$ for each time point because the model fits a common slope.
- The example data set has 7 lots with 54 total observations. Table 7.4 summarizes the number of observations per lot.

TABLE 7.4

Sample Sizes for Example TI Calculation

Lot	A	B	C	D	E	F	G
n	9	9	9	8	7	6	6

- Calculate n_H, where

$$n_H = \frac{7}{\dfrac{1}{9}+\dfrac{1}{9}+\dfrac{1}{9}+\dfrac{1}{8}+\dfrac{1}{7}+\dfrac{1}{6}+\dfrac{1}{6}} = 7.49$$

- Calculate $Z^2_{(1+p)/2} = Z^2_{(1+0.99)/2} = Z^2_{0.995} = (2.5758)^2 = 6.634897$
- The value for Z can be calculated in Excel as "=NORM.INV(0.995,0,1) for a standard normal distribution with mean 0 and standard deviation 1.
- Calculate $\chi^2_{df_{error},\alpha} = \chi^2_{52,0.05} = 36.437093$
- The value for x^2 can be calculated in Excel as "=CHI.INV(0.95,52) for a chi-squared distribution with probability $(1 - \alpha)$ and error degrees of freedom from the regression.
- Calculate $k_{2,\,Fixed} = 3.2761$
- The TI is given as $\bar{x}_T \pm k_2\sqrt{\sigma^2}$, where $\sqrt{\sigma^2}$ = RMSE = 0.454062

Figure 7.27 shows a plot of the data and the calculated lower tolerance bound (TB) and upper TB for each time point, along with tabulated values.

Remember, a TI that does not properly account for lot-to-lot variation may be too narrow. An overly restrictive TI may result in unnecessary investigations of truly expected results. Although the calculations for TIs resulting from a Model 7.5 regression are not explicitly

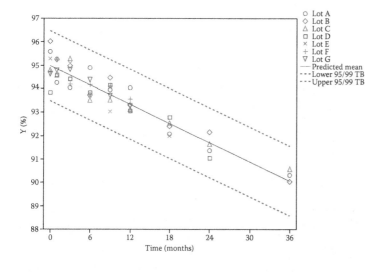

Time (months)	Lower TB	Upper TB
0	93.48	96.46
1	93.34	96.32
3	93.07	96.04
6	92.66	95.63
9	92.25	95.23
12	91.84	94.82
18	91.02	94.00
24	90.20	93.18
36	88.56	91.54

FIGURE 7.27
Plot of tolerance intervals for example calculation.

stated in this chapter, the example shown below illustrates the danger of ignoring random lot-to-lot variation in TI calculations.

- Figure 7.28 shows the output from Model 7.5 where the variance due to Lot is 39.250% of the total.
- The predicted values, $\bar{x}_T$, are the same, regardless of whether Model 7.4 or Model 7.5 is fit to the data.
- The value of $k_{2,Fixed}$ is the same as in the previous example because the number of lots, number of observations per lot, p, and α remain the same for this example.
- For this regression, $\sqrt{\sigma^2} = RMSE = 0.428146$, but $\sqrt{\sigma_L^2 + \sigma_E^2} = \sqrt{0.3017446} = 0.549313$, which is quite a bit larger than the RMSE. Therefore, the true variance in the data set is underestimated by the RMSE.

Figure 7.29 shows a scatter plot of three different TIs:

1. TIs calculated using $k_{2,Fixed}$ (95/99 TB, RMSE in Figure 7.29).
2. TIs calculated using $k_{2,Fixed}$, replacing RMSE with $\sqrt{\sigma_L^2 + \sigma_E^2}$ (95/99 TB, Total Variance in Figure 7.29).
3. TIs calculated using the method described by Hoffman and Kringle (2005) that account for uncertainty in the total variance estimate for random effects models (95/99 TB, Random Lot in Figure 7.29).

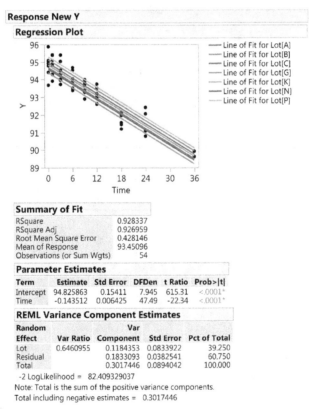

FIGURE 7.28
Output from Model 7.5 for stability trending with random lot variance.

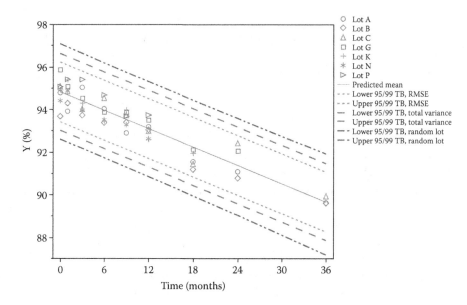

FIGURE 7.29
Comparison of tolerance intervals when random lot variance is present.

From Figure 7.29, it is easy to see that the TIs calculated using $k_{2,\text{Fixed}}$ are narrower than those from (3), regardless of the variance estimate used. Particularly, the TIs from (1) may result in a higher OOT rate than can be expected based on normal process and analytical method variation. In practical terms, if one does not wish to undertake the TI calculation from (3), the TI calculation from (2) may be a sufficient balance between the two extremes. Alternately, one may wish to set a predefined k value, but in the presence of lot-to-lot variation, use of $\sqrt{\sigma_L^2 + \sigma_E^2}$ as the estimate of the variation from the regression model is recommended.

7.6.5 Is a Stability Lot in Trend?

We can also trend the slope parameter for individual lots. Slope trending is useful because it is possible for a lot's individual values to be in trend but its overall slope to be more extreme than the rest of the lots. Slope trending requires a larger number of lots than does trending individual results because the available data set contains only one observation per lot; therefore, it is a good idea to have about 10 to 15 lots before undertaking slope trending.

Since each lot's slope is examined as an individual value, a control chart is most appropriate for slope trending. It is important that calculated limits account for the unequal number of observations per lot used to calculate each lot's slope. Accordingly, control chart limits will have different widths, depending on the number of observations available to calculate the slope. The control limits on the slopes are given by Equation 7.8:

$$\text{Slope Control Limits} = \hat{\beta} \pm 3 * \text{SE}(\hat{\beta}) \tag{7.8}$$

Where
  $\hat{\beta}$ is the average slope for a lot with n time points
  $\text{SE}(\hat{\beta})$ is the standard error of the slope estimate

Before trending the slopes, they must be calculated by fitting a regression to the data. Use Model 7.1 since the slope for an individual lot is viewed as a fixed outcome of the process. Figure 7.30 shows an example of the JMP regression output used to calculate the slopes for each lot using the data in Table 7.5.

1. Notice that although the *p*-value for Lot*Time = 0.8340, it must be retained it in the model to obtain estimated slopes for each lot.

2. Use the **Expanded Parameter Estimates** output to calculate the individual lot slopes, because the **Parameter Estimates** table will not show an estimate for the last Lot in the data set due to the way JMP solves for the regression coefficients.

   • The slope for a lot is given by the estimate for Time plus the estimate for the [specific] Lot*Time. For example, from Figure 7.30, slope for Lot A = −0.148041 + −0.001138 = −0.1469%/mo.

   • Bear in mind that other statistical software may use different parameterization to solve the regression. For example, when using SAS to fit Model 7.1, the parameter estimates for Lot*Time are the difference in slopes compared to the last lot in the data set, not the difference from the average slope as in JMP.

Table 7.6 shows a summary of the slopes created in JMP, including calculated control limits per Equation 7.8.

1. Right click in the Expanded Parameter Estimates table, and select Make into Data Table.

2. Adjust the newly created data table of Parameter Estimates:

   • Retain rows with Parameter Estimates for "Lot[...]*Time" as these are the only estimates needed for subsequent calculations. Note the estimate for Time as it is needed for subsequent calculations.

   • Add a column for "Lot" and enter the lot designation.

   • Add a column for "Slope" and assign a formula where

     Slope = (estimate for Time) + (value in estimate column for Lot[...]*(Time)).

   • Add columns for Lower Control Limit ("LCL") and Upper Control Limit ("UCL") where

     LCL = (estimate for Time) − 3*(value in Std Error column for Lot[...]*(Time)).

     UCL = (estimate for Time) + 3*(value in Std Error column for Lot[...]*(Time)).

Figure 7.31 shows the initial control chart used to trend the slope estimates obtained from Model 7.1. Lots are listed on the x-axis in order of manufacture. The first ten lots used to fit the regression were used to calculate the average slope and the control limits. The control chart limits are dependent on how many and which time points were tested in the stability study.

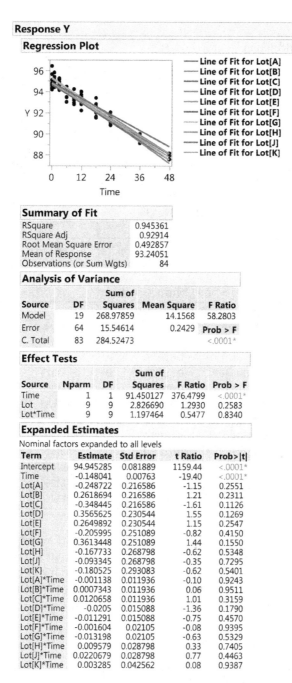

Response Y

Regression Plot

(Line of Fit for Lot[A], Line of Fit for Lot[B], Line of Fit for Lot[C], Line of Fit for Lot[D], Line of Fit for Lot[E], Line of Fit for Lot[F], Line of Fit for Lot[G], Line of Fit for Lot[H], Line of Fit for Lot[J], Line of Fit for Lot[K])

Summary of Fit

RSquare	0.945361
RSquare Adj	0.92914
Root Mean Square Error	0.492857
Mean of Response	93.24051
Observations (or Sum Wgts)	84

Analysis of Variance

Source	DF	Sum of Squares	Mean Square	F Ratio
Model	19	268.97859	14.1568	58.2803
Error	64	15.54614	0.2429	**Prob > F**
C. Total	83	284.52473		<.0001*

Effect Tests

Source	Nparm	DF	Sum of Squares	F Ratio	Prob > F
Time	1	1	91.450127	376.4799	<.0001*
Lot	9	9	2.826690	1.2930	0.2583
Lot*Time	9	9	1.197464	0.5477	0.8340

Expanded Estimates

Nominal factors expanded to all levels

Term	Estimate	Std Error	t Ratio	Prob>|t|
Intercept	94.945285	0.081889	1159.44	<.0001*
Time	-0.148041	0.00763	-19.40	<.0001*
Lot[A]	-0.248722	0.216586	-1.15	0.2551
Lot[B]	0.2618694	0.216586	1.21	0.2311
Lot[C]	-0.348445	0.216586	-1.61	0.1126
Lot[D]	0.3565625	0.230544	1.55	0.1269
Lot[E]	0.2649892	0.230544	1.15	0.2547
Lot[F]	-0.205995	0.251089	-0.82	0.4150
Lot[G]	0.3613448	0.251089	1.44	0.1550
Lot[H]	-0.167733	0.268798	-0.62	0.5348
Lot[J]	-0.093345	0.268798	-0.35	0.7295
Lot[K]	-0.180525	0.293083	-0.62	0.5401
Lot[A]*Time	-0.001138	0.011936	-0.10	0.9243
Lot[B]*Time	0.0007343	0.011936	0.06	0.9511
Lot[C]*Time	0.0120658	0.011936	1.01	0.3159
Lot[D]*Time	-0.0205	0.015088	-1.36	0.1790
Lot[E]*Time	-0.011291	0.015088	-0.75	0.4570
Lot[F]*Time	-0.001604	0.02105	-0.08	0.9395
Lot[G]*Time	-0.013198	0.02105	-0.63	0.5329
Lot[H]*Time	0.009579	0.028798	0.33	0.7405
Lot[J]*Time	0.0220679	0.028798	0.77	0.4463
Lot[K]*Time	0.003285	0.042562	0.08	0.9387

FIGURE 7.30
Regression output to calculate stability lot slopes.

TABLE 7.5

Data for Example TI Calculation

Time	Lot A	Lot B	Lot C	Lot D	Lot E	Lot F	Lot G	Lot H	Lot J	Lot K
0	94.622	95.622	94.771	95.077	94.757	94.334	96.396	94.278	94.586	94.155
1	94.622	94.821	94.385	95.122	95.375	95.112	95.784	94.780	94.499	94.898
3	94.213	94.551	94.765	95.128	94.926	94.337	94.195	94.109	95.239	94.884
6	94.430	93.995	93.006	94.208	94.056	93.440	93.465	94.428	93.924	94.044
9	92.773	93.271	94.206	94.204	93.585	93.477	93.154	93.489	93.401	92.928
12	93.382	93.977	92.201	92.781	93.521	92.905	93.256	93.948	93.689	93.193
18	91.506	93.381	91.993	92.021	92.813	92.572	92.403	91.625	92.453	
24	90.825	91.395	91.376	91.684	91.043	90.813	92.029			
36	89.576	89.997	89.748	89.121	89.449					
48	87.596	87.936	88.170							

TABLE 7.6

Summary of Stability Lot Slopes and Control Chart Limits

Term	Estimate (Difference from Average Slope,%/Mo)	Std. Error	Lot	Slope (%/Mo)	LCL (%/Mo)	UCL (%/Mo)
Lot[A]*Time	−0.001138	0.011936	A	−0.1492	−0.1839	−0.1122
Lot[B]*Time	0.000734	0.011936	B	−0.1473	−0.1839	−0.1122
Lot[C]*Time	0.012066	0.011936	C	−0.1360	−0.1839	−0.1122
Lot[D]*Time	−0.020500	0.015088	D	−0.1685	−0.1933	−0.1028
Lot[E]*Time	−0.011291	0.015088	E	−0.1593	−0.1933	−0.1028
Lot[F]*Time	−0.001604	0.021050	F	−0.1496	−0.2112	−0.0849
Lot[G]*Time	−0.013198	0.021050	G	−0.1612	−0.2112	−0.0849
Lot[H]*Time	0.009579	0.028798	H	−0.1385	−0.2344	−0.0616
Lot[J]*Time	0.022068	0.028798	J	−0.1260	−0.2344	−0.0616
Lot[K]*Time	0.003285	0.042562	K	−0.1448	−0.2757	−0.0204

Future slopes can be calculated by refitting Model 7.1 to an expanded data set. The updated slope can be compared to the control chart limits that are based on the last time point used to calculate the slope. Table 7.7 provides a summary of control chart limits by "last time point tested." Note that there are no limits given for studies shorter than 12 months because they would be too wide to be useful.

7.6.6 How Can I Establish a Stability Trending Program?

Many good references on establishing a stability program are available, including from the PhRMA CMC Statistics and Stability Expert Teams (2003 and 2005) and Hartvig and Kamper (2017). These articles speak to various regulatory and procedural concerns, as well as many ways to perform stability trend analysis, including those not described here. Torbovska and Trajkovic-Jolevska (2013) recommend trending individual results and lot slopes in order to obtain a holistic picture of stability trends.

There are no strict rules on the number of lots required to implement a stability trending program, but it is reasonable to incorporate such a program as a part of commercial process

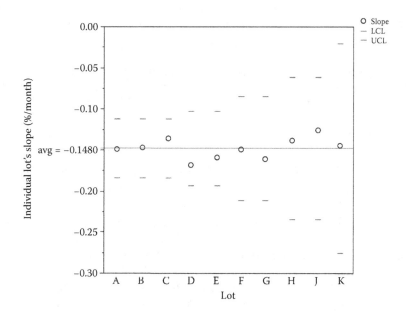

FIGURE 7.31
Initial control chart on stability lot slopes.

TABLE 7.7

Summary of Control Chart Limits by Last Time Point Tested

Last Time Point Tested (Months)	LCL (%/Mo)	UCL (%/Mo)
12	-0.2757	-0.0204
18	-0.2344	-0.0616
24	-0.2112	-0.0849
36	-0.1933	-0.1028
48	-0.1839	-0.1122

verification (CPV). Implementing stability trending assumes that we have a consistent, validated, commercially approved manufacturing process with an established commercial expiry and defined stability acceptance criteria (AC). Regardless of what is monitored, a stability trending program should be developed based on current knowledge, and should be applied to results generated *after* the program is implemented.

The stated purpose of the trending program is to determine if future observations conform to expectations based on current knowledge. In other words, we wish to ensure that the manufacturing process continues to produce lots that are consistent with what we have already observed. It follows, then, that the primary purpose of the trending program is not to monitor how the stability data are performing in relation to the stability AC. How a result relates to the AC may be germane to the impact of an OOT observation, but it is not the best way to determine if an observation is expected. Section 7.7.2 speaks to how to relate the stability trend to the AC.

Some comments on the practical application of trending limits for individual stability results:

- Calculated intervals may be rounded to the reporting precision of the analytical method. However, if TIs are rounded to be narrower than their original width, the stated coverage level will be less than p. Therefore, truncating lower bounds and always rounding upper bounds up will ensure that TIs contain *at least* the stated proportion of future values.

- Care should be taken in setting trending limits for stability at 0 months because the limits calculated using stability data may conflict with control limits used for manufacturing lot release. In practice, it may make sense to implement limits for stability time points only after storage has commenced.

- If based on an adequate data set, calculated TIs define a region containing expected future results. Unless the analytical method or manufacturing process has been changed, the TIs do not require updating whenever new stability data are available because expectations of the general trend should not change too much. A robust trending program may require periodic review of limits (e.g., annually), but the limits should not be recalculated with each new stability time point or each new lot: adding more data will only narrow the TIs.

- Care should be taken when investigating an OOT result. An examination of how the limits were set is part of any thorough investigation. However, just because an OOT result is observed does not mean that the limits should be reset. In fact, limits that will signal unusual observations are the goal of this exercise. Resetting limits blindly each time an OOT result is observed diminishes the effectiveness of the trending program.

- Although two-sided limits are generally preferred regardless of the AC, one must remember to balance usefulness with correctness. For example, a lower OOT limit of 95.1% with a stability AC of 95% may not be practically meaningful. Conversely, maintaining the original purpose, a result may be OOT in either direction, regardless of the AC. For example, if a purity measure that declines over time has a one-sided lower specification of 90% and an upper tolerance bound of 95% at 12 months, then it is of great interest if this method generates a result of 99% at 12 months. It is not important that we don't care if the product is more pure—we care whether we have observed an unusual result.

7.6.7 How Can I Perform an Annual "Trend Analysis" as Required for Commercially Approved Products?

The United States, European Union, and Canada specifically require a "trend analysis" be performed annually for any commercially approved product as outlined in their region-specific regulatory guidelines. However, the guidance is scarcely more specific than that, and may leave us wondering what type of analysis is sufficient and what type of analysis may be excessive.

A stability trend analysis is simply an examination of stability data for evidence of unexpected patterns. A scatter plot of the stability data from active annual lots might reasonably fulfill this requirement. However, simply providing plots of data without some type of quantitative statements leaves any conclusions open to interpretation.

Section 7.6.4 discussed how to determine if individual results are in trend, Section 7.6.5 showed how to determine whether stability lots' slopes were expected, and Section 7.6.6

described how to implement a stability trending program. It makes sense that providing an outline of trending analyses, such as a tabular summary of any observed OOT results and unusual lot slopes, meets the "trend analysis" requirement.

One additional important component of an annual trend analysis is an examination of how each active lot is performing in relation to the established AC and expiry period. Section 7.7.2 speaks to the evaluation of individual lots against the expiry period, and including this information will provide a complete picture of our stability knowledge.

7.7 How Is the Stability Profile Related to the Expiry Period?

The stability profile dictates the expiry period because it quantifies the amount of change expected over the duration of storage at the recommended storage condition (RSC). Not all quality attributes can be analyzed statistically using the methodology described in this section: Only quantitative attributes with established stability acceptance criteria (AC) can use this methodology because it requires comparison of calculated regression values to the AC. We may still be able to make statements about quantitative attributes without AC by providing analysis of the expected stability trends as examined in Sections 7.6.1 through 7.6.3. Additionally, we may be able to exclude some formulation-dependent parameters or nonstability indicating parameters from the statistical expiry evaluation using analyses presented in 7.6.1 through 7.6.3 together with scientific rationale.

Per ICH Q1E, the expiry is determined as the earliest time point where the 95% confidence bound (CB) on the mean intersects the stability AC. For CQAs with one-sided specifications, the one-sided 95% CB on the mean is compared to the AC, and for two-sided specifications, the two-sided 95% confidence interval (CI) on the mean is compared to the AC. These calculations require fitting a regression model to the data.

Expiry may be established or extended by using either Model 7.1—the fixed lot model, or Model 7.2—the random lot model, depending on the number of lots available for analysis. The methodology outlined below follows the guidance outlined in ICH Q1E, although only the fixed lot model is expressly detailed in the guideline. Per ICH Q1E, "the purpose of a stability study is to establish, based on testing a minimum of three batches of the drug substance or product, a retest period or shelf life and label storage instructions *applicable to all future batches manufactured and packaged under similar circumstances.*" Thus, the focus of inference for the random lots model more closely aligns with the Q1E guidance, so the random lot model is preferred because its conclusions can be applied to all future lots.

ICH Q1E provides a decision tree as a guide for how much extrapolation is allowed, depending on the RSC for the product and the extent of the change seen at RSC and accelerated storage conditions (ASC). Q5C states that expiry for biologics at time of registration should be based on real-time data. The regression analysis can be used to make predictions at time points where no real-time data have been collected, but the uncertainty in the prediction increases as the extent of the extrapolation increases.

For small molecules, ASC data can sometimes be used to predict behavior at RSC. The Arrhenius equation expresses a degradation rate as a function of temperature, relies on first order kinetics, and requires the activation energy for the molecule in question (Brady and Holum 1996). In practical terms, observed changes at ASC might be used to make statements about how long it will take to observe the same amount of change at RSC. However, the Arrhenius equation is not necessarily predictive for certain complex formulations (e.g., emulsions or suspensions) or for large molecules where changes at ASC are sometimes never observed at RSC (Roberts 2015). This chapter will not discuss analysis using the Arrhenius equation, but interested readers can refer to Chow (2007) for applications to accelerated stability analysis.

7.7.1 What Is the Appropriate Expiry or Retest Period for My Product?

Establishing expiry using the Fixed Lot Model, Model 7.1

Once Model 7.1 is fit to the data, it is necessary to determine what model to use for the evaluation. In particular, batch-related terms are evaluated for poolability in order to define an appropriate model. The question of poolability is aimed at deciding whether the lots are similar enough in both slope and intercept that they can be considered as one large data set or if each of the lots is different enough that they must be considered separately.

Per ICH Q1E, poolability is established by examining the statistical significance of the batch-related terms (Lot and Lot*Time) at $\alpha = 0.25$; non–batch-related terms like Time are evaluated at $\alpha = 0.05$. In practical terms, $\alpha = 0.25$ is used because there are a limited number of lots when initial expiry is established, so it must be demonstrated with great certainty that the lots are similar before ignoring their potential differences. When the lots display differences, each lot is fit with a separate regression line, and the expiry is set based on the "worst-case lot" (WCL), or the lot with the shortest predicted expiry. Additionally, when multiple CQAs are analyzed, the expiry is set based on the CQA with the shortest expiry.

Following the Q1E model reduction algorithm, there are three possible final models, depending on the statistical significance of the model terms:

1. Separate slopes and separate intercepts model (separate slopes)

   Fitting Model 7.1 without reducing it indicates that the lots are dissimilar in both lot-release value and degradation pattern. The result is that each lot is fit with a separate intercept and slope that are estimated using data from that lot alone. The expiry is based on the WCL, usually the lot with the most extreme slope or release value closest to the stability AC.

2. Common slopes and separate intercepts model (separate intercepts)

   The separate intercepts model is constructed by fitting Model 7.1 without the Lot*Time term, which indicates that the lots have a similar degradation pattern but that they are dissimilar at time 0. The result is that each lot is fit with a common slope estimated from all of the data, and each lot has a unique intercept based on its time 0 value. The expiry is based on the WCL, usually the lot with the time 0 value closest to the specification limit.

3. Common slope and common intercept model (pooled lots)

   The pooled lots model is the fully reduced form of Model 7.1, and is specifically shown in Model 7.4. The model with both common slopes and intercepts indicates that the batches have both a similar degradation pattern and a similar time 0 value. The result of this model is that a single regression line is fit to the entire data set, and the expiry is based on the overall mean.

Note that there is no allowance for a separate slopes and common intercepts model because it is best statistical practice to retain main effects in the statistical model if they are involved in significant higher order interactions. In other words, when the Lot*Time term is significant, the Lot term is also retained because it is part of the Lot*Time term.

The drawbacks to using Model 7.1 to establish expiry are most apparent with the separate slopes model. When a separate regression line is fit to each lot, a point at the beginning or end of the stability time course may be highly influential to the slope, which may result in an expiry estimate that is not truly representative of the expected degradation profile. Additionally, for lots with few time points, the degree of uncertainty in the prediction is large, so the corresponding CI on the regression line is wide and may lead to shortened expiry periods.

Figure 7.32 shows example output from each possible final model, including the initial output from Model 7.1, the reduced models based on the poolability evaluation, and diagnostic pots. Figure 7.33 shows the appropriate estimated value at the proposed expiry period and a plot of the data and regression line as prescribed in ICH Q1E. Data are provided in Table 7.8. Note the following:

- Each example assumes that the intended expiry period is 12 months, based on 6 months of real-time data for 3 lots. The stability AC is 85%, which is a lower limit. Therefore, all conclusions are based on the CB on the mean at 12 months, and the one-sided lower 95% CB is used for each evaluation (i.e., alpha for JMP regression = 0.1).

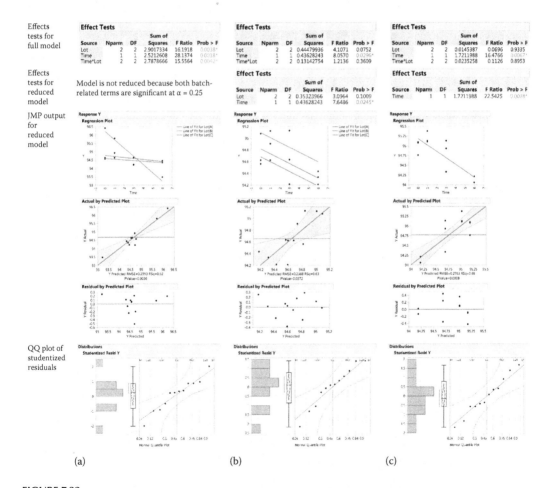

FIGURE 7.32
Example output from fixed lot model: Three possible final models. (a) Separate slopes. (b) Separate intercepts. (c) Pooled lots.

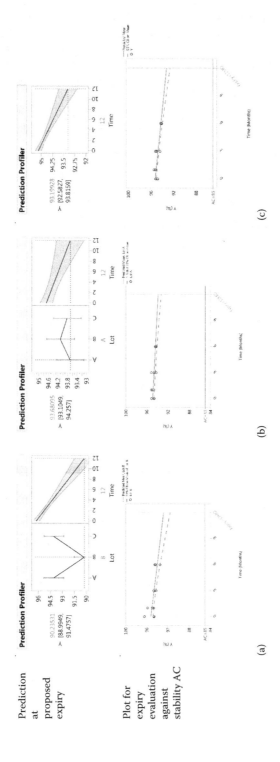

FIGURE 7.33
Example predictions from fixed lot model: Three possible final models. (a) Separate slopes. (b) Separate intercepts. (c) Pooled lots.

TABLE 7.8

Data for Fixed Lots Model Examples

Lot	Time	Separate Slopes	Separate Intercepts	Pooled Lots
A	0	94.622	94.622	95.077
A	1	94.622	94.622	95.122
A	3	94.213	94.213	95.128
A	6	94.430	94.430	94.208
B	0	96.396	95.077	94.757
B	1	95.784	95.122	95.375
B	3	94.195	95.128	94.926
B	6	93.465	94.208	94.056
C	0	94.560	94.560	95.094
C	1	94.905	94.905	95.106
C	3	94.632	94.632	94.329
C	6	94.331	94.331	94.057

- Figure 7.32(a) and 7.33(a)—Separate Slopes Model: Expiry is based on the WCL, Lot B, because it has the steepest slope, and the lowest predicted value at the intended 12 MO expiry. The one-sided lower 95% CB on the mean for Lot B at 12 months is 88.99%, which falls above the stability AC, so the 12 MO expiry period is supported by the analysis.

- Figure 7.32(b) and 7.33(b)—Separate Intercepts Model: Expiry is based on the WCL, Lot A, because it has the lowest intercept, and thus the lowest predicted value at the intended 12 MO expiry. The one-sided lower 95% CB on the mean for Lot A at 12 months is 93.10%, so the 12 MO expiry is supported.

- Figure 7.32(c) and 7.33(c)—Pooled Lots Model: Expiry is based on the pooled data set because there is no evidence that the slopes or intercepts are significantly different between these three lots. The one-sided lower 95% CB on the overall mean at 12 months is 92.58%, so the 12 MO expiry period is supported.

Establishing expiry using the Random Lot Model, Model 7.2

The use of Model 7.2 to make predictions about expiry has been described in Chow (2007) and Shao and Chow (1994), and more recently in Stroup and Quinlan (2016), Burdick et al. (2017), and Capen et al. (2017). Much work has been done to support the use of the random lot model because it more appropriately considers each lot to be a random outcome of a consistent manufacturing process where predictions apply to *all future lots*, which is the preferred focus of inference stated in ICH Q1E.

The random lot model considers the overall trend for every lot in conjunction with the individual trend for each lot. Consequently, regression lines extrapolated far beyond the current real-time data rely more heavily on the historical mean of all lots. As more real-time data are collected, the trend for a given lot is explained more by actual observations gathered on that lot. The random lot model is a corollary to the fixed lots model suggested in ICH Q1E, which acknowledges that other statistical models are appropriate, and specifically cites shao and Chow (1994) that describes an early application of the random coefficients model.

As opposed to the fixed lot model, the random lot model does not test fixed effects Lot and Lot*Time for poolability because these effects are estimated as the random variance components σ_L^2 and σ_B^2, respectively. Instead, each variance component can be examined to determine if it is appropriate to assume that the slopes or intercepts differ considerably from lot-to-lot. Model selection will still result in a final model from three candidate models: Model 7.2 containing σ_B^2, σ_L^2, and σ_E^2, Model 7.5 containing σ_L^2 and σ_E^2, and Model 7.4 containing only σ_E^2. Considering Model 7.2—random slopes, Model 7.5—random intercepts, and Model 7.4—residual only, is analogous to considering the fixed models with separate slopes, separate intercepts, and pooled lots, respectively.

There are several ways to determine which variance components should be included in the final model for setting expiry. In general, any of these methods is statistically acceptable, if the method is stated, justified, and used consistently across all CQAs.

1. F-test for significance of variance components:

   The F-test of variance components tests the hypotheses H_0: $\sigma_L^2 = 0$ vs. H_A: $\sigma_L^2 \neq 0$, and H_0: $\sigma_B^2 = 0$ vs. H_A: $\sigma_B^2 \neq 0$. One may choose to use a significance level of $\alpha = 0.25$ to align with the ICH Q1E guidance for the poolability test. The correct calculations for the hypothesis tests of variance components are conducted using the expected mean square (EMS) values from the regression analysis, and are described in Burdick and Graybill (1992). Note that the CIs and p-values obtained for the random variance components in JMP are not recommended for use in these tests because they are based on large sample approximations that may not be valid for small sample sizes (Park and Burdick 2003).

2. Set a threshold for percent contribution to total variance (TV):

   Setting a threshold for percent contribution to TV does not require any additional calculations. One may choose to say that σ_L^2 and σ_B^2 must each contribute at least, say, 5% to TV before they are large enough to include in the final model. The choice of the threshold percentage is somewhat arbitrary, and this method doesn't consider the quality of the fit of models that contain all variance components compared to the model that contains none. However, it is simple to implement.

3. Use an information criterion to select the most appropriate model:

   The corrected Akaike Information Criterion (AICc) measures the relative quality of a model fit compared to other candidate models with different random effects. The model with the lowest AICc is taken as the model of best fit. AICc is a relative measure, so it cannot be compared across CQAs; it is used for model selection within one CQA alone. To implement model selection using AICc, fit the three candidate models and set expiry using the model with the lowest AICc.

The AICc can be obtained in JMP in the model output window by clicking on the drop-down arrow by **Response → Regression Reports → AICc.**

When σ_B^2 and/or σ_L^2 are non-zero, each lot will have a unique regression line based on the Best Linear Unbiased Predictor (BLUP) for that lot. As with the fixed lot model, set expiry using the WCL, which is the lot with the prediction closest to the AC at the intended expiry.

Figure 7.34 shows example model selection output for three different data sets that result in three different final models. Data are provided in Table 7.9. Note that the % TV and AICc selection methodologies are shown for illustrative purposes, but in practice, only one methodology should be used consistently across CQAs. In these examples, the % TV and AICc model selection methods agree.

Random effects and AICc for model (7.2)

Response y
AICc 43.4867

REML Variance Component Estimates

Random Effect	Var Ratio	Var Component	Std Error	Pct of Total
Lot	4.4038674	0.1713715	0.1181664	76.885
Lot*Time	0.3239684	0.0176069	0.0083196	5.656
Residual		0.0389319	0.0108397	17.459
Total		0.2228923	0.1186435	100.000

-2 LogLikelihood = 31.6096696/1
Note: Total is the sum of the positive variance components.
Total including negative estimates = 0.2228923

Random effects and AICc for model (7.5)

Response y
AICc 102.63

REML Variance Component Estimates

Random Effect	Var Ratio	Var Component	Std Error	Pct of Total
Lot	1.1594549	0.5008714	0.3600211	53.692
Residual		0.4319887	0.1094529	46.308
Total		0.9328602	0.3719156	100.000

-2 LogLikelihood = 93.417915299
Note: Total is the sum of the positive variance components.
Total including negative estimates = 0.9328602

Random effects and AICc for model (7.4)

Response y
AICc 107.7945

Analysis of Variance

Source	DF	Sum of Squares	Mean Square	F Ratio
Model	1	132.28918	132.289	149.69111
Error	36	3181.493	0.884	Prob > F
C. Total	37	164.10411		<.0001*

Final model based on Minimum 5% contribution to TV

Model (7.2) has $\sigma_B^2 \approx 6\%$ of TV and $\sigma_L^2 \approx 77\%$ of TV

Fit σ_B^2, σ_L^2, and σ_E^2

Final model based on AICc

Model (7.2) has lowest AICc = 43.48

Fit σ_B^2, σ_L^2, and σ_E^2

(a)

Random effects and AICc for model (7.2)

Response y
AICc 86.88529

REML Variance Component Estimates

Random Effect	Var Ratio	Var Component	Std Error	Pct of Total
Lot	0.791055	0.1952286	0.1654218	44.064
Lot*Time	0.0042043	0.0010392	0.0012508	0.234
Residual		0.2471745	0.0645858	55.702
Total		0.4437423	0.1745906	100.000

-2 LogLikelihood = 75.010289165
Note: Total is the sum of the positive variance components.
Total including negative estimates = 0.4437423

Random effects and AICc for model (7.5)

Response y
AICc 86.67044

REML Variance Component Estimates

Random Effect	Var Ratio	Var Component	Std Error	Pct of Total
Lot	1.1542292	0.3202346	0.2288449	53.580
Residual		0.2774445	0.0702284	46.420
Total		0.5976791	0.2368769	100.000

-2 LogLikelihood = 77.458315994
Note: Total is the sum of the positive variance components.
Total including negative estimates = 0.5976791

Random effects and AICc for model (7.4)

Response y
AICc 92.25439

Analysis of Variance

Source	DF	Sum of Squares	Mean Square	F Ratio
Model	1	102.66670	102.667	174.8662
Error	36	21.13617	0.587	Prob > F
C. Total	37	123.80287		<.0001*

Final model based on Minimum 5% contribution to TV

Model (7.2) has $\sigma_B^2 \approx 0.2\%$ of TV and $\sigma_L^2 \approx 44\%$ of TV

Fit σ_L^2 and σ_E^2

Final model based on AICc

Model (7.5) has lowest AICc = 86.67

Fit σ_L^2 and σ_E^2

(b)

Random effects and AICc for model (7.2)

Response y
AICc 74.89348

REML Variance Component Estimates

Random Effect	Var Ratio	Var Component	Std Error	Pct of Total
Lot	-0.208554	-0.056219	0.018998	0.000
Lot*Time	0.0051047	0.0013761	0.0010926	0.508
Residual		0.2695656	0.0672078	99.492
Total		0.2709417	0.0674541	100.000

-2 LogLikelihood = 63.018476189
Note: Total is the sum of the positive variance components.
Total including negative estimates = 0.2147228

Random effects and AICc for model (7.5)

Response y
AICc 77.08582

REML Variance Component Estimates

Random Effect	Var Ratio	Var Component	Std Error	Pct of Total
Lot	0.0001435	4.0539e-5	0.0250743	0.014
Residual		0.2825051	0.0698459	99.986
Total		0.2825051	0.0667046	100.000

-2 LogLikelihood = 67.873698127
Note: Total is the sum of the positive variance components.
Total including negative estimates = 0.2825051

Random effects and AICc for model (7.4)

Response y
AICc 64.45557

Analysis of Variance

Source	DF	Sum of Squares	Mean Square	F Ratio
Model	1	67.372985	67.3730	238.4895
Error	36	10.169954	0.2825	Prob > F
C. Total	37	77.542940		<.0001*

Final model based on Minimum 5% contribution to TV

Model (7.2) has $\sigma_B^2 \approx 0.5\%$ of TV and $\sigma_L^2 \approx 0\%$ of TV

Fit σ_E^2 only

Final model based on AICc

Model (7.4) has lowest AICc = 64.46

Fit σ_E^2 only

(c)

FIGURE 7.34
Model selection criteria for random lot model: Three possible final models. (a) Random slopes. (b) Random intercepts. (c) Residual only.

TABLE 7.9

Data for Random Lots Model Examples

Lot	Time	Random Slopes	Random Intercepts	Residual Only
A	0	94.785	95.602	95.023
A	1	94.745	94.809	95.005
A	3	94.177	95.176	95.533
A	6	93.198	95.199	93.418
A	9	92.542	93.380	93.197
A	12	91.857	93.417	92.624
A	18	90.125	91.953	93.193
A	24	88.349	91.651	90.951
B	0	94.601	94.402	95.546
B	1	94.510	94.564	94.230
B	3	93.564	93.684	94.478
B	6	92.398	92.558	92.895
B	9	91.364	92.606	93.295
B	12	90.172	92.211	93.334
B	18	88.325	89.882	91.222
B	24	87.070	89.039	90.083
C	0	94.058	94.636	94.615
C	1	94.324	94.284	94.834
C	3	93.943	93.900	94.628
C	6	93.344	93.530	93.996
C	9	92.713	93.113	92.941
C	12	92.373	92.778	93.114
C	18	91.600	89.682	91.162
C	24	90.578	89.523	90.629
D	0	94.835	95.415	95.298
D	1	94.948	95.656	94.078
D	3	94.824	94.542	95.149
D	6	94.565	93.645	93.948
D	9	94.601	93.083	93.776
D	12	94.192	92.422	91.684
E	0	95.028	95.911	95.372
E	1	94.867	95.284	95.047
E	3	94.025	94.831	94.152
E	6	92.930	93.553	93.405
F	0	95.298	94.996	94.933
F	1	95.453	96.535	94.708
F	3	94.667	94.402	94.567
F	6	93.750	94.603	93.661

Figure 7.35 shows output for the final expiry models determined in Figure 7.34. Figure 7.36 shows the appropriate estimated value at the proposed expiry and a plot of the data with regression line as prescribed in ICH Q1E. Note the following:

- Each example assumes that the intended expiry period is 24 months, based on 6 to 24 months of real-time data for 6 lots. The stability AC is 85%, which is a lower limit. Therefore, all conclusions are based on the prediction at 24 months, and the

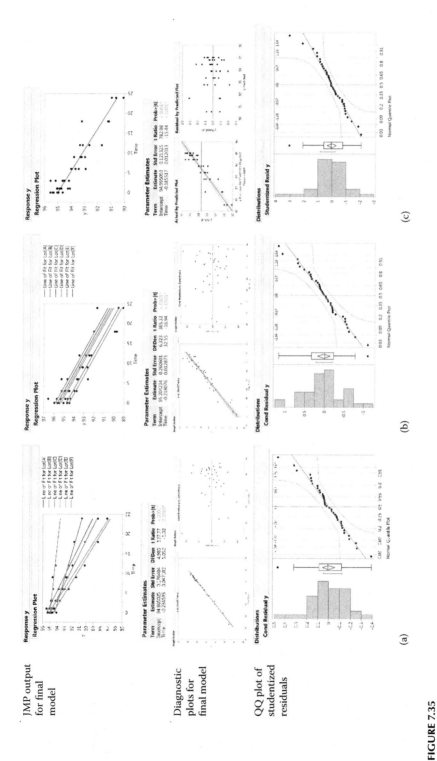

FIGURE 7.35
Example output from random lot model: Three possible final models. (a) Random slopes. (b) Random intercepts. (c) Residual only.

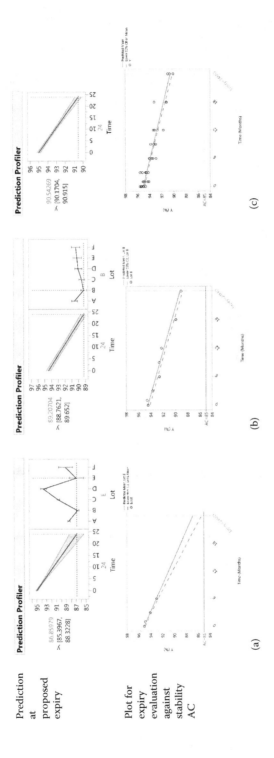

FIGURE 7.36
Example predictions from random lot model: Three possible final models. (a) Random slopes. (b) Random intercepts. (c) Residual only.

one-sided lower 95% CB on the BLUP is used for each evaluation (i.e., alpha for JMP regression = 0.1).

- The data in this example are "unbalanced," that is, lots have differing numbers of observations. Recognize that Model 7.2 predictions for lots with fewer time points are more closely related to the overall average trend.

- Figure 7.34(a), 7.35(a), and 7.36(a): Random Slopes, Model 7.2 is selected as the final model. Diagnostic plots using the conditional predicted values and residuals verify model assumptions. Expiry is based on the WCL, Lot E, because it has the lowest value for the CB on the BLUP at the intended 24 MO expiry period; this value (85.40%) falls above the stability AC (85%), so the 24 MO expiry period is supported by the analysis.

- Figure 7.34(b), 7.35(b), and 7.36(b): Random Intercepts, Model 7.5 is selected as the final model. Diagnostic plots using the conditional predicted values and residuals verify model assumptions. Expiry is based on the WCL, Lot B, because it has the lowest value for the CB on the BLUP at the intended 24 MO expiry period; this value (88.76%) falls above the stability AC, so the 24 MO expiry period is supported by the analysis.

- Figure 7.34(c), 7.35(c), and 7.36(c): Residual Only, Model 7.4 is selected; this model is the same as the most reduced version of the fixed effects model. Diagnostic plots using the predicted values and Studentized residuals verify model assumptions. Expiry is based on the overall mean because there are no random variance components, so neither the slopes nor intercepts differ among the lots. The value for the one-sided lower 95% CB on the mean 24 months is 90.17%; this value falls above the stability AC, so the 24 MO expiry period is supported by the analysis.

7.7.2 Will an Individual Lot Meet Its Intended Expiry Period?

We may ask whether an individual lot will meet its intended expiry period because we are trying to demonstrate that an annual lot supports the current expiry, or because we are investigating a lot that may have an unusual slope. As a commercial stability program matures, it is important to show that each annual stability lot is predicted to meet expiry. Since only one lot is placed on stability every year, this lot represents all others manufactured that year. By examining the trend for each annual stability lot, it can be inferred that all other lots not on stability are probably performing as expected. Conversely, if we observe an unusual trend in an annual stability lot, then the trend for other lots on the market may be in question. Providing the predictions at expiry for each active annual stability lot is the last piece of a robust "trend analysis" to include in an annual product quality review, as discussed in Section 7.6.7.

Given our focus of inference—*to all possible lots*—Model 7.2 is the most appropriate model to answer this research question. As we discovered in Section 7.7.1, the regression line on the WCL (and all the other lots) can be calculated if the statistical model contains terms that allow the slopes or the intercepts to vary among lots. When using Model 7.2 and allowing for nonzero slope variance $\left(\sigma_B^2\right)$ and nonzero intercept variance $\left(\sigma_L^2\right)$, each lot will be fit with a unique regression line (if both σ_B^2 and σ_L^2 are equal to zero, all lots have the same regression line). There is no need to reduce Model 7.2 for this research question because we want the individual prediction at expiry for each lot.

TABLE 7.10

Example Predictions for Individual Lots at Current Expiry

Lot	Predicted Mean at 24 Months (%)	Lower one-Sided 95% CB on Predicted Mean at 24 Months (%)	Meets AC of ≥85% at Expiry of 24 Months?
A	88.464	88.213	YES
B	86.605	86.354	YES
C	90.558	90.307	YES
D	93.569	92.967	YES
E	86.860	85.397	YES
F	89.066	87.603	YES

To answer whether an individual lot is predicted to meet expiry, each lot is evaluated in the same way that a lot is evaluated when establishing expiry: Compare the 95% CB on the conditional mean (i.e., BLUP) to the stability AC at the current expiry period. If the CB lies inside the AC, then the lot is predicted to meet expiry.

Table 7.10 shows the individual predictions from Model 7.2 using the "Random Slopes" data from Table 7.9. Although Lot B has a lower predicted value at 24 months, Lot E has a lower CB value at 24 months because there is more uncertainty associated with the 24-month prediction for a lot with no 24-month data. Each lot's prediction at the current 24-month expiry falls above the stability AC of 85%, so every lot is predicted to meet the expiry period. Figure 7.37 shows regression plots for each individual lot.

There are a few practical considerations when examining predictions for all individual lots in the context of an annual product quality review:

- Actions may be incorporated into procedures when a lot is not predicted to meet expiry. Such actions may be based on the number of time points observed to date, and may include waiting until the next time point is observed, adding additional time points, or removing the lot from the market if the prediction is concerning enough. Remember that drastic actions taken for annual lots may implicate all other lots manufactured in the given year.

- If a given lot has already been tested at the expiry time point and is within the AC, then a prediction outside of the AC has no practical impact. Real-time results that meet the AC support that the lot remains acceptable through expiry.

- When fitting Model 7.2 to the data set, a lot may be included in the analysis even if it has only been tested at time 0. The predicted value for the lot will be based on the overall average trend and the time 0 value for that lot. The prediction at expiry may be useful information if a lot is released at a value that is unexpected but still within lot release specification limits.

- Predictions may be reported to the precision of the method when comparing to the stability AC. Remember, the predicted values are just that—predictions—so if these values were obtained during testing, they would be formatted to the specification precision before they were reported.

- A large number of lots with predictions outside of the AC at expiry signals that the expiry period may need to be re-evaluated.

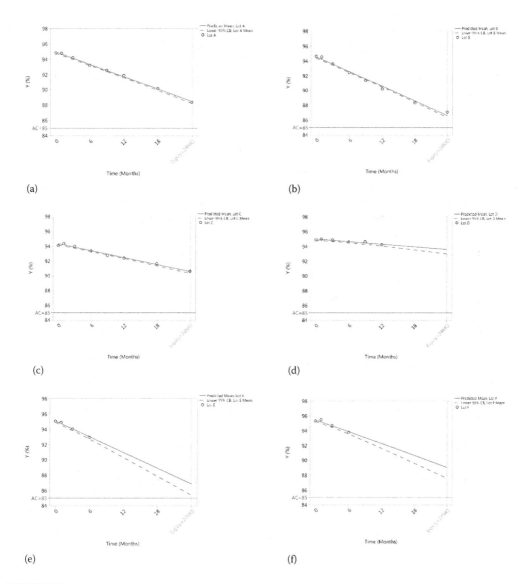

FIGURE 7.37
Example predictions from Model 7.2 for individual lots at expiry. (a) Prediction for lot A. (b) Prediction for lot B. (c) Prediction for lot C. (d) Prediction for lot D. (e) Prediction for lot E. (f) Prediction for lot F.

7.7.3 Can I Extend the Expiry Period?

Although ICH Q1E does not expressly address expiry extensions, an expiry extension analysis is no different in substance from an analysis that establishes the expiry period. We can use the same methodology outlined in Section 7.7.1 to evaluate predictions at a new intended expiry period. In the case of an expiry extension, more lots are likely available, so Model 7.2 should be fit if possible.

If we wish to extend both the DS and DP expiry periods, both product stages can be evaluated together to determine if both extensions are reasonable, as described in Section 7.7.4. We may also wish to ask, "What is the probability on an individual OOS result?" If there is a trend on stability and the shelf life is extended, then the risk for an OOS may increase toward the end of the shelf life. The method for calculating the probability of an individual OOS result is discussed in Section 7.8.3.

7.7.4 How Can I Model Behavior for End-to-End Stability for Multiple Product Stages?

One consideration for a product's overall expiry, particularly with respect to an expiry extension, may be the total change observed when DS and DP trends are considered together. In other words, if DS expiry is extended, will the DP remain within specification at expiry if filled with (almost) expired DS? An end-to-end stability study is one where DS held through expiry is filled into DP, which is then studied through its intended expiry. One can imagine that this type of study could take six years or more to complete. Some simple calculations can help estimate the mean at DP expiry while waiting for the real time end-to-end study data.

Conceptually, the end-to-end behavior on stability can be modeled by taking together the calculated regression lines for DS and DP at RSC. The DS regression line has intercept DS*, and average DS slope, β_{DS}. The calculated DP regression line has intercept DP_0 and average DP slope, β_{DP}. The DP intercept for the end-to-end calculation, DP*, must account for the estimated value at DS expiry, DS_{exp}, and any potential offset between DS* and DP_0. There are two cases to consider when calculating DP*: $DP_0 \geq DS^*$ or $DP_0 < DS^*$.

- Figure 7.38 shows Case 1 where $DP_0 \geq DS^*$ for a parameter that decreases with time. In this case, we can simply shift the DP regression and data down by the total DS change on stability, $DS^* - DS_{exp}$. If $DP_0 > DS^*$, we should also shift the DP regression and data down by $DP_0 - DS^*$.

- Figure 7.39 shows Case 2 where $DP_0 < DS^*$. In practice, DP_0 may be less than DS* because purity is impacted due to filtration at filling, for example. In this case, we must shift the DP regression and data down by the total DS change on stability, $DS^* - DS_{exp}$. However, we must also shift the DP regression and data down by the offset seen between DS* and DP_0 (i.e., $DS^* - DP_0$).

- Note that the relationships are reversed for an attribute that is increasing with time. In any case, the estimates should be adjusted so that the calculation results in the value closest to the stability AC.

Before proceeding, a few items bear mention:

- Notice that Figures 7.38 and 7.39 do not show any CIs on the regression lines. Shao and Chow (2001) provide a method for fitting all of the data in one statistical model and calculating CIs that account for the DS and DP uncertainty in the same model. For simplicity, we will calculate the CIs separately for DS and DP because we wish to make an approximate prediction, not establish expiry as per Q1E. We may choose to calculate DP* based on the CI on DS_{exp} instead of the point estimate of DS_{exp}.

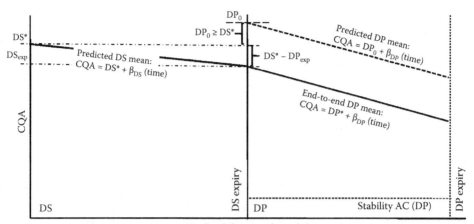

FIGURE 7.38
Case 1: Graphical representation of end-to-end regression when $DP_0 \geq DS^*$.

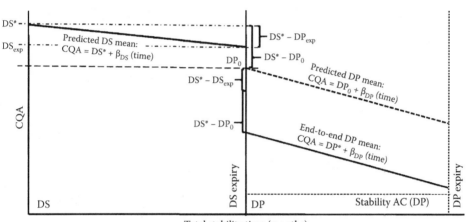

FIGURE 7.39
Case 2: Graphical representation of end-to-end regression when $DP_0 < DS^*$.

- Figures 7.38 and 7.39 show the *average* regression line for DS and DP. This analysis requires the assumption that all lots degrade in approximately the same way. The best way to calculate these regression lines is to fit Model 7.2 and use the average predicted mean (not the conditional predicted means that may vary by lot). Fitting Model 7.2 allows for any potential lot-to-lot variance when calculating CIs on the regression lines.

- This technique assumes that the degradation rate for DP *does not depend on the DS age*. In other words, we assume that DP will degrade at the same rate if it is filled from new DS or from almost expired DS.

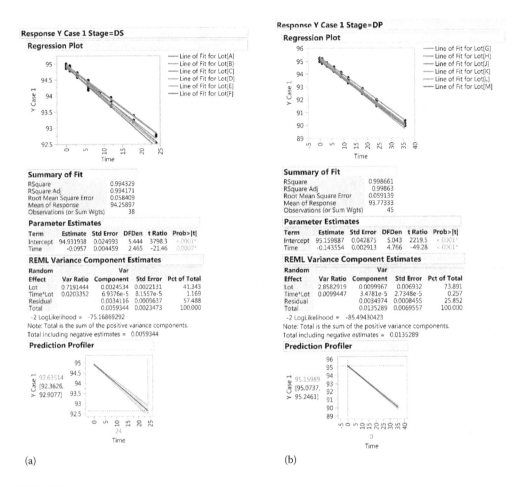

FIGURE 7.40
Case 1: Example analysis when DP0 ≥ DS*. (a) DS regression output. (b) DP regression output.

Figure 7.40 shows example JMP output for Case 1 where $DP_0 \geq DS^*$. The DS intercept, $DS^* = 94.932$, and the DP intercept, $DP_0 = 95.160$, so all DP values should be shifted down by $95.160 - 94.932 = 0.228\%$. The predicted value for DS at the 24-month expiry is 92.635, so all DP values are shifted down by an additional $94.932 - 92.635 = 2.297\%$. In total, DP values are shifted down by $0.228 + 2.297 = 2.525\%$. Figure 7.41 shows the end-to-end regression with the adjusted DP data and predicted values.

Figure 7.42 shows example JMP output for Case 2 where $DP_0 < DS^*$. The DS intercept, $DS^* = 94.932$, and the DP intercept, $DP_0 = 93.002$, so all DP values should be shifted down by $94.932 - 93.002 = 1.93\%$. The predicted value for DS at the 24-month expiry is 92.635, so all DP values are shifted down by an additional $94.932 - 92.635 = 2.297\%$. In total, DP values are shifted down by $1.93 + 2.297 = 4.227\%$. Figure 7.43 shows the end-to-end regression with the adjusted DP data and predicted values.

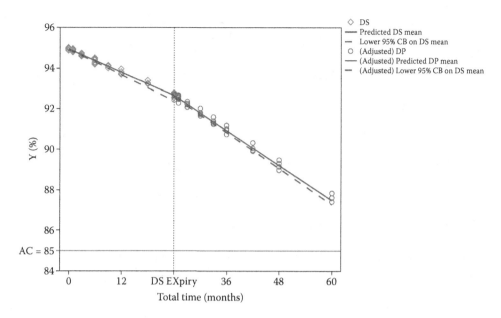

FIGURE 7.41
Case 1: Scatter plot for example analysis when DP0 ≥ DS*. (Note: All DP values have been shifted down by 2.525% to adjust for DS change over time.)

7.8 How Does the Stability Profile Relate to the Specification Limit?

The stability profile is linked to the specification limit in that expiry is based on the intersection of the confidence bound on the regression line with the stability acceptance criterion (AC). Note that this chapter refers to the "specification limit" as the value that a lot must meet at release and the "stability AC" as the value that a lot must meet through its labelled shelf life under recommended storage conditions (RSC). Some companies may use terminology that differs, and some may use internal release limits that are not filed with regulatory agencies.

Specification limits are ideally customer-based; in other words, the specification should be based on some intrinsic requirement of the product. For example, we may know that a gear for a machine should be 10 cm ± 0.5 cm or it won't fit in the machine. However, we frequently do not know the boundary between an acceptable and unacceptable product unless there is a safety-based limit for a given attribute. As such, we can use our data to describe what the process is capable of delivering, and in this way, specifications can be determined as a function of process and method variation. For stability-indicating attributes, the specifications should also consider the stability profile to ensure that allowance for acceptable change over time is built into the stated limit.

No matter how specification limits are calculated, these values should be a starting point for the discussion of an appropriate limit, not the final word on what the limit should be. If a calculated limit seems too restrictive or doesn't make scientific sense, it is likely not appropriate. For example, a data set may be particularly consistent with little variation, resulting in a calculated stability AC of 99.9%. In reality, if results are reported to 1 decimal

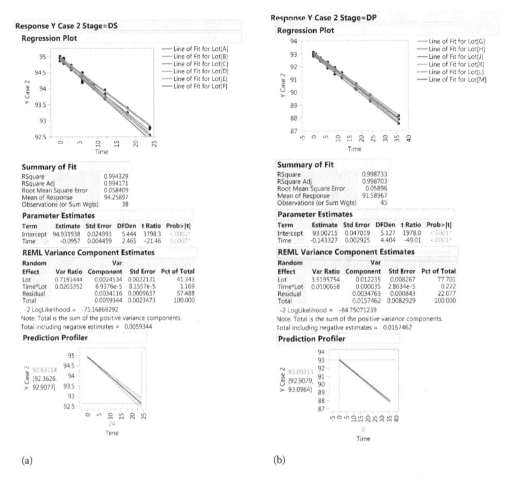

(a)   (b)

FIGURE 7.42
Case 2: Example analysis when DP0 < DS*. (a) DS regression output. (b) DP regression output.

place per the specification, there are only two possible results that will meet the stability AC: 99.9% and 100.0%. When setting the limit for this attribute, consider if it is reasonable to assume that the process will be able to consistently meet such a restrictive limit.

7.8.1 What Is the Appropriate Specification Limit to Achieve a Desired Expiry or Retest Period?

As shown in Section 7.7, the expiry period is determined using calculated CBs on the predicted mean for a stability data set. However, these CBs apply only to the average value, and do not capture a region where individual values are expected to fall. Since specifications apply to individual results, we should set stability AC such that we expect all results to meet the AC when the product is truly safe and efficacious.

As described in Section 7.6.4, a TI on individual results applies to *all future results* generated under current process conditions. A TI describes the region expected to contain a certain proportion of future results (*p*) with a specified level of confidence $(1 - \alpha)\%$.

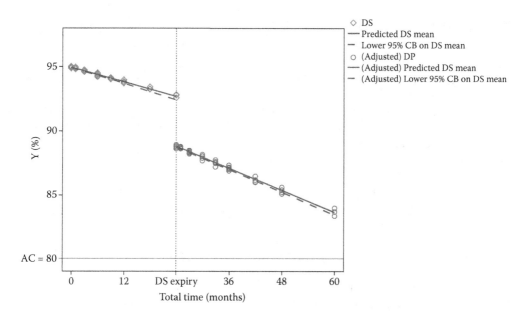

FIGURE 7.43
Case 2: Scatter plot for example analysis when DP0 < DS.* (Note: All DP values have been shifted down by 4.227% to adjust for DS change over time.)

For example, a 95% confidence, 99% coverage TI (95/99 TI) is expected to contain *at least* 99% of future observations with 95% confidence. In practice, we may choose to set specifications using TIs that are expected to cover most of the future results, such as a 95/99.73 TI.

As in Section 7.6.4, a TI can be calculated with stability data that accounts for change over time at RSC. For example, from the calculated 95/99 TIs shown in Figure 7.27, the lower tolerance bound at 36 months is 88.56%. Therefore, a value of 88% or 88.5% could be appropriate for use as a stability AC for a product that has a 36-month shelf life, depending on the reporting precision for the analytical method. Note that rounding a tolerance bound away from the middle of the interval ensures that it contains *at least* the stated proportion of the population. Remember, the calculated TI merely captures the limit that the process is capable of meeting, not a limit that necessarily represents safe or efficacious product.

Recall that Section 7.6.4 describes the potential for stability data to exhibit estimable lot-to-lot, or process, variability. TIs calculated without considering substantial process variability may be too tight, which is especially concerning if using the TIs to set stability AC. Although the calculations are not shown explicitly in this chapter, TIs are most appropriately calculated per Hoffman and Kringle's method (2005) when there is considerable lot-to-lot variability. As an example, Figure 7.29 shows that the correctly calculated TI at 36 months is closer to 87%, compared to the estimated 88.56% when lot-to-lot variation is not considered in the calculation.

A stability AC set using TIs has one inescapable flaw: Setting the AC as the calculated TI at a given expiry period may preclude us from extending the expiry by a considerable amount. Although the regression analysis to set or extend expiry considers only CBs on the mean, we know that the probability of an OOS result [Pr(OOS)] will increase if the expiry is extended beyond the time point used to calculate the limit. Therefore, we want to set the stability AC by considering the calculated TI in conjunction with future business needs, process capability, and patient safety.

7.8.2 Is It Appropriate to Have a Tighter Specification Limit at Lot Release?

For many attributes, the lot release specification limit and the stability AC are equal; this may present a problem if a lot is released close to the limit and the attribute is expected to change on stability. As such, we may decide to set a more stringent limit at lot release compared to the stability AC. As in Section 7.8.1, we can calculate a TI on the entire stability data set and use the value(s) of the interval at time 0 to help with decisions about appropriate lot release limits. For example, from Figure 7.27, the lower 95/99 tolerance bound at 0 time is 93.48%, so a value of 93% or 93.4% could be appropriate for use as a lot release limit, depending on the reporting precision for the analytical method.

The stability data include only a subset of all lots manufactured, so calculating a TI on only the lot release data provides a good comparison for the TI from the stability data. Because the stability data are generated as repeated measures on the same lots over time, we can explicitly estimate the lot-to-lot variation $\left(\sigma_L^2\right)$—something we cannot do using the lot release data since there is no replication at release. If there is substantial process variability, we may be able to get a better measure of expected future variation from the correctly calculated TI on stability data at 0 time.

Implementing a release limit can be done in a number of ways, from using it as an internal control limit to filing it as a formal lot release specification limit. For expiry extensions, especially those beyond 48 or 60 months, implementing a formal release limit may provide assurance that product will remain within the stability AC through the requested expiry period.

7.8.3 Does Changing the Specification Limit Impact the Expiry?

Since the expiry is determined by the earliest intersection of the 95% CB on the mean with the stability AC, any change to the AC could impact the expiry period. Clearly, tightening the specification could potentially shorten the expiry, but for practical purposes, we would probably not tighten a specification if it would shorten our expiry.

Model 7.1 or Model 7.2 can be fit to the stability data to evaluate the expiry using a different value for the stability AC. If the current expiry is still supported with the updated specification limit, the change doesn't impact the expiry. However, we may wish to determine if the likelihood of observing an individual OOS result would increase if a more stringent AC were implemented, as described in Section 7.8.4. An increased probability of an OOS result would need to be factored into any decision to tighten specification limits.

7.8.4 What Is the Probability of an Individual OOS Result on Stability?

Although the expiry period is based on the CI on the *mean*, it does not speak to the expectation for the result from an individual measurement. Since individual results are evaluated against stability AC, it is of interest to determine the probability that each result may fall outside of the AC. This question becomes of particular interest when considering expiry extension or revision to specification limits.

The probability of an OOS stability result [Pr(OOS)], can be related to a TI on individual results as Pr(OOS) = 1 − p where p is the coverage of the TI as defined in Equation 7.7 for $k_{2,\text{fixed}}$. A CI on Pr(OOS) can be computed as described in Chapter 4 of Hahn et al. (2017) and Chapter 2 of Burdick et al. (2017), but will not be discussed in this chapter. However, it is a good idea to compute a CI on any quantity that is used to make a decision because it allows us to ascertain how widely our estimate may vary. Burdick et al. (2017) describe the potential shortcomings of this approach due to the assumptions required to calculate the TIs and provides an alternative approach based on Bayesian methodology. So, proceed with the subsequent calculations of Pr(OOS), bearing in mind that there is uncertainty associated with the result, and that it is best to use the results as only a part of the assessment of risk associated with extending expiry or changing stability AC.

The Pr(OOS) can be calculated by solving the equation for a two-sided TI for the coverage level using known limits. First, solve Equation 7.7 for $Z_{(1+p)/2}$, depending on whether the limit of concern is an upper (USL) or a lower (LSL) limit (Equations 7.9 or 7.10, respectively):

$$Z_{(1+p)/2} = \sqrt{\frac{\chi^2_{df_{error},\alpha}\left(\dfrac{USL - \bar{x}_T}{\sqrt{\sigma^2}}\right)^2}{\left(1 + \dfrac{1}{n_H}\right) \times df_{error}}} \tag{7.9}$$

$$Z_{(1+p)/2} = \sqrt{\frac{\chi^2_{df_{error},\alpha}\left(\dfrac{\bar{x}_T - LSL}{\sqrt{\sigma^2}}\right)^2}{\left(1 + \dfrac{1}{n_H}\right) \times df_{error}}} \tag{7.10}$$

Pr(OOS) is calculated as

$$Pr(OOS) = 1 - (2{}^{*}Z_{calc} - 1) \tag{7.11}$$

Where Z_{calc} is area to the left of $Z_{(1+p)/2}$ from a standard normal distribution.

Table 7.11 presents the results of a few calculations evaluating different values for the LSL at the intended expiry time points of 36 and 48 months, using the results for the regression example from Figure 7.26b and data from Table 7.3. It is apparent that if the intended expiry

TABLE 7.11

Example Calculations for Pr(OOS) for Different AC and Expiry Periods

Intended Expiry (Months)	LSL,%	Predicted Mean at Expiry,% $(\bar{x}_T)$	$Z_{(1+p)/2}$	Pr(OOS)
36	85	90.0661	8.7724	0%
36	86	90.0661	7.0408	0%
36	87	90.0661	5.3092	0%
36	88	90.0661	3.5777	0.03%
36	89	90.0661	1.8461	6.49%
48	85	88.4317	5.9422	0%
48	86	88.4317	4.2106	<0.01%
48	87	88.4317	2.4790	1.32%
48	88	88.4317	0.7474	45.48%

is 36 months, an LSL of 88% gives an acceptable Pr(OOS), but an LSL of 89% is probably too restrictive. Similarly, if targeting a 48-month expiry, an LSL of 87% may be acceptable, but it is probably desirable to calculate an upper CI on the Pr(OOS) because Pr(OOS) = 1.32% may be close to a risk-based decision threshold.

Recall from Figure 7.26b that

- $n_H = 7.49$
- $df_{error} = 52$
- $\chi^2_{df_{error},\alpha} = \chi^2_{52,0.05} = 36.437093$
- $\sqrt{\sigma^2} = RMSE = 0.454062$
- $\bar{x}_T = (estimated\ intercept) + (estimated\ slope)*T = 94.969584 + (-0.136207)*T$
- The value for Z_{calc} can be calculated in Excel as "=NORM.DIST(*calculated* $Z_{(1+p)/2}$,0,1,TRUE) for a standard normal distribution with mean 0 and standard deviation 1.

7.9 How Much Exposure to a Particular Condition Can Be Allowed without Impacting the Shelf Life?

Different conditions of real-world use require support from stability studies, particularly for refrigerated or frozen products. Several special studies may be conducted as one-time studies, and results simply compared to AC. Statistical analysis can help to establish limits for exposure.

7.9.1 What Is an Appropriate Limit for Exposure to Temperatures above Recommended Storage?

Exposure to elevated temperatures can be supported with analysis like that shown in Section 7.7.4, where trends at RSC are considered in conjunction with trends at the elevated temperature. Such analysis may support temperature excursions or a room temperature label claim for a refrigerated or frozen product. The additional exposure can be evaluated with or without considering the DS shelf life or other exposures at other product stages.

For elevated temperatures, the assumption that aged DP degrades at the same rate as fresh DP may be untenable, or at least require validation. A well-designed study can be conducted where DP is aged for certain periods of time prior to ASC exposure and the slopes of the different ASC conditions are compared. Table 7.12 shows a study designed to evaluate DP degradation at ASC as a function of DP age. Once the data are collected, the slopes of the ASC data can be evaluated as shown in Section 7.9.3 using DP age as a categorical variable. Friedman and Shum (2011) propose an alternative analysis technique that fits all of the data in a single model.

TABLE 7.12

Example Study Design to Evaluate ASC Degradation
as a Function of DP Age

DP Age (Months)	ASC Time Points Tested (Months)
0	0, 0.25, 0.5, 1, 2.5, 2.75, 3
3	0, 0.25, 0.5, 1, 2.5, 2.75, 3
6	0, 0.25, 0.5, 1, 2.5, 2.75, 3
9	0, 0.25, 0.5, 1, 2.5, 2.75, 3
12	0, 0.25, 0.5, 1, 2.5, 2.75, 3

7.9.2 How Much Light Exposure Is Acceptable?

Light exposure limits are evaluated differently than most other stability questions: The study is typically conducted once, the x-axis is usually amount of light exposure rather than time, and the evaluation is often more of a binary question where we demonstrate "acceptable change" or "appreciable change."

Per ICH Q1B, products are subjected to a minimum amount of exposure from light sources with wavelengths from both the UV and visible light spectra, either mirroring sunlight or 1.2 million lux-hr of cool white light and 200 watt-hr/m^2 of UV light. Beginning with directly exposed product, additional layers of packaging are added until the results show "acceptable change," which in practical terms can be interpreted as "no appreciable change." For some products, the minimum exposure levels required by Q1B cause appreciable change to product in its minimal packaging (directly exposed or in vials). Although we can usually show that the product is protected from light when stored in its marketed packaging, we may need to establish light exposure limits for unpackaged product since the product must be removed from its package for some period before it is administered.

So how much light exposure is acceptable in a real-world setting? Suppose that the packaging line at the manufacturing facility has windows that expose the product to natural sunlight for some period of time. In most cases, the DP in a stability study has already been exposed to any light at the manufacturing plant, so we have indirectly supported that the typical exposure is acceptable, but we may need to support additional exposure in the case of delays during packaging. Suppose we know that the product may be unpackaged and at room temperature for up to 24 hours at the pharmacy or clinic. How intense is the light in these settings? For a photosensitive product, we must establish that exposure to "ambient light" is acceptable, or we will have to implement controls to ensure that there is no negative product impact.

Short of directly measuring light intensity levels at a specific location, many sources provide general recommendations for light intensities in a medical setting. For example, the U.S. Veterans Affairs Guidelines (2015) recommend that pharmacies have fluorescent lighting with an average maintained illumination of 1000 lux. We may choose to assume that indoor lighting typically does not contain a UV component, although that may not be true in a setting where sunlight is part of the light exposure.

A few assumptions are made when designing a photostability study to support ambient fluorescent lighting:

- The units for fluorescent light exposure are lux-hours. We can calculate the time points for the study by measuring the intensity of the light source and determining the total exposure amounts that we wish to study where: Time (hours) = Total Light Exposure (lux-hours)/Light Source Intensity (lux)
- Each study should include dark controls where samples are wrapped in foil and exposed to the light source side-by-side with test samples. By studying the dark controls, adjustments can be made for any potential degradation due to temperature or humidity exposures. Dark controls and exposed samples are tested at each time point.
- A light source may cause increased temperature during the study. Temperature-controlled photostability chambers are available. For refrigerated products, studies can be conducted at both refrigerated and room temperature conditions in case there is some interaction between elevated temperature exposure and light exposure.

The photostability study is aimed at showing the acceptable amount of change, so analysis is conducted on delta, the difference between the exposed sample and the dark control (DC). Model 7.4 is fit to the data because the study is typically conducted on one lot. One must determine the amount of acceptable change, which is based on some reasonable definition of an acceptable change, such as a percentage of the AC.

Table 7.13 shows an example of a photostability study design to support ambient lighting conditions, including example data for analysis. If the ambient lighting conditions are

TABLE 7.13

Example Photostability Study Design with Exposed Samples and Dark Controls Tested at Each Time Point

Total Light Exposure (Lux-Hours)	Study Time Point Using Light Source of 2000 Lux (Hours)	Duration of Exposure if Ambient Light Is 1000 Lux (Hours)	Exposed Samples (%)	Dark Controls (%)	Delta (%)
0	0	0	94.888	95.147	−0.260
500	0.25	0.5	95.158	94.961	0.198
1000	0.5	1	94.930	94.929	0.002
2000	1	2	94.887	95.016	−0.129
4000	2	4	94.944	95.056	−0.112
8000	4	8	94.905	95.020	−0.115
12,000	6	12	94.799	95.094	−0.295
18,000	9	18	94.688	94.869	−0.181
24,000	12	24	94.448	95.148	−0.700
36,000	18	36	94.192	95.075	−0.883
48,000	24	48	93.696	95.005	−1.309
60000	30	60	93.618	94.791	−1.173
72000	36	72	93.177	94.805	−1.628
84000	42	84	92.925	94.905	−1.979
96000	48	96	92.722	94.762	−2.039

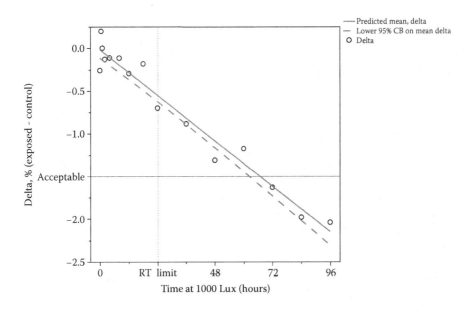

FIGURE 7.44
Example photostability analysis plot.

around 1000 lux, then any allowed ambient temperature exposure must be considered in the study design. For the Table 7.13 example, suppose we need to support 24 hours at ambient conditions, which would be 24 hours * 1000 lux = 24,000 lux-hr. The proposed study incorporates exposures up to four times this amount to support the allowed exposure and potential excursions.

Figure 7.44 shows an example plot from an analysis of a photostability study conducted at room temperature (RT) following the design in Table 7.12. Similar to an expiry analysis, the lower one-sided 95% CB on the average delta is evaluated against the acceptable amount of change. In this example, the stability AC is 80%, and the initial value is 95%, so an acceptable change is defined as 10% of the possible change before reaching the AC, or 10% of (95% − 80%) = 1.5%. The lower CB on the average delta is greater than 1.5% at the current allowed 24 hours RT exposure time, so the product can be exposed to ambient light conditions for the allowed 24 hours at RT without negative impact. Further, up to 60 hours at ambient conditions is supported before the estimated delta exceeds the acceptable change of 1.5%.

7.9.3 Does Temperature Cycling Impact My Product?

Temperature cycling studies support real-world product use and temperature or shipping excursions. Many different study designs may be used, and the specific temperatures, number of cycles, and cycle durations will depend on the product and likely exposures requiring support. Temperature cycling could be from frozen to ASC, refrigerated to ASC, or refrigerated to frozen conditions. For our purposes, we assume that the cycling is a pretreatment, and that data are collected on samples returned to RSC after cycling.

The analysis is conducted by fitting Model 7.3—the qualitative predictor model. In this analysis, the qualitative predictor is the "number of cycles," which is treated as a categorical variable. The temperature cycling study is typically a one-time study conducted on one lot; as such, the model does not have a Lot term. After fitting Model 7.3, the output is examined to determine if there is a difference in the intercepts or slopes between the groups based on the number of cycles. In general, this analysis uses hypothesis testing to test whether there is a difference between the groups, but we do not prove that temperature cycling causes no product impact.

Providing estimates of differences between the control and other conditions affords definitive statements of the effects of temperature cycling. Differences could be estimated between any two groups at any combination of time points. However, computing all possible pairwise differences can lead to an increased Type I error rate, implying the possibility of declaring a difference to be significant when, in fact, it is not. In the temperature cycling study, we are not truly interested in all possible comparisons. The comparisons of real interest are of cycled samples to uncycled samples. Dunnett's test controls for the Type I error rate associated with multiple comparisons when we are only interested in comparing every group to a control group.

Table 7.14 shows a possible study design and example data. The study includes a few time points that are not typically studied on stability (0.5 and 5.5 months), so that the slopes can be better estimated. Figure 7.45 shows output resulting from the Model 7.3 fit. The p-value for the "# of Cycles" term is < 0.0001, which means that at least one of the groups has a different intercept than the others. The Prediction Profiler shows that the product that was cycled 5 times clearly has a lower intercept than the product subjected to 0, 1, or 3 cycles. The p-value for the "# of Cycles*Months after Cycling" term is 0.7856, indicating that there is no evidence that the slope depends on the number of cycles.

Figure 7.46 shows how to obtain results from Dunnett's test at Time 0 from JMP:

- From the Model Output, click the drop-down arrow, and select **Estimates → Multiple Comparisons → User Defined Estimates**.
- Enter the Time Point of Interest in **Months after Cycling**, then **Add Estimates**. Continue adding estimates of interest (e.g., Number of Cycles = 5, Months after

TABLE 7.14

Example Temperature Cycling Study and Data

Duration of RSC Storage after Temperature Cycling (Months)	0 Cycles	1 Cycle	3 Cycles	5 Cycles
0	94.904	94.830	95.185	94.079
0.5	94.878	94.863	95.003	94.097
1	95.073	94.787	94.842	94.279
3	94.763	94.790	95.265	94.042
5.5	94.957	94.596	94.966	93.883
6	94.718	94.807	94.802	93.851

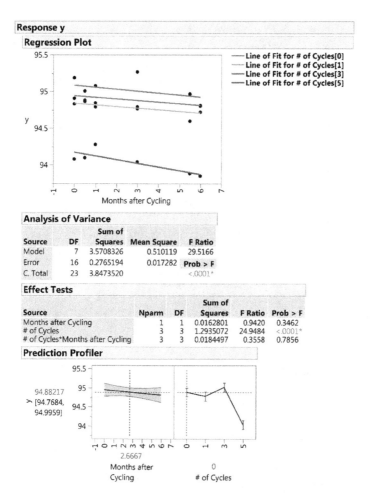

FIGURE 7.45
Example temperature cycling analysis.

Cycling = 0). It is best to limit comparisons to control to those within the same time point (e.g., 0 cycles at 6 months vs. 3 cycles at 6 months).

- Click **Comparison with Control—Dunnett's**. The next screen asks you to select the control group: Select 0 cycles.

Output from the comparisons with control using Dunnett's test is shown in Figure 7.47. The difference between the value for 0 cycles versus 5 cycles at Time 0 is −0.7681%, with 95% CI = (−1.06, −0.47), which is a statistically significant difference at the 95% confidence level. We can state that cycling the product 5 times leads to a loss of at least 0.5%, and we can decide if that is a practically important difference in the context of the particular CQA and the stability AC.

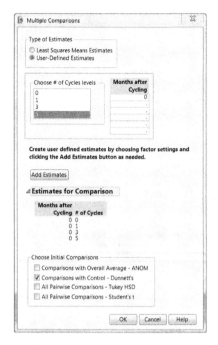

FIGURE 7.46
JMP dialogue to conduct Dunnett's test at Time 0.

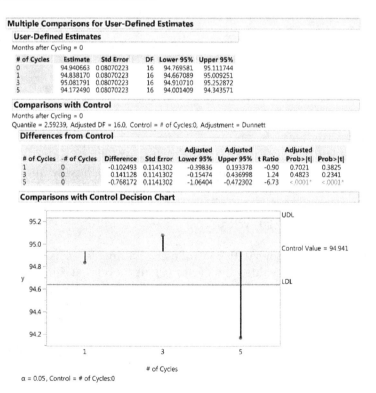

FIGURE 7.47
JMP output from Dunnett's test at Time 0.

7.10 Do Two (Or More) Different Permutations of My Molecule Change the Same Way over Time?

Many products have more than one configuration of some sort: Multiple strengths, different containers, different formulations, and so on. We may also wish to study the product after some type of change has been made, such as an excipient, formulation, container, manufacturing process, or manufacturing site change. Although we can study these changes at the time of product manufacture, small changes that are undetected at the time of release may be detected after storage on stability.

7.10.1 Can I Apply a Bracketing Approach to Several Different Configurations of the Same Product Formulation?

A bracketing approach may be used for a stability program for a product with multiple strengths, fill volumes, or container sizes, where only the low and high levels are monitored on stability. The bracketing approach can save many resources by eliminating testing of batches at intermediate configurations, but it assumes that all configurations have similar stability profiles. Before moving forward with a bracketing approach, it is best to establish that the bracketing approach is valid.

Model 7.3 can be fit to a data set with data for multiple configurations of the same product formulation. The qualitative predictor, X, is a variable representing "configuration." Model output is examined for statistical significance of the X and X*Time terms. For this application, the qualitative predictor is actually a continuous variable, such as strength or fill volume, and the analysis can treat X as either continuous or categorical:

- Treating X as continuous answers whether a unit change in X is related to a unit change in the intercept or the slope. Tests of X and X*Time will be statistically significant if the intercept or slope (respectively) differ as a function of changes in the value of X. For example, we may ask if the degradation rate increases as the strength increases.

- Treating X as categorical answers whether at least one level of X has a different intercept or slope than the other levels of X. Treating X as a categorical variable does not examine the relationship between the numerical value of X and the linear change in intercept or slope, but it allows estimates of differences between each level of X.

Table 7.15 shows an example design with data for a product formulated at five different strengths; each lot is studied at the same time points. The data are plotted with fitted regression lines by strength in Figure 7.48. In this design, it is assumed that the program's bracketing strategy will study three lots at each end of the strength range with no intermediate strengths. We may wish to analyze ASC data to observe a measurable slope in a 12-month period.

The JMP analysis shown in Figure 7.49 fits Model 7.3 to the data from Table 7.15 with Strength as the variable of interest.

- The Figure 7.49(a) analysis treats X as a continuous variable. The p-value for Strength is 0.3002, so there is no evidence that the average value at Time 0 differs by Strength. The p-value for Time*Strength is < 0.0001, so there is evidence that

TABLE 7.15

Example Bracketing Study and Data

Time (Months)	Lot A 0.25 mg	Lot B 0.25 mg	Lot C 0.25 mg	Lot D 0.5 mg	Lot E 1.0 mg	Lot F 2.5 mg	Lot G 5.0 mg	Lot H 5.0 mg	Lot J 5.0 mg
0	94.780	95.919	94.858	95.061	95.435	95.706	94.411	94.479	94.974
1	94.710	95.579	94.554	94.919	95.499	95.681	94.440	94.621	95.072
3	94.193	95.049	94.112	94.751	95.267	95.312	94.597	94.579	95.050
6	93.752	94.777	93.749	94.288	94.999	94.926	94.074	94.324	94.928
9	93.377	94.019	93.252	94.012	94.699	94.983	93.956	94.254	95.047
12	92.987	93.392	92.693	93.785	94.401	94.568	93.855	94.273	94.851

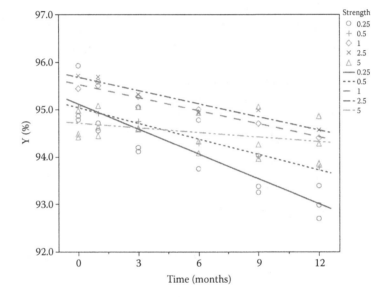

FIGURE 7.48
Plot of example data for bracketing study analysis.

the slope depends on Strength. Because X is treated as continuous, we can say that the slope gets steeper as the Strength changes, and based on Figure 7.48, the lower strengths have a steeper slope.

- The Figure 7.49(b) analysis treats X as a categorical variable. Treating X as a categorical variable allows estimation of the slope for each Strength. The slope for each strength is estimated by adding the estimate for the (particular) Time*Strength to the estimate for Time. For example, the estimated slope for the 2.5 mg strength is $-0.074703 + -0.100096 = -0.174799\%/$month. The slope estimate for the 5 mg strength is the Time estimate minus the sum of the other Time*Strength estimates: $-0.100096 - (-0.074703 + -0.009297 + 0.0084595 + 0.0076946) = -0.0322501\%/$month.

Based on the results of the example analysis, the different strengths do not degrade in the same manner, but there is a relationship between the strength and the slope. The bracketing strategy may be valid: If we study the lowest and highest strengths, then there

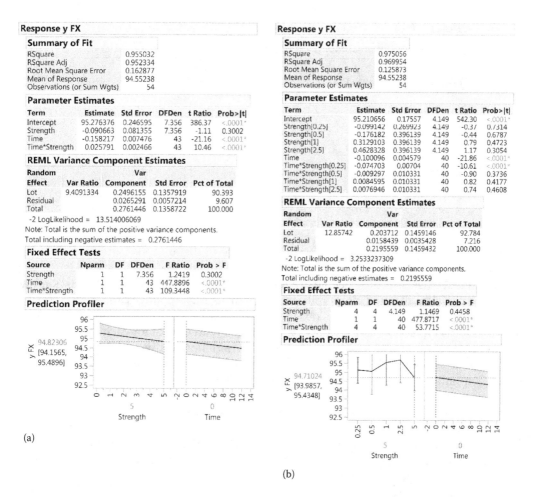

FIGURE 7.49
Example bracketing study analysis. (a) X as continuous. (b) X as categorical.

is evidence that the intermediate strengths' degradation rates will fall somewhere within the range represented by the ends of the bracketed range. However, different degradation rates may require different stability AC for each strength.

7.10.2 Is One Formulation, Container, or Configuration More Stable at a Given Temperature?

We can fit Model 7.3 to examine the differences in degradation rates based on any qualitative predictor, X, such as formulation, container, or configuration. In this type of analysis, we examine the Time*X interaction to determine if there is evidence that at least one of the levels of X has a different slope than the others. If there is one current level of X that should be treated as a control, we can proceed with this analysis as for the temperature cycling study in Section 7.9.3. If the X variable is continuous, we can proceed with the analysis as

TABLE 7.16

Example Container Comparison Study and Data

Time (Months)	Amber Vial	Clear Vial	Lyophilized	Syringe
0	0.662	0.576	0.556	0.496
0.25	0.686	0.645	0.609	0.566
0.5	0.663	0.550	0.443	0.556
1	0.738	0.822	0.548	0.781
2	0.890	0.867	0.712	0.878
2.5	0.887	0.864	0.676	0.911
2.75	0.950	0.923	0.777	0.909
3	0.993	1.045	0.691	1.129

in Section 7.10.1. If the X variable is strictly categorical, the analysis can be conducted as shown in Figure 7.49(b).

Note that studies seeking specifically to examine the differences in degradation rates should be run at accelerated temperatures so that measurable change can be observed over the life of the study. If no change is observed, then there is no way to examine differences in slopes. This type of study may only be conducted with one lot for each level of X, especially if we are seeking to select a container or formulation. If this is the case, it is best to use the same DS lot to fill the different DP configurations so that lot-to-lot differences will not be confounded with potential configuration differences.

When examining the X*Time term for statistical significance, if there is no evidence that the levels of X have different slopes, then there is, by extension, no evidence that one configuration is more stable. If the X*Time term is statistically significant, then the slope estimates can be examined to see which level of X has the least extreme slope. Pairwise comparisons can be made between the slopes for the different levels of X, but care must be taken to only make comparisons of interest so that the Type I error rate is not inflated.

Table 7.16 shows an example design and data for a study comparing four different container/formulation combinations; all DP lots were filled from the same DS lot. In this example, there is concern about a specific impurity increasing over time, and seek a container/formulation combination that will minimize the impurity. Based on the JMP analysis output shown in Figure 7.50, the Time*Container p-value is 0.0071, so at least one container has a different slope than the others. Based on the regression plot, lyophilized vials have the least steep slope, and the estimated slope is 0.1240309 + −0.052179 = 0.0719%/month. Therefore, the lyophilized vial is the container that minimizes formation of the impurity of concern. Understand that these conclusions apply only to the particular DS lot filled into these four container types, studied at this temperature. If further evidence is required to support the conclusion on container type, more lots should be studied.

7.10.3 Is the Stability Profile the Same after a Manufacturing or Process Change?

We can use the qualitative predictor model in Model 7.3 to analyze stability data from pre- and post-change product, where the qualitative predictor, X, is some categorical variable such as "status." Although we can examine p-values for the model terms representing the categorical variable, the standard hypothesis test structure results in conclusions such as, "There is no evidence of a difference between pre- and post-change product." However, when making a change to a commercial manufacturing process, we would like to make

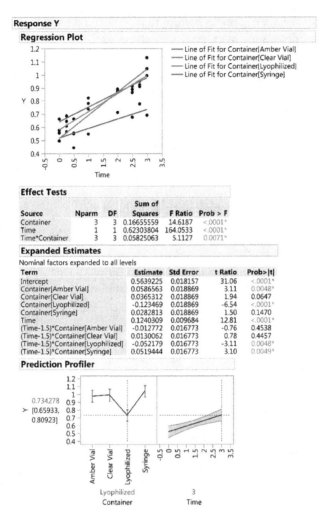

FIGURE 7.50
Example container comparison study analysis.

the strongest statement possible, which is something more like, "The pre- and post-change product are the same." In order to make strong statements of similarity, the best approach is an equivalence analysis, such as that described in Section 7.6.3.

When comparing products that differ by a qualitative predictor, we are examining the estimate for the difference in slopes between the levels of X, which comes from the X*Time term in Model 7.3. When conducting an equivalence test of the difference between pre- and post-change product using the X*Time term, the equivalence limit (EL) is defined by an acceptable difference in degradation rates between the two products. As with any equivalence test, the practically important difference should be scientifically defined when possible.

In the absence of scientific rationale, the EL may be mathematically defined by analyzing prospectively the data from the prechange product using Model 7.2. Fitting Model 7.2 allows for separate estimation of variance components due to lot-to-lot differences. Equation 7.12 for the EL considers the residual variance observed in the pre-change product with respect to the spread in time values as described in Burdick and Sidor (2013).

If considerable slope variance is present, Equation 7.13 can be used to account for the additional variance that impacts the average slope estimates.

$$EL = ES \times \sqrt{\frac{\sigma_E^2}{SST}}$$
(7.12)

$$EL = ES \times \sqrt{\sigma_B^2 + \frac{\sigma_E^2}{SST}}$$
(7.13)

Where
   ES is the effect size, or the allowable multiple of the error

$$SST = \sum_{j=1}^{T}\left(t_j - \bar{t}\right)^2 \quad \text{and} \quad \bar{t} = \sum_{j=1}^{T} t_j/T$$

T is the number of time points for each lot in the study
   σ_E^2 and σ_B^2 are estimates from Model 7.2 of residual variance and slope variance, respectively

TABLE 7.17

Example Stability Comparability Study and Data

Lot	Time	Y	Status	Lot	Time	Y	Status
A	0	94.783	Prechange	G	0	95.869	Postchange
A	0.5	93.914	Prechange	G	0.5	95.081	Postchange
A	1	95.028	Prechange	G	1	94.530	Postchange
A	2	94.034	Prechange	G	2	93.880	Postchange
A	2.5	92.901	Prechange	G	2.5	93.862	Postchange
A	3	93.188	Prechange	G	3	93.507	Postchange
B	0	93.680	Prechange	K	0	94.928	Postchange
B	0.5	94.291	Prechange	K	0.5	95.390	Postchange
B	1	93.727	Prechange	K	1	94.310	Postchange
B	2	93.379	Prechange	K	2	93.461	Postchange
B	2.5	93.402	Prechange	K	2.5	93.997	Postchange
B	3	93.047	Prechange	K	3	92.604	Postchange
C	0	95.080	Prechange	N	0	94.408	Postchange
C	0.5	94.837	Prechange	N	0.5	94.872	Postchange
C	1	94.009	Prechange	N	1	93.963	Postchange
C	2	94.530	Prechange	N	2	93.519	Postchange
C	2.5	93.725	Prechange	N	2.5	93.283	Postchange
C	3	92.984	Prechange	N	3	92.626	Postchange
			Prechange	P	0	95.061	Postchange
			Prechange	P	0.5	95.408	Postchange
			Prechange	P	1	95.396	Postchange
			Prechange	P	2	94.677	Postchange
			Prechange	P	2.5	93.685	Postchange
			Prechange	P	3	93.736	Postchange

An example analysis evaluating the practically important difference between the stability slopes for pre-change and post-change product was conducted using the data in Table 7.17.

- Figure 7.51 shows the calculation of the EL using the pre-change lots only. There is measurable lot-to-lot variance (~23% of total), but the average slope is not impacted by the intercept variability, so only residual variance is considered in this example.
- The residual variance is 0.1990841. SST = 7 (calculated using excel). Suppose ES = 2. Then EL = 2*SQRT(0.1990841/7) = 0.3373%/mo. If equivalence is passed, the conclusion signifies that the stability slopes differ by no more than two times the expected prechange variation.
- Figure 7.52 shows the output from Model 7.3 fit to the entire data set from Table 7.17. The 90% CI for the Status*Time parameter is (−0.2005, −0.0041)%/month. The difference in slopes is not practically significant because the 90% CI falls entirely inside of the EL interval from −0.3373 to 0.3373%/month.

Parameter Estimates

Term	Estimate	Std Error	DFDen	t Ratio	Prob>|t|
Intercept	94.626955	0.229695	5.288	411.97	<.0001*
Time	-0.472035	0.097366	14	-4.85	0.0003*

REML Variance Component Estimates

Random Effect	Var Ratio	Var Component	Std Error	Pct of Total
Lot	0.3069424	0.0611074	0.0951184	23.486
Lot*Time	0	0		0.000
Residual		0.1990841	0.0752467	76.514
Total		0.2601915	0.1132353	100.000

-2 LogLikelihood = 27.605256228
Note: Total is the sum of the positive variance components.
Total including negative estimates = 0.2601915

FIGURE 7.51
Calculation of EL for stability comparability exercise.

Response Y

Parameter Estimates

Term	Estimate	Std Error	DFDen	t Ratio	Prob>|t|	Lower 90%	Upper 90%
Intercept	94.946972	0.161953	9.642	586.26	<.0001*	94.652328	95.241615
Time	-0.574309	0.058012	33	-9.90	<.0001*	-0.672487	-0.476132
Status[PostChange]	0.3200162	0.161953	9.642	1.98	0.0774	0.0253726	0.6146597
Status[PostChange]*Time	-0.102274	0.058012	33	-1.76	0.0872	-0.200452	-0.004097

REML Variance Component Estimates

Random Effect	Var Ratio	Var Component	Std Error	Pct of Total
Lot	0.6252782	0.1010071	0.0811813	38.472
Residual		0.1615394	0.0397683	61.528
Total		0.2625465	0.0874342	100.000

-2 LogLikelihood = 61.575315796
Note: Total is the sum of the positive variance components.
Total including negative estimates = 0.2625465

Fixed Effect Tests

Source	Nparm	DF	DFDen	F Ratio	Prob > F
Time	1	1	33	98.0065	<.0001*
Status	1	1	9.642	3.9045	0.0774
Status*Time	1	1	33	3.1081	0.0872

FIGURE 7.52
Model output to evaluate stability comparability of pre- and post-change product.

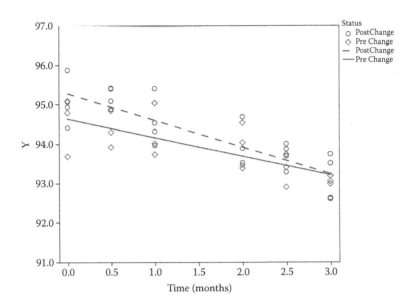

FIGURE 7.53
Scatter plot of stability data used to evaluate pre-change and post-change equivalence.

- Figure 7.53 shows a scatter plot of the data marked by status with fitted regression lines based on the conditional predicted values from the model. The regression lines appear approximately parallel, so the conclusion of "equivalent" seems reasonable.

As in Figure 7.25 in Section 7.6.3, Figure 7.52 also shows the *p*-values for Status*Time because the same model can be used to test for either practical significance or statistical significance. Again, it is best practice to state only one conclusion in case the conclusion about statistical significance conflicts with the conclusion about practical significance. In this analysis, we choose to state the equivalence conclusion because we want to make the claim that the difference in pre-change and post-change slopes is not practically significant with respect to the stated EL.

7.11 Conclusion

This chapter described statistical methodologies that can be applied to most research questions that may be addressed in a pharmaceutical stability program, including questions that extend beyond the typical analysis of expiry periods. Questions about stability trends may be best addressed as a stability program matures in order to leverage previous process knowledge to predict future behavior. Many one-time studies may be conducted to address specific storage or handling questions, and results from these studies may benefit from statistical analysis so that more objective, data-driven decisions can be made to support conclusions. Stability studies may also be used to compare degradation patterns of different product configurations or to compare stability profiles observed after manufacturing changes. Of course, the stability analysis can always be applied to examine appropriate expiry periods, and two different statistical models may be employed, depending on the focus of inference and amount of stability data available.

References

Berger, R. L. and Hsu, J. C. 1996. Bioequivalence trials, intersection-union tests and equivalence confidence sets. *Statistical Science*, 11:283–319

Bluman, A. G. 2014. *Elementary Statistics: A Step By Step Approach*, 9th edition. New York: McGraw-Hill.

Borman, P. J. and Chatfield, M. J. 2015. Avoid the perils of using unrounded data. *Journal of Biomedical Analysis*, 115: 502–508.

Box, G. and Cox, D. 1964. An analysis of transformations. *Journal of the Royal Statistical Society, Series B*, 26(2): 211–252.

Brady, J., and Holum, J. 1996. *Chemistry: The Study of Matter and its Changes*, 2nd ed. New York: John Wiley & Sons.

Burdick, R. and Graybill, F. 1992. *Confidence Intervals on Variance Components*. New York: Dekker, Inc.

Burdick, R. and Sidor, L. 2013. Establishment of an equivalence acceptance criterion for accelerated stability studies. *Journal of Biopharmaceutical Statistics*, 23:730–743.

Burdick, R., LeBlond, D., Pfahler, L. et al. 2017. *Statistical Applications for Chemistry, Manufacturing and Controls (CMC) in the Pharmaceutical Industry*. Switzerland: Springer.

Capen, R., Forenzo, C. et al. 2017. Evaluating current practices in shelf life estimation. *AAPS Pharm SciTech*, 18: 1–13. Accessed from https://doi.org/10.1208/s12249-017-0880-4.

Chow, S. 2007. *Statistical Design and Analysis of Stability Studies*. Durham, NC: Chapman & Hall.

EMA Guidelines on the Requirements for Quality Documentation Concerning Biological Investigational Medicinal Products in Clinical Trials. Effective April 15, 2012.

EU Guidelines to Good Manufacturing Practice for Medicinal Products. Part I, Chapter, 1, Section 1.10, vii.

FDA Center for Veterinary Medicine. 2008. Guidance for Industry: Drug Stability Guidelines, December 9, 2008.

FDA Office of Regulatory Affairs (ORA) Laboratory Manual. Section 4.3, Volume III. Data Handling and Presentation. Accessed October 18, 2017, from https://www.fda.gov/downloads/Science Research/FieldScience/LaboratoryManual/UCM092179.pdf.

Freeman, M. and Tukey, J. 1950. Transformations related to the angular and the square root. *Annals of Mathematical Statistics*, 21(4): 607–611.

Friedman, E. and Shum, S. 2011. Stability models for sequential storage. *AAPS PharmSciTech*, 12(1): 96.

Hahn, G., Meeker., W., Escobar, L. 2017. *Statistical Intervals: A Guide for Practitioners and Researchers*, 2nd edition. New York: Wiley & Sons.

Hartvig, N. and Kamper, L. 2017. A statistical decision system for out-of-trend evaluation. *Pharmaceutical Technology*, 41(1): 34–43.

Health Canada. Guidance for Sponsors: Lot Release Program for Schedule D (Biologic) Drugs, Section 5.1.1.3.

Health Canada. Guidance Document, Post-Notice of Compliance (NOC) Changes: Quality Document. Effective September 30, 2009.

Hoffman, D. and Kringle, R. 2005. Two-sided tolerance intervals for balanced and unbalanced random effects models. *Journal of Biopharmaceutical Statistics*, 15:283–293.

Huynh-Ba, K. et al. 2009. *Handbook of Stability Testing in Pharmaceutical Development*. New York: Springer.

International Conference on Harmonization (ICH). 1995. Q5C, Stability Testing of Biotechnological/ Biological Products.

International Conference on Harmonization (ICH). 1996. Q1B, Stability Testing: Photostability Testing of New Drug Substances and Products.

International Conference on Harmonization (ICH). 2002. Q1D, Bracketing and Matrixing Designs for Stability Testing of New Drug Substances and Products.

International Conference on Harmonization (ICH). 2003. Q1A (R2), Stability Testing of New Drug Substances and Products.

International Conference on Harmonization (ICH). 2003. Q1E, Evaluation for Stability Data.

JMP® 13 Fitting Linear Models, 2nd edition. 2017. Cary, NC: SAS Institute.

Kutner, M., Nachtsheim, C., Neter J., and Li, W. 2005. *Applied Linear Statistical Models*, 5th ed. New York: McGraw-Hill/Irwin.

NIST/SEMATECH e-Handbook of Statistical Methods. 2012. Section 7.2.6.3. Tolerance Intervals for a Normal Distribution. Accessed from http://www.itl.nist.gov/div898/handbook/prc/section2/prc263.htm.

Ott, L. and Longnecker, M. 2001. *An Introduction to Statistical Methods and Data Analysis*, 5th ed. Pacific Grove, CA: Duxbury.

Park, D. and Burdick, R. 2004. Confidence intervals on total variance in a regression model with an unbalanced onefold nested error structure. *Communications in Statistics—Theory and Methods*, 33:11.

PhRMA CMC Statistics and Stability Expert Teams. 2003. Identification of out-of-trend stability results. *Pharmaceutical Technology*, 27(4): 38–52.

PhRMA CMC Statistics and Stability Expert Teams. 2005. Identification of out-of-trend stability results, part II. *Pharmaceutical Technology*, 29(10).

Roberts, A. 2015. Maintaining the stability of biologics. *BioPharm International*, 28(3): 38–41.

Shao, J. and Chow, S. 1994. Statistical inference in stability analysis. *Biometrics*, 50: 753–763.

Shao, J. and Chow, S. 2001. Two-phase shelf-life estimation. *Statistics in Medicine*, 20: 1239–1248.

Stroup, W. and Quinlan, M. 2016. Statistical considerations for stability and the estimation of shelf life, in *Nonclinical Statistics for Pharmaceutical and Biotechnology Industries*, ed. Zhang, L., pp. 575–604. Switzerland: Springer.

Therapeutic Goods Administration (TGA). 2003, July. Australian Regulatory Guidelines for OTC Medicines.

Torbovska, A. and Trajkovic-Jolevska, S. 2013. Methods for identifying out-of-trend results in ongoing stability data. *Pharmaceutical Technology*, 37(6).

U.S. Code of Federal Regulations. Title 21, Chapter I, Part 211, Section 211.180.e.

U.S. Department of Veterans Affairs. 2015. Office of Construction and Facilities Management, Lighting Design Manual, Section 4.2.18, Pharmacy. Accessed from https://www.cfm.va.gov/til/dManual/dmLighting.pdf.

Wasserstein, R. and Lazar, N. 2016. The ASA's statement on p-values: Context, process, and purpose. *The American Statistician*, 70:2, 129–133.

Wheeler, D. 2011. What is chunky data? *Quality Digest*, 15:58.

8

Continued Process Verification

Tara Scherder and Katherine Giacoletti

CONTENTS

8.1 Introduction

According to the FDA's 2011 Guidance for Industry Process Validation: General Principles and Practices, Stage 3 of the Process Validation Lifecycle, Continued Process Verification (CPV), is intended to provide "continual assurance that the process remains in a state of control (the validated state) during commercial manufacture." These activities must be part of a prospectively defined program that identifies the what, when, who, and how of attribute and parameter monitoring, including criteria for requisite actions "… to correct, anticipate, and prevent problems so that the process remains in control" [1].

Statistical process control (SPC) tools, such as control charts and capability analyses, form the analysis backbone of CPV. These tools aren't new to any biopharmaceutical manufacturer, as they are very likely part of annual product review. However, meeting the goals for CPV detailed in the guidance will require more evaluation of process behavior, including possibly more thorough exploration of trends, additional parameters, different personnel, and more frequent review. These changes should lead to better process understanding, more opportunities for continuous improvement, and (thereby) fewer supply interruptions and overall lower costs across the life cycle.

In any application of statistics, the choice of a specific methodology depends on the goals of the statistical analysis. The most successful solutions depend on an understanding of goals and a comparison of alternatives that enable those goals. The goals of CPV, as stated in the guidance, are to (1) *understand* routine variability, (2) *detect* unusual variability, and (3) enable process *improvement*. Unlike typical application of SPC, this activity is most often performed retrospectively in biopharmaceutical manufacturing, and *immediate* or real-time assessment and process adjustments are not sought. Recognition of this difference in application, and the failure to meet statistical assumptions, are crucial to the choice and interpretation of common SPC tools such as control charts and process capability indices in the context of CPV.

This chapter provides further discussion of these characteristics and relevant examples, and is organized as follows: (1) Introduction to the statistical tools most frequently used in CPV; (2) considerations for the use of these tools during CPV of biopharmaceutical processes; (3); and review of several advanced charting tools, and considerations for their use.

It will be shown that using the simplest SPC tools is often the optimal approach, for both patient and business, to meet the goals of CPV. Success is dependent on interpretation and action in context of the nuances of biopharmaceutical processes.

8.2 Statistical Tools for CPV

SPC is a powerful collection of problem-solving tools to assess and improve process stability and capability (defined later) through the reduction of variability [2]. As stated in the introduction, the goals of CPV are to detect unusual variation, ensure product quality, and enable process improvement. Clearly the goals of SPC and CPV are very similar. However, there are differences, most notably the time frame of review and action. Unlike the typical application and goals of SPC, control chart review during CPV is not performed in real-time, nor are immediate adjustments to maintain performance sought. Additionally, product quality data in CPV typically fail several assumptions for simple interpretation of statistical results, the foremost being independence.

It is critical that these differences between classical SPC applications and the use of SPC tools in CPV be recognized; otherwise, interpretation and action can be sorely misguided and wasteful. Additional insight is provided in the following discussion and examples.

8.2.1 SPC Phases, Control Charts and Process Monitoring

A control chart is the most common tool used to assess the state of control of a manufacturing process, to understand its routine variability, and to detect unusual variability. This extremely powerful tool provides a visual representation of process performance over time, allowing process engineers to readily identify and (when needed) investigate and determine the root cause(s) of any changes in performance.

There are many types of control charts, and the best chart for a given measurement depends primarily on the type of measurement (continuous vs. attribute, for example); however, the context—that is, the manufacturing practices, goals of the analysis, and related decision-making—must also be considered in the selection and interpretation of control charts.

Woodall [3] describes two phases of a typical SPC program and emphasizes important distinctions between the use of control charts in these phases. In Phase 1 SPC, historical data are evaluated using a control chart to determine if a process is in a state of statistical control. A process in a state of statistical control exhibits only chance, or common, causes of variation. Woodall further adds that control charts in Phase 1 SPC resemble a tool of exploratory data analysis. This use is quite different than Phase 2 SPC, when control charts are used prospectively after every measurement to detect changes as quickly as possible so that process adjustments can be made in real- or near–real-time to maintain the state of control. In classic Phase 2 SPC, large assignable causes have been removed and the emphasis is on real-time process monitoring of a stable process to detect and react to small shifts.

Mention SPC and most people will think only of the scenario of Phase 2 SPC. However, the activities of CPV align most closely to a Phase I SPC scenario, since evaluation is retrospective, quick corrective action is not sought, and large sources of variability are present. This has significant implications for the design of a CPV program, and the use and interpretation of statistical tools within that program. Shewhart control charts are very effective in Phase 1 SPC because of their simplicity, and because patterns are easy to interpret and have direct physical meaning. Since evaluation and action do not occur in real-time and multiple consecutive data points are typically evaluated retrospectively, average run length (ARL), the average number of points that must be plotted before a point indicates an out-of-control condition, is not as critical in Phase 1 as in Phase 2 SPC applications. Sensitizing rules (such as Nelson or Western Electric rules) discussed in the following section are effective at reducing ARL and identifying changes in process behavior. False alarms associated with these rules do not have the same repercussions in Phase 1 SPC as they may have in a Phase 2 SPC application. In fact, the probability that an assignable cause of variability is detected is of more interest in Phase 1 SPC than is reducing the occurrence of false alarms. Thus, the use of sensitizing rules is effective for process understanding and improvement in Phase 1 SPC [2].

Thus, for many CQAs and process parameters included in a CPV program for a biopharmaceutical process, where (1) a single continuous measurement is taken from each batch, and (2) the charts will be reviewed *periodically* and *retrospectively* (every quarter, or after every campaign, for example), a simple Shewhart chart for individuals will be the appropriate choice. The statistical basis, assumptions, and interpretation of these charts is discussed in detail in the next several subsections. Examples of several more complex charts and their possible implementation during CPV are discussed later in this chapter.

8.2.2 Shewhart Control Chart for Individual Measurements

An example Shewhart control chart for individual measurements ("Individuals—Moving Range Chart or I-MR") is shown in Figure 8.1.

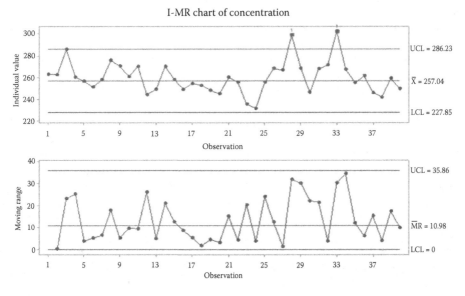

FIGURE 8.1
Example I-MR chart.

The x-axis displays the lot numbers, manufacturing dates, or some other unique identifier in time order from oldest to newest. The top chart y-axis displays the individual measurements, and the bottom chart displays the moving range, which is the absolute difference between two consecutive measurements. In each, the average across all the values is indicated by the solid center line. The top chart, therefore, provides a visual representation of the process measurements over time, allowing the reviewer with process knowledge to immediately link the pattern on the chart to other information they may have, specifically any process input or parameter changes that may have occurred. The moving range (MR) is used as the measurement of variability in the I-Chart, and the bottom chart gives a visual indication of any changes or trends in process variability over time. Caution must be exercised in the interpretation of MR charts given the correlation between measurements and the effect of changes in the mean of the process on the MR chart, leading some experts to recommend against construction of the MR chart [2,3]. As long as the analyst understands the limitations and relies primarily on the individuals chart, there is no harm in evaluating both.

In the I-MR chart, the moving range provides the estimate of short-term process variability and is used to calculate the control limits for both the I and MR charts. Formulas for the control limits can be found in SPC texts [2], or in the help files of statistical software such as Minitab® or JMP®. The control limits bracket the expected range of measurements from the process due to inherent, expected/routine, random variability—often called *common cause variation*. Common cause variation typically includes such sources as measurement variability, sampling variability, and the typical part-to-part variability. When atypical variability occurs, referred to as "special cause variation," the process measurements or moving ranges may fall outside of control limits.

The point on the chart outside of control limits in Figure 8.1 is identified with a distinct marker from the other points and a numerical label. These labels typically reference the Nelson rules [4]. As noted previously, this set of sensitizing rules can be used on control charts to highlight nonrandom behavior that may indicate special cause variation is present. The most commonly used four of the eight Nelson rules are summarized in Table 8.1 below.

The presence of behavior meeting one of the Nelson Rule criteria, *for data meeting the assumptions underlying the control limits and the rules*, is an indication that special cause variation may be present, and the process is no longer in a state of control. It is critical to note that the typical interpretation of these rules as an indication of a lack of process control relies on certain assumptions which, as will be discussed later in this chapter, are frequently violated in biopharmaceutical processes.

A common rule of thumb is to require at least 25–30 data points before calculating control limits in order to obtain a reasonable estimate of the distribution (mean and variance) of the process data. Control charts can be evaluated prior to accumulating this minimum amount of data, and in fact, can be quite useful, particularly in a Phase 1 SPC application. Note that for any process it is important to consider not only the *number* of data points, but also how much manufacturing activity is needed to capture all sources of routine, expected variability that act on a process such as raw material lots, equipment train, and seasonal effects. This assessment must recognize that the effects of some sources of variability may require more time to observe than others. If control limits are used on charts prior to having enough data to have a thorough estimate of process variability, they should be treated as tentative or preliminary, and reactions to points outside of limits should be made with this understanding. This will be discussed in more detail later in the chapter, in the context of implementing control charts in CPV for biopharmaceutical processes.

TABLE 8.1

Nelson Rules 1–4

Rule & Description	Example	Possible Cause
Rule 1: One point more than 3σ from the mean	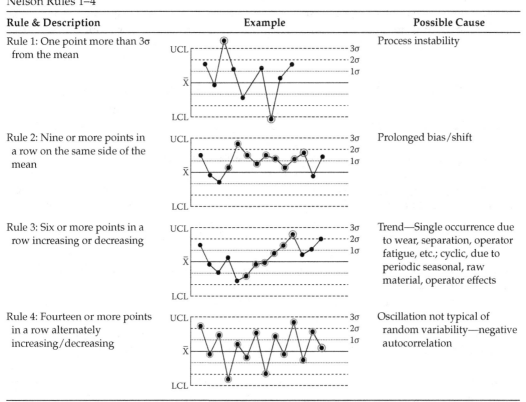	Process instability
Rule 2: Nine or more points in a row on the same side of the mean		Prolonged bias/shift
Rule 3: Six or more points in a row increasing or decreasing		Trend—Single occurrence due to wear, separation, operator fatigue, etc.; cyclic, due to periodic seasonal, raw material, operator effects
Rule 4: Fourteen or more points in a row alternately increasing/decreasing		Oscillation not typical of random variability—negative autocorrelation

Part of what makes a Shewhart control chart such a powerful tool for monitoring, understanding, and improving processes in a Phase 1 SPC application is its simplicity and ease of interpretation. The few calculations required are simple to perform and understand, and the assumptions are few. In fact, the only assumptions underlying the conventional interpretation of a Shewhart chart for either subgroups ($\bar{X} - S$ or $\bar{X} - R$) or individuals (I or I-MR) are (1) the measurement to be charted is continuous (charts for discrete measurements/attributes are discussed later in this chapter), (2) the observations to be charted are independent and random outputs from the process, and (3) the data are normally distributed (Gaussian distribution).

Note, assumptions (2) and (3) are not required to create the chart; instead, they form the basis for evaluating statistical performance and interpreting behavior. In fact, charting data can provide information regarding independence and distribution, particularly in Phase 1 SPC. The normality assumption is the one most often debated, emphasized, and agonized over. Indeed, the theoretically derived α-risk (probability of a point outside three control limits from an in-control process) for a Shewhart chart is based on a Normal distribution, yet it can be shown that control limits of the $\bar{X}$ chart are robust to all but extreme departures from normality [2] and three-sigma limits bracket greater than 97.5% of data, even for variables following distributions having high skewness or kurtosis [5]. Also, the decrease in ARL_0 (the average run length when a process is in a state of control) as non-normality increases does not have the consequences in a Phase 1 SPC application compared to a Phase 2 application. The most critical concepts for proper interpretation of control charts are randomness and independence—properties that are frequently violated in practice, especially in biopharmaceutical processes. Thus, the overall success of a CPV program depends on the design and interpretation of these charts, considering these violations of the assumptions for the charts. The nuances of application for biopharmaceutical manufacturing, and elements of a successful program are further discussed in Section 8.3.

8.2.3 Process Capability

The term *process capability* refers to the magnitude of the inherent variability of an *in-control* process relative to the specifications or requirements for the outputs of the process. Thus, as the term indicates, process capability is a measure of the ability of a process to meet its requirements. If a process is not in a state of control, any assessment of capability must be considered tentative or unreliable, since a stable estimate of its mean and/or variability cannot be made.

Process capability is typically summarized using one of several *capability indices*, each of which is a ratio of the spread of the process specifications to the spread of the expected process outputs. All estimate the spread of the process outputs to be six standard deviations (6σ). The most commonly used are summarized in Table 8.2. The distinction between these two indices is the formula for the standard deviation estimate; C_{pk} reflects short-term (e.g., batch to batch) variability, while P_{pk} reflects long-term (overall) variability. Shifts in the process mean is a common reason for C_{pk} to be greater than P_{pk}. For any of these indices, larger values are better and a value <1 indicates that the spread of the process is greater than the spread of the specifications, a signal that the process is not capable.

Figure 8.2 is a histogram of measurements with the specifications indicated by dashed reference lines. The estimated process spread is indicated by the fitted Normal distribution curve overlaid on the histogram. The fact that the distribution is entirely contained within the specifications, with a sizable margin in either direction, is an indication that the process is quite capable of producing product that meets specifications.

Target minimum values of capability indices are often used to support product quality claims and to prioritize efforts to reduce process variability. It is common to target a minimum of 1.33; however, in biopharmaceutical processes, the maximum achievable capability for some attributes may actually be even lower because specifications were derived from process performance. The practice of using product performance to define specifications results from the challenge to define clinically relevant specifications for some parameters of a biopharmaceutical product. But this also means that the process performance will be close to those specifications, resulting in inherently limited capability. Furthermore, like Shewhart charts, simple interpretation of process capability indices depends on the

TABLE 8.2

Commonly Used Capability Indices

Index	Formula	Interpretation
C_{pk}	$min\left(\dfrac{(\mu - LSL)}{3\sigma_{ST}}, \dfrac{(USL - \mu)}{3\sigma_{ST}}\right)$	Short-term capability
P_{pk}	$min\left(\dfrac{(\mu - LSL)}{3\sigma}, \dfrac{(USL - \mu)}{3\sigma}\right)$	Long-term capability

Note: LSL = lower specification limit; USL = upper specification limit; μ = sample mean; σ_{ST} = short-term (also known as within) standard deviation; σ = long-term (overall sample) standard deviation.

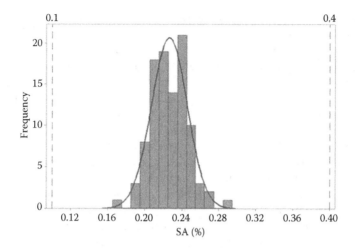

FIGURE 8.2
Histogram with specifications to assess capability visually.

assumptions of normality and independence, which are often not met. The implications of these issues, and recommendations for using capability analyses to meet the goals of CPV, are further discussed in the next section.

8.3 Special Considerations for CPV in the Biopharmaceutical Industry

As alluded to in earlier sections, there are aspects of biopharmaceutical manufacturing that pose challenges for a simple "textbook" application of statistical process control tools such as Shewhart control charts and capability analyses. This section will describe the issues in detail and suggest some practical approaches to address them for efficient and value-added implementation of CPV. While there are many ways to address these challenges, it is critical to keep two principles in mind: (1) Interpretation and activities should incorporate risk-based decision-making as advised in the FDA guidance (" ...the variation should be controlled in a manner commensurate with risk...") [1], and (2) to provide the most value to both the patient and the biopharmaceutical business, CPV should not be treated solely as a compliance exercise; rather, the goals of CPV are to ensure that the process remains in a state of control (and thereby consistently delivers quality product to patients) *and* to enable continuous process improvement by increased process understanding. Interpretation of the phrase "state of control" is discussed in more detail in the following section.

8.3.1 Randomness, Independence, and Normality—Lack Thereof

A process in a state of control is often described as being subject only to common cause variation, resulting in points on a control chart varying over time in a random and predictable pattern around a singular mean. Interpretation of $\pm 3\sigma$ control limits and the sensitizing Western Electric or Nelson rules in this scenario commonly assumes two process data attributes: (1) They are normally distributed and (2) they are independent. (The combined assumptions are sometimes referred to as the data being "iid," or independent and identically distributed—in other words, that the data are independent and have a common distribution [in this case normal], that is, a common mean and variability across time.) Biopharmaceutical data quite often violate one, if not both, of these assumptions, which has important implications for the interpretation of Shewhart charts and capability indices in CPV. Of the two, violation of the independence assumption is more prevalent and has more practical impact in the context of CPV than violation of the normality assumption. In fact, the prerequisite of normality for use of control charts is debated [5,6,7]; however, understanding the implications of both assumptions is critical to an effective CPV program.

A *random* variable is one whose possible values are numerical results of a random phenomenon. In the context of a manufacturing process operating under statistical control, randomness would mean that all variability of the measured results around the process average is due to *random* variation due to measurement, sampling, part-to-part, and so on (i.e., common cause variability). Thus, the statistical basis for typical creation and interpretation of control charts is that the measurements from the process vary randomly around a single process mean and therefore any nonrandom behavior is a sign of (potential) special cause variability. An example of a frequent violation of the randomness assumption in biopharmaceutical processes is trending of in-process controls. Process adjustments are deliberately made if values exceed predefined alert/action limits; thus, these values are not random. Although this manufacturing condition does not preclude the use of control charts, lack of randomness renders the usual simple interpretation of control charts invalid. Similarly, interpretation of capability assessments and metrics, such as C_{pk} or P_{pk}, warrants careful attention, since the process is allowed to drift in between the alert/action limits, but deliberate adjustments are made before results fall outside of specification or alert limits. Prediction of the outside-of-specification (OOS) rate made assuming a random variable will therefore be erroneously high, compared to the true rate.

A closely related and critical assumption of control charts is that the points on the chart represent *independent* measurements of the process. Two measurements are independent if the value of one does not depend on the value of another. It is often easiest to understand the concept of independence of samples or measurements by considering examples where independence does not hold. The example above of an in-process control, where an earlier sample measurement may affect the measurement of a later sample measurement through adjustments to the process exhibits both nonrandomness and lack of independence. However, there are myriad other examples of violations of independence in biopharmaceutical manufacturing. Non-independence arises routinely in biopharmaceutical manufacturing due to the simple fact that the sources of *routine, expected* variability (such as raw material lots, operators, equipment, multiple analytical lab factors, etc.) are not applied randomly to the process. As a simple example, consider the impact of variability between lots of drug substance on a CQA on the finished drug product. A single lot of drug substance may be used in multiple lots of drug product, all of which will be more similar to each other than to a group of drug product lots made from a different lot of drug substance. On the Shewhart chart shown in Figure 8.3, this appears as groupings of data which may be identified as potential special cause variability, when in fact it is due to inherent variability of the in-control process.

This non-independence has multiple implications for interpretation of a Shewhart chart. Most importantly, it must be considered in the evaluation of process control. Because an increase in sensitizing rule violations is expected with non-independence, the absence of statistical signals or special cause variation in general cannot be used as the criterion to deem that a process is in an acceptable state of control. In other words, process control cannot be thought of as equivalent to statistical control. Indeed, it is a goal of CPV to reduce

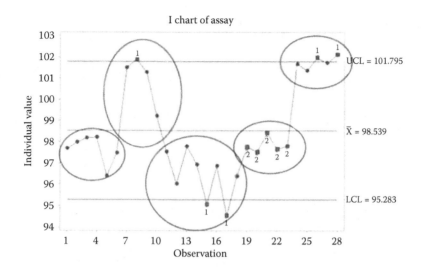

FIGURE 8.3
Shewhart chart of assay with drug product batches from the same drug substance lot, indicated by circles.

variability over time; however, the decision to remove sources of variability is based on risk–benefit–cost analysis. In a Phase 1 SPC scenario of a capable process, removing every source of variability may not be desirable from this perspective. Thus, in the context of non-independent results in CPV, variability patterns do not necessarily translate to an out-of-control process that warrants attention. Predictability in this common scenario is not as accurate or straightforward as the case of a homogenous distribution; assessment of process control depends heavily on understanding the historical variability pattern. These concepts are described further in the next section and by Scherder and DiMartino et al. [8,9].

In addition to the effect of non-independence on the designation of process control, it is important to recognize that more results are expected to fall outside of Shewhart control limits derived from the average moving range when non-independence exists, compared to the theoretical amount for independent results. Because the variability within each cluster is smaller than the variability between clusters, the average moving range that reflects short-term variability will underestimate the long-term variability, and limits may be too narrow. For this reason, many manufacturers choose to compute the control limits of an individuals chart using the sample standard deviation, which reflects long-term process variability. Figure 8.4 displays the assay data above using this approach.

Because the sample standard deviation includes the variability between drug substance lots (the shifts in the mean), the limits derived from the sample standard deviation are wider compared to those derived from the average moving range. In contrast to limits computed using the average moving range, this simple combination of the within and between subgroup variability often results in an overestimate of variability, which must be considered in both interpretation and effectiveness of control charts and process capability. Statistical modeling of the between and within variance components is an option; however, this is likely a challenging exercise as it may necessitate that both random and nonrandom process practices and constraints be identified and modelled. If necessary, a Bayesian solution could be used to address this complexity.

In some cases, staging the control chart, as in Figure 8.5, is a sensible approach to the treatment of non-independence. The optimum method for computation and interpretation

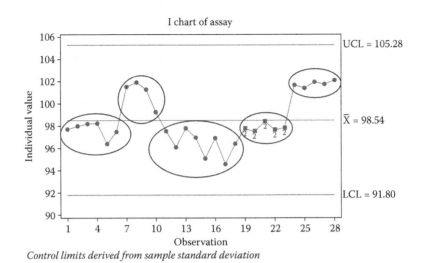

FIGURE 8.4
Individuals chart of Figure 8.3 assay results using sample standard deviation to compute control limits.

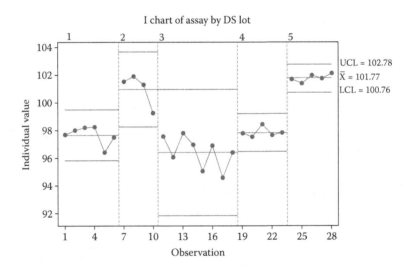

FIGURE 8.5
Individuals chart of Figure 8.4 assay results staged by drug substance lot.

of control limits depends on multiple criteria, including: (1) the data structure, which is inherently tied to manufacturing practices and attribute characteristics; (2) the manner of use of the control chart (determined by the goals of analysis); and (3) risk vs. benefit.

As discussed briefly, the normality assumption is also frequently violated in biopharmaceutical data. Transformation of data to a more normal distribution should not be considered a panacea to this situation. Indeed, there are attributes with underlying distributions that are truly non-normal, such as bounded distributions like impurities; or a lognormal distribution, for some potency measurements. In these cases, evaluation of transformed data may be appropriate. However, quite often the apparent non-normality exists because of nonhomogeneity; that is, the data set includes multiple subpopulations resulting from the non-independence described previously. The observed non-normal distribution in this case is happenstance, and a different (normal or non-normal) distribution will be observed with the next data set. Transformation in this case is not only nonvalue added, it is statistically inappropriate. In these cases, it is most important to recognize the reason for non-normality, potentially exploring the causes of the subpopulations if a risk assessment warrants it.

In practice, non-normality should not have significant consequences, particularly considering the context of CPV as a Phase 1 SPC application. That is, any increase in ARL_0 or Nelson rule violation due to non-normality does not have the same consequences in CPV that it would in a Phase 2 application of SPC. This assumes that a risk-based approach to evaluation of signals is in place. Nelson rules that result from non-normality should not be immediately interpreted as a process out of control; instead the underlying nature of the data, for instance a nonhomogenous distribution, should be understood and acted upon within a risk-based framework. Also, as mentioned earlier, three-sigma limits bracket greater than 97.5% of data from many non-normal distributions. In other words, points outside of control limits occur infrequently even for non-normal distributions, thus signaling a likely change in variability to be evaluated according to the risk-based procedure. Thus, in most cases a Shewhart chart is a reasonable, and even recommended, choice for non-normal data, considering its overall utility in meeting the goals of CPV.

8.4 Business Considerations for Implementation of CPV

For most biopharmaceutical manufacturing organizations, implementation of an effective CPV program will require considerable changes to business processes, resources, and culture. However, if well-designed, the time and effort to establish and maintain it will be far outweighed by the benefits to patients/customers and the business. The key to a well-designed and executed CPV program is to keep in mind the goals of CPV. The procedures, systems, and training that become part of the CPV program must all be designed to evaluate process performance, and take appropriate action commensurate with risk and business benefit. A risk-based approach should be used to design the following elements of a CPV program:

- Parameters (CQAs, CPPs, CMAs, IPCs) to include.
- Level of monitoring to implement.
- Type of charts to use for each parameter.
- Frequency of trending and reporting.
- Sampling plans.
- Criteria for computation of control limits and capability.
- Persons responsible to review charts/metrics and perform any additional evaluations if needed.
- Rules to apply to control charts and reaction to control chart signals.
- Triggers and procedures to change aspects of a CPV plan for a given product.

Manufacturers may choose to standardize elements across all products, or by platform, or to tailor some or all elements to each product. A risk-based approach would align with the latter. Whatever the choice, the greatest benefit from a CPV program will be realized if these decisions are made in a way that enables ongoing learning about process variability, rather than simply an exercise in compliance. There is no single correct or justifiable approach to any of the elements above, though a few recommendations follow.

Parameters to include: In most cases, all critical quality attributes should be monitored. Note, however, that monitoring is not synonymous with control charting, or even run charting (a run chart is simply a plot of consecutive data points over time, with no associated limits or trending alarms). For instance, quality attributes that are consistently below the limit of detection (LOD) may be better summarized in a simple statement and monitored for results above the LOD.

Not all process parameters need to be included in CPV monitoring and trending. Inclusion can be based on risk-based criteria such as the level of process/platform knowledge, process understanding developed during Stages 1 and 2 of the PV lifecycle, process capability, and parameter criticality. Additionally, if the control strategy maintains variation of a parameter within a range that is known to pose negligible patient risk, ongoing trending is not required (this assumes that variation outside that range will be appropriately identified).

Some companies choose to use capability metrics, such as C_{pk}, to prioritize the parameters and choose only to include those with capability below some threshold. While capability estimates can be useful to aid in these decisions, a statistical capability index estimate must be considered carefully, and along with other performance details. Not only are these indices only estimates, often based on a limited or nonhomogenous data set, they do not capture information about the criticality of the parameters to the patient, the basis of specifications (e.g., particularly in biopharmaceutical processes many parameters may have specifications determined based on process capability, thus ensuring low capability indices), or the influence of the control strategy.

Level of monitoring: All attributes and parameters included in a CPV program need not be monitored or trended with the same frequency and rigor. Some parameters may merit sampling beyond release requirements and scrutiny on a frequent basis—for example, a CQA with capability index close to 1, or in the case of a product with little manufacturing experience, for instance during Stage 3A of CPV (baseline performance). Others, for example, an attribute with demonstrated high capability, may only require trending of release results. If varying levels of monitoring and trending are utilized in a CPV program, risk-based criteria and procedures should be used to define and choose those levels, and to trigger any changes to them.

Frequency of trending and reporting: The frequency of review of process data may be one of the most substantial changes from previous practice in implementing CPV. The charts included in an annual product review may not suffice to show that the process has remained in a state of control, assess its capability, and provide for adequate understanding of process variability. While CPV for traditional batch processes (and even elements of continuous processes) is not expected to be real-time SPC trending, the ability to identify and understand the magnitude of sources of variability generally decreases with decreasing frequency of data review and trending. Cumbersome, lengthy reports should not inhibit timely review. Like other elements, the frequency of trending and reporting should be determined using a risk-based approach, with the goal of deeper, ongoing, process understanding.

Types of charts, sampling plans: Ideally a statistician, or someone with extensive statistical training and experience with manufacturing processes and data, should be involved in determining the types of charts to be used and design of sampling plans (when more than routine release testing is deemed appropriate). For most platforms, it is possible to proceduralize the types of charts to be used for typical CPV parameters. The CPV procedures should allow for flexibility in sampling plans, utilizing risk-based decision criteria and expert input.

When to calculate control limits and capability: As noted in Section 8.2.2, some minimum amount of data is required before reasonable control limits can be calculated—and considerations for determining an appropriate minimum must include not only numerical requirements (25–30 data points), but also knowledge regarding routine sources of variability that act on the process over the long term. For example, the variability introduced from multiple lots of a key raw material is routine variability, but may only be observed once multiple batches are manufactured from each lot of raw material. Other such long-term sources of routine variability include seasonal effects, personnel changes, equipment changes, and analytical reference standards. The sources relevant for a given product are determined based on development data and process knowledge. Once these sources are identified, the minimum amount of time, in addition to a minimum number of data points, before computation of long-term control limits and capability can be established. During this time, the process can be considered to be in Stage 3A of the process validation life cycle, gathering information necessary to establish baseline performance. CPV procedures should include these requirements, guidelines for monitoring the process during the period before long-term limits have been set (e.g., use of tentative control or alert limits or run charts), and triggers for recalculating control limits (e.g., process improvements, site-transfers).

Persons Responsible: While it is beneficial and recommended to have a statistician involved in the design of many elements of a CPV program, analysis of charts and metrics is best performed by process subject matter experts, with input from a statistician as needed. Process experts are best able to interpret and understand any patterns or signals on the control charts and to make the risk-based assessments that are key to a value-added and effective CPV program. That said, it is also essential that these process experts be trained in and knowledgeable about the statistical tools they will use (control charts and capability analyses), including the impact of non-independence and nonrandomness on the charts, and that they have access to someone with statistical expertise to assist with complex situations.

Rules to apply to control charts and reaction to control chart signals: Application of a selection of sensitizing rules such as those in Table 8.1 can enhance the ability to understand process variability. Because of the non-independence described above, violation of these rules is expected more often than if the independence assumption were met. It may therefore be tempting to conclude that they should not be used at all. This conclusion is often rooted in a fear of signals (commonly identified with red dots) on charts, because they are immediately translated to a process that is not in control. Or because the signals are identified as undesirable "false positives," and resources will be wasted evaluating them. Each of these reactions is misguided in a scenario of known non-independence. These signals do not necessarily indicate that the process is out of control, nor are they truly false positive signals. In fact, there likely is a change, and the signals enable process understanding. Indeed, there may be situations where the use of multiple signals does not provide much insight, and is not value-added, as in a mature process where sources of variability are well understood, and process capability is broadly acceptable. Otherwise, omission of signals or avoidance through data manipulation or more complicated trending tools can result in missed opportunities for deeper process understanding and improvement. Instead, if process control is interpreted in context of non-independence, and a risk-based approach is used to respond to signals, overreaction is prevented, resources are used wisely, and the signals can potentially be a rich source of information regarding process variability. This enables process improvement, a benefit to both patients and manufacturers. Elements of a risk-based approach is discussed by Scherder and DiMartino et al. [8,9].

Note that the lack of signals does not mean no change has occurred. The ARL for small changes in a Shewhart chart using one or two rules is large. Better ARL performance can be obtained if more rules are applied or by using other charts; the latter comes at the price of ease and interpretation. The next section provides more details and an example. No matter which chart is used, the eyes of a process subject matter expert are a critical tool to maximize the information available.

8.5 Other Control Charts

As noted above, in the context of CPV (aligns with a Phase 1 SPC scenario), a simple Shewhart control chart will often be the appropriate choice for monitoring attributes and parameters. The Shewhart chart is easy to understand, implement, and interpret; this last point being especially important, since more complex charts which don't present the raw data values are harder for the process experts—the people best suited to identify unusual behavior and what might be causing it—to interpret. There are some types of data, however, for which the standard I, I-MR or Xbar-R chart is not an appropriate choice. Recommended charts for some commonly encountered parameters are discussed in this section, along with several other control charts which have superior qualities for specific situations.

Three-way chart (I-MR-R/S): It is common to use an Xbar-R or Xbar-S chart when measurements are taken in subgroups; however, it is also quite common to find that the control limits do not function well to bracket the expected variability, even when a process is completely stable and predictable. This occurs because the within-subgroup variation, which is directly used to compute the limits of the Xbar chart, underestimates the between-subgroup variability. This can be misinterpreted as a process that is out of control, when in fact the relationship between the two variance components (within- and between-subgroup) is expected. In this situation, a three-way chart, also called an I-MR-R/S or between/within chart, is most appropriate. Common examples of parameters for which this type of chart is applicable include multiple measurements at each time point for uniformity of dosage units (UDU), fill weights, and tablet measurements such as hardness. It can also be appropriate when there are samples from multiple pieces of equipment such as dissolution baths or filters. A comparison of the two types of charts to monitor the flux through three separation columns used within a batch is given in Figure 8.6.

The points plotted in the top chart of the XBar chart on the left are the subgroup (batch) averages; that is, the average flux of the three filters used within a batch. The range of the three filters, the within-batch variability, is plotted in the bottom chart. The average range within the batches is used to compute the control limits of the Xbar chart. The multiple out of control points in the Xbar chart result because the average variability *within* a batch does not describe expected variability *between* batches, and the limits on the Xbar chart fail to bracket expected between-batch variability. This can be remedied with the I-MR-R/S chart shown on the right. The points plotted in the top chart are identical to the point in the Xbar chart; that is, they are the batch averages. However, these averages are treated as individual results, and the top two charts are an I-MR chart of the batch average. Accordingly, the control limits of the top chart are derived from the average moving range of the batch

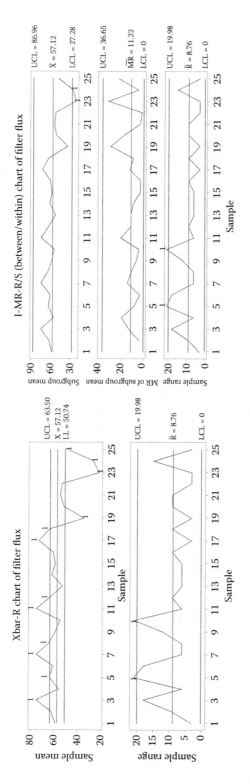

FIGURE 8.6
Example Xbar-R chart (left) and three-way (I-MR-R/S) control chart (right).

average, thus bracketing the expected between-batch (subgroup) variability. The bottom chart is identical to the R-chart in the Xbar-R chart.

Differences in the two variance components may be completely expected, often supported by scientific reasoning, and not necessarily an indication of a process control issue. Failure to recognize the differences in the expected between- and within-subgroup variability can lead to poor chart performance, resulting in either overreaction or underreaction to between-subgroup variability.

Charts for attribute (pass/fail) or count data: As discussed above, I, I-MR, or I-MR-R/S charts may be used for the vast majority of continuous data measurements. They are in fact recommended in the context of CPV due to their simplicity and ease of interpretation even for parameters that do not follow a normal distribution. However, there are some exceptions, the most common being counts or proportions of defective units (binomial data) or counts of defects per unit (Poisson data). The charts appropriate for these types of data are summarized in Table 8.3. Note that even for count or proportions data, if the values are far enough from 0 (counts) or from both 0 and 1 (proportions), then a chart intended for normally distributed data may be used, but a statistician should be involved in this decision.

CUSUM and EWMA charts: One critique of Shewhart charts often cited is that the average run length to detect small changes is greater than other available charts, specifically cumulative sum (CUSUM) and exponentially weighted moving average (EWMA) charts. For instance, the CUSUM chart will detect a 1σ shift about four times as fast as a Shewhart chart when only the first sensitization rule (outside of control limit) is applied. For large shifts, CUSUM and EWMA charts are less sensitive compared to a Shewhart chart; combined CUSUM-Shewhart or EWMA-Shewhart procedures can address this limitation [2]. The detection of smaller shifts using Shewhart charts can be improved to the levels of the other charts by applying sensitizing rules in addition to Rule 1. The concern with this action is the subsequent increase in false positive signals; that is, a signal of a change when there has not been any change in distribution.

The increased sensitivity of CUSUM and EWMA charts could lead practitioners to swiftly choose them as a preferred chart for CPV. However, like other elements of a CPV program, a comparison of chart characteristics and, ultimately, the choice of chart must account for the goals and typical environment of CPV (aligned with Phase 1 SPC). For instance, immediate response to a process change is not sought, and large sources of variability remain, and are often deemed acceptable. Also, the consequences of false positive signals in a Phase 2 environment are not relevant in CPV, as retrospective review allows careful interpretation of signals in context of risk (assuming there is a risk-based procedure to respond to signals). As noted above, in a Phase 1 SPC application, such as CPV, the identification of assignable causes is more important than occurrence of false alarms. Assignable causes can be easiest to identify on a Shewhart chart given patterns have direct physical meaning.

TABLE 8.3

Control Charts for Counts or Proportions

Data Type	Type of Chart
Proportion defective units (Binomial)	P Chart
Number of defective units (Binomial)	NP Chart
Number of defects (Poisson)	C Chart
Number of defects per unit (Poisson)	U Chart

Indeed, there may be situations where prompt identification of small changes is critical and CUSUM or EWMA charts are the optimal chart choice. However, basing the choice on this quality alone, overlooking the CPV environment, resources, ease of deployment, and loss of interpretability may inhibit the goals of CPV. The benefit of detecting small shifts more rapidly must be weighed against these elements.

Cumulative sum (CUSUM) control charts display the cumulative sum of the subgroup mean or individual value differences from the target value, rather than the values themselves. Thus, while in a Shewhart chart each new point reflects the information in only that sample, in a CUSUM chart each new point is calculated using all the samples up to and including the current one. CUSUM can be represented in two ways: (1) tabular CUSUM and (2) V-mask form. Montgomery provides several reasons to choose tabular CUSUM instead of the V-mask form [2], and discussion here is limited to tabular CUSUM. In tabular CUSUM form, the control limits are typically set as a multiple of the process standard deviation σ, referred to as the decision interval. The performance of tabular CUSUM depends on both the width of the decision interval (often 4 or 5σ), and a slack value, k.

Exponentially weighted moving average (EWMA) charts display the weighted average of all subgroup means or individual values including the current sample, with the weights decreasing exponentially going backward in time through the samples. The ARL performance of EWMA charts can approximate that of CUSUM charts. Performance depends on the choice of two parameters, L (the multiple of sigma used in the control limits) and λ (the weighting constant). ARL_0 performance of EWMA charts is robust to non-normality.

Figures 8.7–8.9 illustrate Shewhart, CUSUM, and EWMA charts for a parameter that includes a 1.5σ process shift at observation 21, followed by a brief return to previous conditions beginning at observation 31.

It is clear that the sensitivity of the Shewhart chart to a shift of this magnitude using only Nelson Rule 1 is inferior to the CUSUM and EWMA (detection at batch 35 vs 26). However, the application of the additional Nelson rules increased the sensitivity of the Shewhart chart to the level of the other two charts. Immediate interpretation of the variability

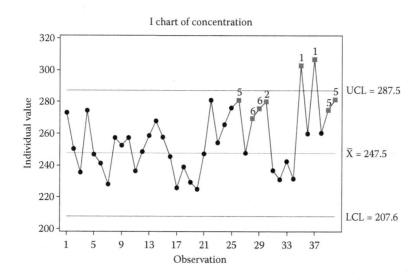

FIGURE 8.7
Shewhart individuals chart with all Nelson rules applied; 1.5σ process shift at observation 21, with temporary return at batch 31.

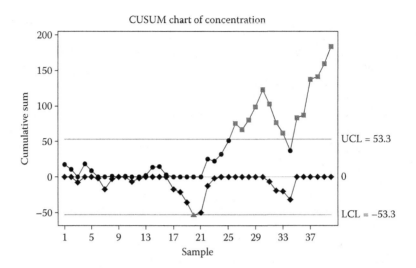

FIGURE 8.8
CUSUM chart (h = 4, k = 0.5) of Figure 8.7 data; 1.5σ process shift at observation 21, with temporary return at batch 31.

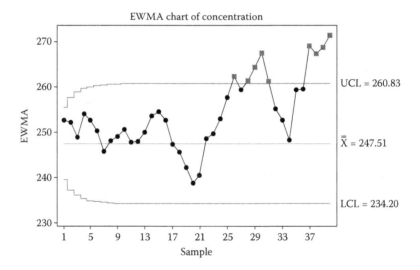

FIGURE 8.9
EWMA chart (λ = 0.2) of Figure 8.7 data; 1.5σ process shift at observation 21, with temporary return at batch 31.

pattern (exact timing and magnitude in raw terms), which is essential to identification and practical significance of process changes, is most straightforward in the raw data/scale of the Shewhart chart. Also, no matter what chart is chosen to identify process changes, a chart of raw data is often necessary to fully and practically interpret the pattern for potential causes.

Multivariate Control Charts: One challenge biopharmaceutical manufacturers face in implementing CPV is the large number of measured parameters (CQAs, CPPs, CMAs, and in-process data) from some processes. The resources required if many parameters are to be collected/trended/reported is daunting. Also, the Type I error and probability of a point correctly plotting inside limits when the process is in control for the collection of charts is not equal to the values for each chart treated independently. The Type I error is inflated due to the simultaneous evaluation of many charts. Furthermore, quality may be better described by the joint behavior of two or more parameters, instead of the independent behavior of each parameter. In such situations, the use of multivariate process monitoring, such as Hotelling T^2 charts, or principal components, may be an option. Practitioners are encouraged to have more than a cursory understanding of these methods and to seek expert advice before implementation. Discussion here is limited to general considerations.

Although multivariate monitoring can provide superior performance to univariate monitoring in some situations, it should not be construed as a magical solution to the issue of many variables or correlation among variables. The potential advantages come at the price of increased complexity and associated consequences. Proper implementation and evaluation of multivariate monitoring is challenging; thus, the risk of erroneous conclusions regarding process behavior can actually be greater compared to a univariate evaluation of correlated variables. The increased difficulty to interpret multivariate charts and signals can result in a loss in the process knowledge gained from chart review, and an increase in resources required to evaluate charts—the exact opposite of the expected advantage of a multivariate approach.

Before choosing a multivariate solution, the underlying need and expected advantages should be warranted from both statistical and scientific perspectives. It may be possible to reduce the number of monitored parameters through risk assessment that incorporates process knowledge and the control strategy. This approach will often be more effective to meet the goals of CPV than trending a multivariate combinations of parameters.

References

1. U.S. Food and Drug Administration (FDA). Guidance for Industry. Process Validation: General Principles and Practices. Revision 1, January 2011.
2. Montgomery, D. C. *Introduction to Statistical Quality Control*, 7th ed. John Wiley & Sons, Inc, 2013.
3. Woodall, W. H. Controversies and contradictions in statistical process control. *Journal of Quality Technology*, 32, 4, October 2000.
4. Nelson, L. S. Technical aids. *Journal of Quality Technology*, 16, 4, October 1984.
5. Wheeler, D. J. Are you sure we don't need normally distributed data? *Quality Digest*, November 2010.
6. Wheeler, D. J. Avoiding statistical jabberwocky. *Quality Digest*, October 2009.
7. Balestracci, D. Four control chart myths from foolish experts. *Quality Digest*, March 2011.
8. Scherder, T. Embrace special cause variation during CPV. *Pharmaceutical Engineering*, 37, 3, May/June 2017.
9. DiMartino, M., Zamamirim, A., Pipkins, K., Heimbach, J., Hamann, E., Adhibhatta, S., Falcon, R., Legg, K., Payne, R. CPV signal responses in the biopharmaceutical industry. *Pharmaceutical Engineering*, 37, 1, January/February 2017.

9

Multivariate Analysis for Bioprocess Understanding and Troubleshooting

Jianchun Zhang and Harry Yang

CONTENTS

9.1 Background

Bioprocess development is a complex process due to the nature of manufacturing living cells. In general, it consists of development of both upstream and downstream processes. The former involves selection of host cell line, development of culture medium, design of bioreactor and its operating conditions. The latter encompasses several filtration and purification steps to maximize yield and reduce impurities. During the process development, vast amounts of online and offline data are generated. These data, however, are often highly correlated, making the process understanding, optimization, and control a daunting task. The increasing acceptance of quality-by-design (QbD) and process analytical technology (PAT) to biopharmaceutical industry provides an important opportunity for better process understanding, optimization, and control. The objective of QbD initiatives by the U.S. FDA (FDA 2004a) and ICH (ICH 2006) is to use systematic risk-based lifecycle approaches to manufacturing process development. QbD begins with predefined objectives and emphasizes product and process understanding and process control based on

273

scientific risk management. PAT (FDA 2004b), on the other hand, is a system for designing, analyzing, and controlling pharmaceutical manufacturing processes through measurements of critical raw and in-process materials and process parameters that affect critical quality attributes. Among the PAT tools are some statistical techniques of multivariate data analysis (MVDA) and multivariate statistical process control (MSPC).

Multivariate data-based statistical methods play a critical role in providing valuable insight during the life cycle of biopharmaceutical process development. Product development starts with defining the quality target product profile (QTPP) in terms of its desired clinical benefits and quality standard. This is followed by identification of critical quality attributes (CQAs), which should be within appropriate limits or distribution to warrant product quality. After the CQAs are defined, process development becomes the central focus. To develop a manufacturing process that produces a product in line with the QTPP, experiments are designed and carried out to understand process parameters and their interactions. These experiments are multivariate in nature both with respect to input variables and response measures. To determine the optimal operating condition and design space, multivariate analysis becomes necessary.

As discussed in Chapter 6, the safety, efficacy, and quality of a biological product is warranted through a set of effective control strategies. Understanding the relationships between CQAs and raw material attributes/process parameters enables the development of such control strategy. However, due to the large number of variables, their interactions, and potential collinearity, it is challenging to effectively extract information from such complex data. *Principal component analysis* (PCA) provides a means of reducing the dimensionality of the data and coping with collinearity and possible missing data. Through decomposing the covariance matrix of the data, it projects the high-dimensional data set onto a low dimension space spanned by so-called principal components, which represent the directions of major variability in the data. The concept of PCA is illustrated in Figure 9.1. The data in the graph show that the three quality attributes are highly correlated as evidenced by the fact that their measured values vary in a flat plane spanned by two perpendicular lines, u_1 and u_2. Therefore, each of the measurement (x_1, x_2, x_3) can be expressed as a linear combination of u_1 and u_2. That is, there exist two constant a and b

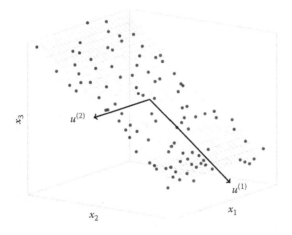

FIGURE 9.1
Principal component analysis reduces dimensionality of data by projecting the original data to two principal components which represent the directions of largest variability in the data.

such that $(x_1, x_2, x_3) = a \times u_1 + b \times u_2$. This is to say that the three-dimensional measurement (x_1, x_2, x_3) can be expressed as a point (a, b) in the two-dimensional space. This transformation or projection only reduces the dimensionality of the data but also remove the interdependence among the original three CQAs as the perpendicularity of the two axis lines u_1 and u_2 implies the independence between the transformed variables a and b. Since the number of principal components needed to explain the overall process variability is often much less than the number of original variables, such reduction simplifies data analysis and interpretation, making it easier for process understanding, outlier identification, and root cause analysis.

When the data set contains both the product quality variables and process parameters, it is often difficult to describe the data using the traditional regression techniques because of high dimensionality and multicollinearity. *Partial least square* (PLS) is a useful alternative method. It reduces the dimensionality for both process variables and response variables by projecting these two sets of variables to their respective spaces spanned by their corresponding sets of latent variables while maintaining the information contained in the original data. This is accomplished through maximizing the covariance matrices between the process variables and response variables. It also effectively removes the multicollinearity within the data. In addition, possible missing data can be nicely handled by the PLS method.

Statistical process monitoring and control (chart) is an integral part of the overall control strategy to ensure manufacturing consistency. However, control charts designed for univariate analysis are less effective in monitoring multivariate process quality or parameter variables. On one hand, using univariate statistical process control charts may greatly inflate the Type I error as the number of variables to be monitored increases. In other words, the probability of falsely detecting an out-of-control event will be much greater than the nominal Type I error rate. On the other hand, because some of the variables could be highly correlated, an out-of-control event might be missed by univariate control charts. This problem is illustrated in Figure 9.2, where each of the two univariate control charts does not indicate the points marked by "*" as out-of-control. However, it is captured in the multivariate control chart because these points are beyond the ellipse, which is the control limit of the multivariate control chart. The reason for this is that univariate control

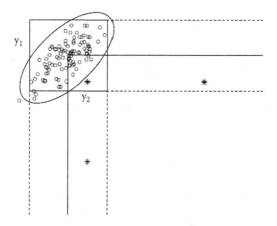

FIGURE 9.2
Performance of multivariate control chart versus univarite control charts. (Adapted from Kourti, T. and MacGregor, J.F., Process analysis, monitoring and diagnosis, using multivariate projection method, *Chemometrics and Intelligent Laboratory Systems*, 28(1), 3, 1995.)

charts fail to account for the positive correlation between the two variables and use the squared region at the upper left-hand corner as the acceptable limit for both variables when in fact the acceptable region is the ellipse established based on the joint distribution of the two variables. Traditional multivariate control charts such as Hotelling's T^2 chart is used for multivariate process monitoring. The Hotelling's T^2 statistics follows a scaled F-distribution and thus a single one-sided control limit is sufficient to control the overall Type I error for the many correlated variables. Montgomery (2008) gave an introduction to multivariate control charts. As Montgomery (2008) points out, the average run-length (ARL) performance to detect a specified shift increases, making the traditional control charts ineffective as monitoring tools when the number of variables is large. PCA and PLS are two useful dimension reduction methods that can be used for process control and monitoring.

Over the past decade, driven by the regulatory quality initiatives (FDA 2004a; ICH 2006, 2007a, 2007b, and 2011), multivariate analysis techniques have been used extensively for bioprocess development, optimization, and monitoring. For example, several case examples on bioprocessing are provided by Johnson et al. (2007). LeBrun (2012) presents examples on how to use multivariate analyses for analytical development. A thorough discussion of determining Bayesian design space can be found in Peterson (2008) and Stockdale and Cheng (2009). The intent of this chapter is to provide an in-depth discussion of the currently available multivariate methods and illustrate their applications using examples in the published literature. The remaining of this chapter is organized as follows: Section 9.2 gives a general technical description of multiple regression, PCA, and PLS, followed by multivariate process control in Section 9.3; Section 9.4 provides four examples to illustrate how these multivariate tools are applied to bioprocess optimization, batch comparability assessment, process control, and fault detection; concluding remarks are given in Section 9.5.

9.2 Multivariate Analysis

9.2.1 Multiple Regression

Multiple regression is one of the most widely used methods in process development and optimization. It models the relationships between a set of CQAs of the product and process parameters. Let $\mathbf{Y} = (Y_1, \ldots, Y_p)'$ be a $p \times 1$ vector of measures of p CQAs, A the set of joint acceptable ranges of the CQAs, and $\mathbf{x}$ a $k \times 1$ vector of process parameters and other controllable inputs, such as material attributes. Suppose that the relationship between $\mathbf{Y}$ and $\mathbf{x}$ can be characterized through the following model:

$$\mathbf{Y} = \mathbf{f}(\mathbf{x}; \boldsymbol{\theta}) + \boldsymbol{\varepsilon} \tag{9.1}$$

where $\mathbf{f}(\mathbf{x}; \theta)$ is a mathematical function, θ are model parameters, and ε are measurement errors.

There are several applications of the multiple regression model in Equation 9.1. One is to determine the joint operating range which gives rise to outputs meeting certain specifications. The other is to identify the optimum operating condition. This can be accomplished through the desirability function approach as described below. Furthermore, coupled with prior knowledge of the model parameter θ, one may determine the design space of process parameters as follows:

$$DS = \left\{ \mathbf{x} : \Pr\left[\mathbf{Y} \in A | \mathbf{x}, data\right] \right\} \tag{9.2}$$

where $\Pr[\mathbf{Y} \in A | \mathbf{x}, data]$ is the posterior predictive probability (Peterson 2008; Stockdale and Cheng 2009).

9.2.1.1 Overlapping Response Surfaces

Let $\hat{\boldsymbol{\theta}}$ be the vector of estimates of the model parameters. Then the predicted mean values of the CQAs at $\mathbf{x}$ is given by $\hat{E}[\mathbf{Y} | \mathbf{x}] = \mathbf{f}(\mathbf{x}; \hat{\boldsymbol{\theta}})$. The idea of the overlapping mean approach is to identify a common set of $\mathbf{x}$ values or space, denoted as Ω, such that the predicted values of the CQAs are within their acceptable limits. That is,

$$\Omega = \left\{ \mathbf{x} : \hat{E}[\mathbf{Y} | \mathbf{x}] \in A \right\}. \tag{9.3}$$

Figure 9.3 illustrates the idea of overlapping mean surfaces for a cell culture system with two CQAs, yield and cell viability, and two critical parameters, temperature and pH. The shaded region of temperature and pH represent the normal operating region, in which both the yield and cell viability meet their specifications.

In the literature, the overlapping response surfaces have been used to determine design space for process parameters (CMC Biotech Working Group 2009; Ng and Rajagopalan 2009; and CMC Vaccine Working Group 2012) and normal operating range for analytical methods (Sivakumar and Valliappan 2007; LeBrun 2012). In Section 9.4, we provide a detailed discussion of an application of the overlapping response surfaces to develop a chromatography assay provided by Sirvakumar and Valliappan (2007).

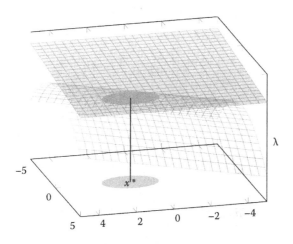

FIGURE 9.3
Operation region determined based on two overlapping mean response surfaces.

9.2.1.2 Desirability Approach

In process development, it is often desired to find operating conditions at which the process assumes maximum performance such as highest yield and lowest impurities. However, the conditions that result in the highest yield does not necessarily produce the product of least amount of impurities. Therefore, optimization of one quality attribute is often achieved at the expense of others. To ensure a viable process that produces quality product, there is always a trade-off. One way to make such trade-off is through the use of so-called desirability function. First introduced by Harrington (1965), the desirability function provides a means of measuring closeness of each response to its objective. The optimum operating condition is one such that the desirability function achieves its maximum value. For each response, Y_i, $i = 1,...,p$, the desirability function $d(Y)$ assumes values in the range of 0 and 1, with 0 and 1 corresponding to the least and most desirable values, respectively. These functions are then combined to give rise to an overall desirability function, using geometric mean:

$$D(\mathbf{Y}) = \left[\prod_{i=1}^{p} d(Y_i) \right]^{1/p} .$$

Since the objectives of quality attributes are different, as some are to be maximized, some are to be minimized, and others are to be maintained around target values, it is critical to define the individual desirability functions commensurate with their objectives. For this purpose, Derringer and Suich (1980) proposed a set of desirability functions. We define L_i, U_i, and T_i as the lower, upper, and target values, respectively, for the quality attribute Y_i such that $L_i \leq T_i \leq U_i$. Depending on whether the objective is to meet target, maximization, or minimization, the following desirability functions $d_T(Y_i)$, $d_T(Y_i)$, or $d_L(Y_i)$ may be used:

$$d_T(Y_i) = \begin{cases} 0 & \text{if } Y_i < L_i \\ \left(\dfrac{Y_i - L_i}{T_i - L_i} \right)^s & \text{if } L_i \leq Y_i \leq T_i \\ \left(\dfrac{Y_i - U_i}{T_i - U_i} \right)^t & \text{if } T_i < Y_i \leq U_i \\ 0 & \text{if } Y_i > U_i \end{cases}$$

with the parameters s and t being chosen to reflect the importance to meet the target,

$$d_U(Y_i) = \begin{cases} 0 & \text{if } Y_i < L_i \\ \left(\dfrac{Y_i - L_i}{T_i - L_i} \right)^s & \text{if } L_i \leq Y_i \leq T_i \\ 1 & \text{if } Y_i > T_i \end{cases}$$

with T_i being a value deemed to be large enough,

$$d_L(Y_i) = \begin{cases} 1 & \text{if } Y_i < T_i \\ \left(\dfrac{Y_i - L_i}{T_i - L_i}\right)^s & \text{if } T_i \le Y_i \le U_i \\ 0 & \text{if } Y_i > U_i \end{cases}$$

with T_i being a value deemed to be small enough.

9.2.1.3 Bayesian Approach

As noted by several researchers (Peterson 2008; Stockdale and Cheng 2009; LeBrun 2012), the overlapping mean surfaces method suffers several deficiencies. Chief among those is that it only warrants that the response values of the CQAs, on the average, are within their acceptable limits when the process parameters are within the design space. This obviously does not provide sufficient quality assurance. Second, it does not account for the variability in the model parameters, nor does it take into account the potential correlations among the multivariate CQAs. As a remedy, Bayesian analysis was suggested (Peterson 2008; Stockdale and Cheng 2009; LeBrun 2012), which is briefly described in the following.

Assume the function $\mathbf{f}(\mathbf{x};\theta)=\mathbf{Bz}(\mathbf{x})$, where $\mathbf{B}$ is a $p \times q$ matrix of regression coefficients, $\mathbf{z}(\mathbf{x})$ is a $q \times 1$ vector of function of $\mathbf{x}$."; Let Σ be the variance–covariance matric of the measurement errors ε in Equation 9.1. We further assume that the parameters $\mathbf{B}$ and Σ have a noninformative joint prior distribution. That is,

$$p(\mathbf{B}, \Sigma) \propto |\Sigma|^{-(p+1)/2}. \tag{9.4}$$

The posterior predictive distribution is a multivariate-t with degrees of freedom $\nu = n - p - q + 1$, that is,

$$\tilde{\mathbf{Y}}|\mathbf{x}, data \sim t_\nu\left(\hat{\mathbf{B}}\mathbf{z}(\mathbf{x}), \mathbf{H}\right) \tag{9.5}$$

where $\mathbf{H} = [1 + \mathbf{z}(\mathbf{x})'\mathbf{D}^{-1}\mathbf{z}(\mathbf{x})]\hat{\Sigma}$ and $\mathbf{D} = \sum_{i=1}^{n} \mathbf{Z}_i\mathbf{Z}_i'$, where $\mathbf{Z}_i = \mathbf{Z}(x_i)$, $i = 1,...,n$. $\hat{\mathbf{B}}$ and $\hat{\Sigma}$ are the least squares estimates of $\mathbf{B}$ and Σ given by $\hat{\mathbf{B}} = (\mathbf{Z}'_{exp}\mathbf{Z}_{exp})^{-1}\mathbf{Z}'_{exp}\mathbf{Y}_{obs}$ and $\hat{\Sigma} = [\mathbf{Y}_{obs} - (\hat{\mathbf{B}}\mathbf{Z})']'[\mathbf{Y}_{obs} - (\hat{\mathbf{B}}\mathbf{Z})']/\nu$, respectively, with $\nu = n - p - q + 1$, where $\mathbf{Y}_{obs} = (\mathbf{Y}_1,...,\mathbf{Y}_n)'$ be an $n \times p$ matrix consisting of n observations of the $1 \times p$ response vector $\mathbf{Y}$ and $\mathbf{Z}_{exp} = (\mathbf{Z}_1,...,\mathbf{Z}_n)'$ be an $n \times q$ matrix.

A design space can be obtained by determining $\mathbf{x}$ such that

$$\left\{\mathbf{x} : \Pr\left[\mathbf{Y} \in A | \mathbf{x}, data\right] \ge R\right\}. \tag{9.6}$$

where R is a preselected positive value between 0 and 1. Figure 9.4 shows an example of Bayesian design space. It consists of combinations of process parameters, pH and protein load, such that the posterior predictive probability $\Pr[Y \in A | x, data]$ exceeds 99%.

As previously discussed, it is advantageous to apply the Bayesian approach to determine the design space. In addition, because of readily available software packages such as WinBUGS (Ntzoufras 2008), implementation of computation-intensive Bayesian approach becomes straightforward. Several excellent examples of using multivariate Bayesian analysis to optimize multiple response surfaces and determine multivariate design space were given by Peterson (2004, 2008) and Stockdale and Cheng (2009). Lebrun (2012) provided case examples for analytical method optimization based on multivariate analysis.

9.2.2 PCA

PCA can be viewed as a method to obtain a new coordinate system formed by a smaller number of orthogonal latent variables which contains the most informative dimensions. For a sample data matrix X with n observations each having K variables, it can be decomposed as follows:

$$X = TP' \tag{9.7}$$

where T is the score matrix and P is the loading matrix. Denote $P = (p_1, p_2, \cdots, p_K)$ and $T = (t_1, t_2, \cdots, t_K)$. The first principal component p_1 is the line (or coordinate axis) in the K-dimensional space that best approximates the data in terms of variability. Mathematically, p_1 is chosen to maximize:

$$Var(Xp_1) \text{ subject to } p_1'p_1 = 1. \tag{9.8}$$

The score vector t_1 is the coordinate of X projected to p_1, such that $t_1 = Xp_1$. The second principal component p_2 is the line in the K-dimensional space that best approximates the data while being orthogonal to p_1. Mathematically, p_2 is to maximize:

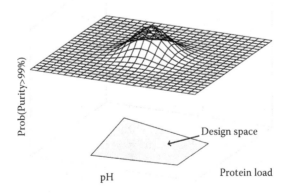

FIGURE 9.4
Design space (DS) based on Bayesian predictive modeling that links input process parameters **x** and material attribute **z** with CQAs **Y**. The DS is determined such that there is a high probability that the CQAs jointly meet their acceptance criteria when the process parameters and material attributes are within the DS.

$$Var(Xp_2) \text{ subject to } p_2'p_2 = 1 \text{ and } p_1'p_2 = 0. \tag{9.9}$$

In general, the k-th principal component is the k-th line in the K-dimensional space that best approximates the data while being orthogonal to the space expanded by the previous $(k-1)$ principal components. Computationally, however, one does not need to do the calculation one by one. In fact, the previously mentioned maximization problem can be solved with decomposing the covariance matrix of X, say S, to

$$S = P\Lambda P' \tag{9.10}$$

where the loading matrix P is orthonormal with its columns being referred to as eigenvectors; and $\Lambda = (\lambda_1, \lambda_2, \cdots, \lambda_K)$ is a diagonal matrix with elements being the eigenvalues of S sorted in descending order. It is not difficult to show that the variance of the k-th score vector is λ_K.

Usually, only a few principal components are needed, say r components. The data matrix X can then be reconstructed using the first r PCA scores and loadings, that is,

$$X = T_r P_r' + E \tag{9.11}$$

where T_r and P_r are the score and loading matrices from the first r principal components, and E is the residual matrix by not using all the K principal components. The objective of dimension reduction for PCA is to use as few principal components as possible to explain the variability of the original data matrix X. A natural question is how many principal components are needed. There are several techniques to determine the optimal number of principal components to be used. A popular graphic technique is called *scree plot*. A scree plot is a plot of ordered eigenvalues from the largest to smallest. The appropriate

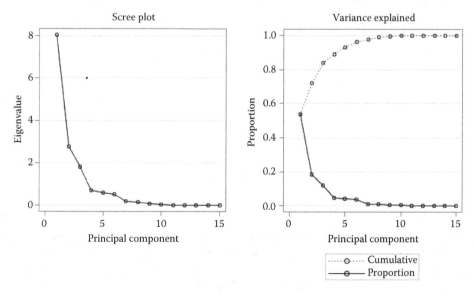

FIGURE 9.5
Scree plot and cumulative variance for number of PCA components.

number of principal components is taken to be the point at which the remaining eigenvalues are relatively small. Figure 9.5 shows a scree plot, an "elbow" occurs in the plot at about $r = 4$ in this example. That is, the first four principal components effectively summarize the total variance. Another popular method is cross-validation in which a PCA model is developed based on $n - 1$ batches, and the response value of the left-out batch is predicted from the model and compared to its observed value. Ultimately, the number of latent vectors is chosen to optimize a cross-validation statistic such as predicted residual sum of squares.

When performing PCA, it would be intuitive for interpretation purposes if no data transformation is performed. However, data transformation is often necessary as the variables of data matrix represent very different attributes of interest and may have substantially different numerical ranges. Without transformation, a variable with large variance is more likely to be given more weight than the low-variance variable. Prior to principal component analysis, it is a common practice to transform the data into a form such that each variable has equal "weight" to form the principal components unless there is prior knowledge that transformation may have undesirable effect. Usually, each column of X is first subject to mean-centering by subtracting the column mean and then to scaling by dividing by the column standard deviation. After mean-centering and scaling, each column of X will have mean 0 and variance 1.

9.2.3 PLS

PLS stands for partial least squares, or more specifically, projection to latent structures by means of partial least squares. Instead of finding hyperplanes of maximum variance between the response and explanatory variables, it first projects both the explanatory variables and the response variables to new spaces of low dimensions spanned by latent variables and then tries to find the maximal covariance of the latent variables.

Formally, assume that X is an $n \times m$ data matrix of explanatory variables and Y is an $n \times q$ data matrix of response variables, so that each row of X and Y represents a joint data point. Also assume that X and Y are properly centered and possibly scaled as in principal component analysis. Rather than to find the linear relationship between X and Y directly, both X and Y are modeled by linear latent variables according to the following PCA-like expressions:

$$X = TP' + E \tag{9.12}$$

and

$$Y = UQ' + F, \tag{9.13}$$

where T and U are called score matrices, P and Q are the loading matrices, while E and F are the respective residual matrices. The x-scores T are linear combinations of x-variables; y-scores U are linear combinations of y-variables. Let $U = T + H$ with H as the residual matrix; Y can be written as $Y = TQ' + F$, with new residual matrix F (with a bit of abuse of notation). Finally, let t_i, u_i, p_i, q_i denote the i-th columns of $T, U, P,$ and Q, respectively.

The algorithm of PLS starts with finding the first component by maximizing the covariance of $t_1 = Xw_1$ and $u_1 = Yc_1$ with restrictions $t_1't_1 = 1$ and $u_1'u_1 = 1$. Mathematically, the maximum is attained when w_1 and c_1 are corresponding to the largest singular value of $X'Y$. Then the first score vectors t_1 and u_1 are readily available. The PLS method predicts X and Y by regressing on t_1, that is

$$\hat{X} = t_1 p_1' \text{ where } p_1 = (t_1't_1)^{-1}t_1'X$$
$$\hat{Y} = t_1 q_1' \text{ where } q_1 = (t_1't_1)^{-1}t_1'Y$$

(9.14)

where p_1 and q_1 are the loading vector for X and Y, respectively.

The residual matrices, $X_1 = X - \hat{X}$ and $Y_1 = Y - \hat{Y}$, are called *deflated matrices*. The second component is obtained in the same way by replacing X and Y with X_1 and Y_1 to obtain the score vectors t_2 and u_2 as well as loading vectors p_2 and q_2. The process of extracting score vectors and loading vectors and deflated matrices is repeated for as many latent components as desired. Finally, vectors t, u, p, and q are saved as columns in matrices T, U, P, Q. Similar to PCA, the optimal number of latent components is often determined using methods such as cross-validation.

9.3 Multivariate Process Control

9.3.1 Process Control

Statistical process control charts such as the Shewhart chart, CUSUM chart, and EWMA chart are well-established procedures for monitoring univariate processes. The Hotelling's T^2 chart (Montgomery, 2008) represents a natural extension of the univariate Shewhart chart to multivariate situations. Multivariate process control techniques reduce the dimensionality of data generated from process development, optimization, and monitoring down to one or two metrics through the application of multivariate statistical modeling. As with univariate statistical process control, development of multivariate control encompasses two phases. In Phase I, historical data are collected to retrospectively construct an in-control process by excluding out-of-control data. In Phase II, the control limits derived from in-control process from Phase I are then applied to monitor incoming process data.

Assume that a PCA is constructed based on historical data and the first r principal components are considered important using methods such as scree plot or cross-validation. For an individual data x, the score vector is $t = x'P_r = (t_1, \cdots, t_r)$, the PCA-based multivariate control chart in terms of Hotelling's T^2 can be plotted based on the first r principal components, that is,

$$T_r^2 = \sum_{k=1}^{r} \frac{t_k^2}{\lambda_k}.$$

(9.15)

Tracy et al. (1992) pointed out that, for Phase I, T_r^2 follows a (scaled) Beta-distribution with parameters $r/2$ and $(n - r - 1)/2$. Thus, the upper control limit (UCL) for this chart is given by

$$T_{r,UCL}^2 = \frac{(n-1)^2}{n} B_{1-\alpha}\left[r/2, (n-r-1)/2\right] \tag{9.16}$$

where $B_{1-\alpha}[r/2, (n - r - 1)/2]$ is the lower $(1 - \alpha)$ quantile of the Beta distribution with parameters $r/2$ and $(n - r - 1)/2$. A control limit for Phase II, however, is given by

$$T_{r,UCL}^2 = \frac{r(n^2-1)}{n(n-r)} F_{1-\alpha}(r, n-r), \tag{9.17}$$

where $F_{1-\alpha}(r, n - r)$ is the lower $(1 - \alpha)$ quantile of F distribution with degrees-of-freedom r and $n - r$. Although a control chart based on the first few principal components can capture the majority of out-of-control events, abnormal effects due to variation orthogonal to the plane formed by the first few principal components are unable to be detected if they occur. Therefore, it is also necessary to monitor the residual variation not explained by the first r principal components. This residual variability is called *squared prediction error* (SPE). SPE is calculated as

$$Q = (x - \hat{x})'(x - \hat{x}) \tag{9.18}$$

where $\hat{x}$ is the vector of predicted value using the first r principal components, that is, $\hat{x} = tP_r'$.

When the process is "in-control," the Q value should be small. The $100(1 - \alpha)\%$ upper control limit of Q can be computed using approximate result from the distribution of quadratic forms (Jackson, 1991), and is given by

$$Q_{UCL} = \theta_1 \left[\frac{z_{1-\alpha}\sqrt{2\theta_2 h_0^2}}{\theta_1} + \frac{\theta_2 h_0(h_0-1)}{\theta_1^2} + 1 \right]^{1/h_0} \tag{9.19}$$
$$\text{where } h_0 = 1 - \frac{2\theta_1\theta_3}{3\theta_2^2}; \ \theta_i = \sum_{k=r+1}^{K} \lambda_k^i \text{ for } i = 1, 2, 3.$$

When a data point is beyond the T_r^2 or Q control limit, the process is declared to be out-of-control. Possible root-cause needs to be found to restore the process back to normal. With PCA, process variables or product quality attributes are transformed and it is difficult to ascertain which variable contributes to the out-of-control. Miller et al. (1998) proposed to use a contribution plot to decompose the t-score into K terms, corresponding to the K variables. A contribution plot is a bar chart of the contributions of each of the process variables to the statistic. The contribution to the T_r^2 statistic from the jth variable is the jth entry of $x'P_r\Lambda_r^{-1}P_r'$, where Λ_r is the diagonal matrix of the first largest r eigenvalues. For the Q statistic, the contribution of the jth variable is the jth entry of the vector $x - \hat{x}$.

Similar to PCA, PLS can also be used for process control. Write $Y = TQ' + F$ as $Y = XM + F$. The score matrix T and coefficient matrix M can be calculated as $T = XR$, $M = RQ'$, where $P'R = R'P = I_r$, with I_r being identity matrix with r latent variables to be used. The Hotelling's T^2 statistic is

$$T_r^2 = x'R\left(\frac{T'T}{n-1}\right)^{-1} R'x \qquad (9.20)$$

and the SPE statistics is calculated as

$$Q = (x - \hat{x})'(x - \hat{x}) \qquad (9.21)$$

with $\hat{x} = PR'x$. Control limits for these statistics are similar to those used for PCA monitoring; see Yin et al. (2011).

9.3.2 Batch Process Monitoring

Monitoring batch processes is important to ensure that process operation is smooth and resultant products are of high quality. Thanks to the advanced technologies and low-cost computers that are connected to the processes, real-time data of process conditions can be collected nowadays without much difficulty. The advantage of real-time or online process monitoring is that abnormal batches can be found in a timely manner for decision-makers. Multivariate statistical methods have been extended to online monitoring and fault detection of batch processes (Nomikos and MacGregor 1995). For typical batch processes, the data is multivariate at each measured time point for each batch/unit operation. Let $\mathbf{X}$ denote all the measurements of process variables throughout the duration of the process and $\mathbf{Y}$ the measurement of final product quality. The $\mathbf{X}$ matrix is an $I \times J \times K$ array, where I is the number of batches or runs, J is the number of variables, and K is the number of time points the measurements are taken.

To apply multivariate analysis method, the three-dimensional array data $\mathbf{X}$ has to be unfolded into a two-dimensional matrix. One unfolding strategy is to put each of $I \times J$ matrix side by side (Gunther et al. 2006) such that the $\mathbf{X}$ assay is unfolded as a $I \times (JK)$ matrix. As in Section 9.2, to apply the PCA or PLS method, the data matrix will be mean-centered and scaled to have unit standard deviation. Assume data from all the I batches are in good operating condition and a new batch x_{new} is incomplete and the data are up to K' time points ($K' \le K$). Let $x_{new}(k)$ denote the new batch data available up to time k; Nomikos and MacGregor (1995) proposed that for PCA method, it only uses the portion of the loading matrix up to elapsed time k to calculate the new score vector, that is, $t_{new}(k) = x_{new}(k)P_{Jk}(P'_{Jk} P_{Jk})^{-1}$. Note that the term $P'_{Jk} P_{Jk}$ is not an identity matrix. Similar to offline monitoring in Section 9.3.1, denote the score matrix of normal operating data up to time k as $T_k = X_{Jk}P_{Jk}(P'_{Jk} P_{Jk})^{-1}$, the Hotelling-type statistic is $T_{new}^2(k) = t_{new}(k) S_k^{-1} t_{new}(k)$, where $S_k = \dfrac{T'_k T_k}{I-1}$. The squared prediction error, $SPE_{new}(k) = \displaystyle\sum_{j=1}^{J} e_{new}^2(k) - \sum_{j=1}^{J} e_{new}^2(k-1)$, where $e_{new}(k) = x_{new}(k) - t_{new}(k) P'_{Jk}$. The SPE only involves the latest online measurements at time point k. Control limits are calculated similar to those used in off-line monitoring (Nomikos and MacGregor 1995). Similar to offline applications, the online PLS method can also applied to areas such as process characterization (Kirdar et al. 2007), outlier detection (Gunther et al. 2006), scale-down model (Tang et al. 2014), to name a few. Separately, Gunther et al. (2009) proposed an evolving PLS method, which builds PLS model at each time point throughout the batch process instead of at the end of process only. The method is computationally intensive but has a better Type I error control.

9.4 Applications

9.4.1 Operating Ranges of Chromatography Assay

Consider the example by Sivakumar and Valliappan (2007) regarding optimization of a reversed-phase high-performance liquid chromatographic method for separation of the enantiomers of ketoprofen in formulations and plasma matrices. Although the intent of the study was to optimize the method, we use the data to show how the design space based on the overlapping mean method is determined. The data were generated using a central composite design with two independent variables, MeCN concentration and mobile phase flow rate, and two dependent variables, retention time of probenecid (IS) (t_{R3}) and resolution of S-ketoprofen from the IS ($R_{S2,3}$). The design and experimental results are given in Table 9.1. The factor levels are coded with −1 and 1 corresponding to 45% and 58% for MeCN concentration and 0.8 and 1.2 mL/min for mobile phase flow rate, respectively. The contour plots of the response surfaces are shown in Figure 9.6.

Suppose the acceptance region A for the responses is given as

$$A = \left\{ \left(t_{R_3}, R_{S_{2,3}} \right) : t_{R_3} \leq 4.246,\ R_{S_{2,3}} \geq 3.435 \right\} \tag{9.22}$$

As depicted in Figure 9.6, the design space for MeCN and mobile phase flow rate is the area between the two contours, $t_{R_3} \leq 4.246$ and $R_{S_{2,3}} \geq 3.435$.

TABLE 9.1

Results from a Central Composite Experiment

MeCN Conc.	Flow Rate	t_{R3}		$R_{S2,3}$	
		Replicate 1	Replicate 2	Replicate 1	Replicate 2
−1	−1	10.025	9.971	6.811	6.646
1	−1	5.423	5.473	3.645	3.608
−1	1	7.589	7.531	6.408	6.606
1	1	4.183	4.174	3.428	3.364
−1.414	0	10.132	10.085	7.108	7.109
1.414	0	4.285	4.24	3.085	3.035
0	−1.414	7.514	7.513	5.018	5.0000
0	1.414	5.122	5.061	4.636	4.619
0	0	6.129		4.843	
0	0	6.123		4.839	
0	0	6.101		4.871	
0	0	6.088		4.815	

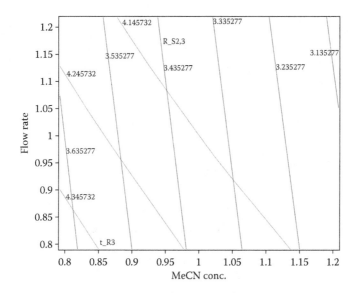

FIGURE 9.6
Design space determined as the "sweet spot" of settings in which the mean responses for retention time of probenecid (IS) (t_{R3}) and resolution of S-ketoprofen from the IS ($R_{S2,3}$) meet acceptance criteria.

9.4.2 Optimization of Cell Culture System

In this section, we discuss optimization of a cell culture system from a case study of applying QbD to vaccines (CMC Vaccines Working Group 2012). The vaccine consists of five serotypes of polysaccharide conjugated to a carrier protein (VLP) and adsorbed to an adjuvant (aluminum salt). The five serotypes account for 80% of the target infectious disease. The process parameters and experimental ranges are given in Table 9.2.

The experiment involves seven response variables, which are listed along with their corresponding objectives as follows:

- Minimal residual peptidoglycan content.
- Targeted molecular size of 200 kD.
- O-acetyl content > 1.6 mole/mole RU.
- Maximal Ps yield.

TABLE 9.2

Process Parameters and Experimental Setting

Factor	High	Middle	Low
Temperature	37	28.5	20
pH	8.8	8.4	8
Enzyme Concentration	200	112.5	25

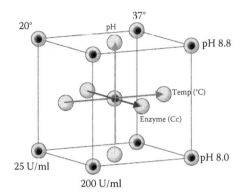

FIGURE 9.7
Face-centered composite design for cell culture system optimization. (From CMC Vaccines Working Group 2012.)

- Filterable extract.
- Minimal response variability.
- Minimal enzyme concentration to reduce process costs.

The optimization experiment used a face-centered composite design shown in Figure 9.7.

The desirability function approach described in Section 9.2.1 was used. For each response variable, the desirability function was defined to reflect its objective. It was calculated for each of the experimental conditions listed in Figure 9.7. These desirability functions were then combined using geometric mean to produce one single desirability function. Figure 9.8 displays a three-dimensional plot of the desirability function with respect to temperature and enzyme concentration with pH = 8.3. The condition that optimizes the desirability function was determined and presented in Table 9.3 and shown in Figure 9.8.

9.4.3 Quantification of Scale-Down Model for Bioreactor

Small-scale models are often developed and used to support the development of commercial process. When well designed, operating conditions developed using these models can be extrapolated across multiple scales, thus reducing costs and shortening development time while maintaining quality of the product produced by the scaled-up processes. However, regardless of the scientific considerations in developing the small-scale models, it is necessary to verify them when batches produced through commercial manufacturing become available. This is in keeping with the concept of continued process verification as recommended by regulatory guidance (FDA 2011). Verification of the small-scale model can be carried out by comparing the performance of both the small-scale process and large commercial process. Because of the large number of output variables such as percent of purity, viable cell density, percent viability, osmolality, which are used to characterize the performance of a process, it is necessary to employ multivariate analysis technique to reduce the dimensionality of the data.

To demonstrate, we use an example from the A-Mab case study (CMC Biotech QbD Working Group 2009). The example concerns demonstration of the applicability of a scale-down model to predict large-scale production bioreactor performance. For this purpose, data from a previous product was used. Thirteen performance variables were

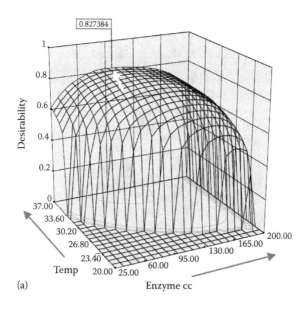

(a)

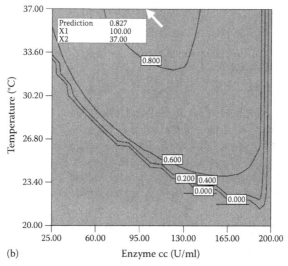

(b)

FIGURE 9.8
Three-dimensional plot (a) and contour plot (b) of desirability function with respect to temperature and enzyme concentration and pH of 8.3. (From CMC Vaccines Working Group, 2012.)

TABLE 9.3

Optimum Conditions for Cell Culture System

Enzyme Concentration	100 U/mL
Temperature	37°C
pH	8.3

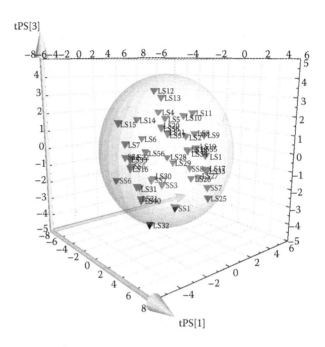

FIGURE 9.9
Scale comparison based on PCA with black and blue triangles corresponding to small and production scales, respectively. (Adapted from CMC Biotech Working Group, 2009.)

measured for batches from both 2 L (N = 8) and 15k L (N = 40) bioreactors. They include Peak VCD, Final Viability, Culture pH, Glucose, Lactate, Peak Lactate, Titer, Final IVC, and product quality attributes P5, P6, P7, P5/P6, and P5/P7 (galactosylation, afucosylation, and acidic variants). These variables were chosen based on their significance for process performance and product quality as established through process characterization studies and represented by the design space model (CMC Biotech QbD Working Group 2009).

A PCA using large scale data was performed, and the results indicated that 99.4% of the variability in the data set was explained by the first five principal components. To demonstrate the comparability between the two scales, a 95% confidence ellipsoid for the five principal components was constructed based on the production scale data set and is shown in Figure 9.9. The corresponding principal components of the small-scale batches are plotted and shown to be within the confidence ellipsoid, indicating comparable performance between the two scales. Therefore, it is justifiable to use the 2 L bioreactor as scale-down model for 15,000 L production bioreactor.

9.4.4 PCA-Based Process Control

PCA-based quality control methods are very useful for process understanding. Identification of batches that appear to be performing abnormally can either lead to corrective action or provide data about the source of the abnormality. For example, Gunther et al. (2006) applied the PCA method to successfully detect abnormal batches and diagnose the root causes. The PLS method can be used for comparison of batches across scales. More applications can be found in Rathore et al. (2015).

To facilitate the understanding, consider the following cell culture example involving the process development of a monoclonal antibody production. In this experiment, twenty 2 L bioreactors were operated with controlled process conditions such as seeding density, pH, temperature, and so on. The process performance variables include peak VCD, final viability, titer, and twelve more related to purity, N-glycan, and charge variants. It is known that the first eighteen batches were run under normal operating conditions (NOC) and the other two were not. A PCA model was constructed using all the process performance data from the twenty batches.

An initial PCA model was constructed with twelve principal components. A scree plot indicated that three principal components may be sufficient. These three principal components explained 84% of the total variability. Thus, a PCA model with three principal components was selected. The score plot in Figure 9.10 showed that batch 19 and batch 20 were separated from the majority and these two batches were potentially outliers. After constructing the PCA model, T_r^2 and Q statistics can be plotted with their upper control limits. Figure 9.11 indicates that batch 19 and batch 20 were outliers. The SPE chart shows that the residuals were under control, indicating that the PCA model based on three principal components captures the variability well.

As shown in Figure 9.12, the contribution plot for batch 20 implied that man5, titer, and viability explain the unusual high value of T_r^2.

In practice, one would like to monitor the process variables instead of product quality attributes so that abnormal conditions can be detected much earlier.

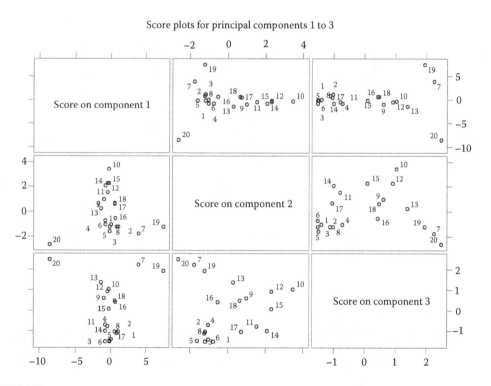

FIGURE 9.10
Score matrix for PCA model with three principal components.

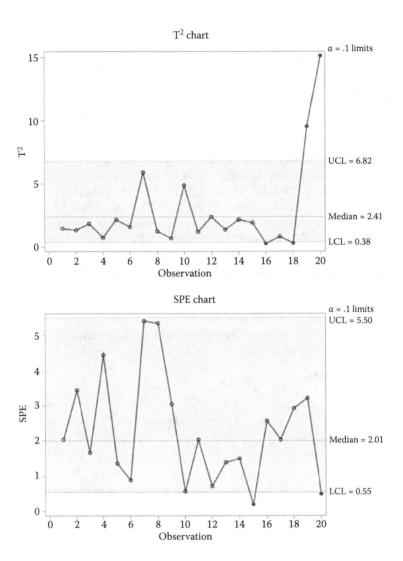

FIGURE 9.11
T^2 and SPE control charts for PCA model with three principal components (upper control limits with 5% type one error were given on the plots by neglecting the lower control limits).

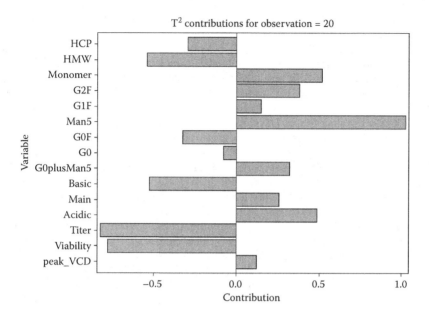

FIGURE 9.12
Contribution plot for batch 20.

9.5 Concluding Remarks

Multivariate data analysis methods such as multiple regression, PCA, and PLS provide essential tools for multivariate process understanding, process monitoring, and control. Determination of process design space, process optimization, process comparability (including scale-down model), and fault detection are notable applications of these methods. In this chapter, the statistical techniques of response surface, PCA, and PLS methods detection are described in detail and illustrated through various examples. The advances in statistical computation tools greatly facilitate the applications of these statistical treatments. Readers are also encouraged to refer to Rathore et al. (2011) and Rathore et al. (2014) for some recommendations on how to perform some of the said analyses using the popular SIMCA P+ software. Other packages such as SAS/QC and R can also perform these tasks.

References

Bersimis, S., Psarakis, S., and Panaretos, J. (2007). Multivariate statistical process control charts: An overview. *Quality and Reliability Engineering International*, 23(5), 517–543.

CMC Biotech Working Group. (2009). A-Mab: A Case Study in Bioprocess Development. Accessed on April 15, 2016, from www.casss.org/associations/9165/.../A-Mab_Case_Study_Version_2-1.pdf.

CMC Vaccine Working Group. (2012). A-VAX: Applying Quality by Design to Vaccines. Accessed on April 15, 2016, from www.ispe.org.

Derringer, G., and Suich, R. (1980). Simultaneous optimization of several response variables. *Journal of Quality Technology*, 12, 214–219.

FDA. (2004a). Pharmaceutical cGMPs for the 21st Century: A Risk-Based Approach. Final Report.

FDA. (2004b). Guidance for Industry: PAT—A Framework for Innovative Pharmaceutical Development, Manufacturing, and Quality Assurance.

FDA. (2011). Guidance for Industry on Process Validation: General Principles and Practices.

Harrington, E.C., Jr. (1965). The desirability function. *Industrial Quality Control* 21, 494–498.

ICH. (2006). Q8(R2) Pharmaceutical Development. Accessed on September 14, 2017, from http://www.fda.gov/downloads/Drugs/.../Guidances/ucm073507.pdf.

ICH. (2007a). Q9 Quality Risk Management. Accessed on September 14, 2017, from http://www.ich.org/fileadmin/Public_Web_Site/ICH_Products/Guidelines/Quality/Q9/Step4/Q9_Guideline.pdf.

ICH. (2007b). Q10 Pharmaceutical Quality Systems. Accessed on September 14, 2017, from http://www.fda.gov/downloads/Drugs/.../Guidances/ucm073517.pdf.

ICH. (2011). Q11 Concept Paper. Accessed on September 14, 2017, from http://www.ema.europa.eu/docs/en_GB/document_library/Scientific_guideline/2011/06/WC500107128.pdf.

Gunther, J.C., Conner, J.S., and Seborg, D.E. (2009). Process monitoring and quality variable prediction utilizing PLS in industrial fed-batch cell culture. *Journal of Process Control*, 19(5), 914–921.

Gunther, J.C., Seborg, D.E., and Conner, J.S. (2006). Fault detection and diagnosis in industrial fed-batch cell culture. *IFAC Proceedings Volumes*, 39(2), 203–208.

Jackson, J.E. (1991). *A User's Guide to Principal Components*. John Wiley & Sons.

Johnson, R., Yu, O., Kirdar, A. O., Annamasai, A., Ahuja, S., Ram, K., and Rathore, A. (2007). Applications of multivariate data analysis in biotech processing, in *Elements in Biopharmaceutical Production Series*, ed. Rathore, A. Bioharm International.

Kirdar, A.O., Green, K.D., and Rathore, A.S. (2008). Application of multivariate data analysis for identification and successful resolution of a root cause for a bioprocessing application. *Biotechnology Progress*, 24(3), 720–726.

Kourti, T., and MacGregor, J.F. 1995. Process analysis, monitoring and diagnosis, using multivariate projection methods. *Chemometrics and Intelligent Laboratory Systems*, 28(1), 3–21.

LeBlond, D. (2015). Applied non-clinical Bayesian Statistics. Presented at 2015 Nonclinical Biostatistics Conference, Villanova, PA.

LeBrun, P. (2012). Bayesian design space applied to pharmaceutical development. Unpublished dissertation. University de Liege. Accessed from http://bictel.ulg.ac.be/ETD-db/collection/available/ULgetd-12192012-155142/unrestricted/thesis.pdf.

Miller, P., Swanson, R.E., and Heckler, C.E. (1998). Contribution plots: A missing link in multivariate quality control. *Applied Mathematics and Computer Science*, 8(4), 775–792.

Montgomery, D.C. (2008). *Introduction to Statistical Quality Control*, 6th ed. John Wiley & Sons.

Ng, K., and Rajagopalan, N. (2009). Application of quality by design and risk assessment principles for the development of formulation design space, in *Quality by Design for Biopharmaceutical: Principles and Case Studies*, ed. Rathore, A.S., and Mhatre, R. John Wiley & Sons.

Nomikos, P., and MacGregor, J.F. (1995). Multivariate SPC charts for monitoring batch processes. *Technometrics*, 37(1), 41–59.

Ntzoufras, I. (2008). *Bayesian Modeling Using WinBUGS*. John Wiley & Sons.

Peterson, J.J. (2004). A posterior predictive approach to multiple response surface optimization. *Journal of Quality Technology*, 36, 139–153.

Peterson, J.J. (2007). A review of Bayesian reliability approaches to multiple response surface optimization. In *Bayesian Statistics for Process Monitoring, Control, and Optimization*, ed. by Colosimo, B. M. and del Castillo, E. Chapman and Hall/CRCPress, Inc.

Peterson, J.J. (2008). A Bayesian approach to the ICH Q8 definition of design space. *Journal of Biopharmaceutical Statistics*, 18, 959–975.

Rathore A.S., and Singh, S.K. (2015). Use of multivariate data analysis in bioprocessing. *BioPharm International*, 28(6).

Rathore, A.S., Bhushan, N., and Hadpe, S. (2011). Chemometrics applications in biotech processes: A review. *Biotechnology Progress*, 27(2), 307–315.

Rathore, A.S. et al. (2014). Guidance for performing multivariate data analysis of bioprocessing data: Pitfalls and recommendations. *Biotechnology Progress*, 30(4), 967–973.

Stockdale, G., and Cheng, A. (2009). Finding design space and a reliable operating region using a multivariate Bayesian approach with experimental design. *Quality Technology and Quantitative Management*, 6(4), 391–408

Tracy, N.D., Young, J.C., and Mason, R.L. (1992). Multivariate control charts for individual observations. *Journal of Quality Technology*, 24(2), 88–95.

Tsang, V.L., Wang, A.X., Yusuf-Makagiansar, H., and Ryll, T. (2014). Development of a scale-down cell culture model using multivariate analysis as a qualification tool. *Biotechnology Progress*, 30(1), 152–160.

Yin, S., Ding, S.X., Zhang, P., Hagahni, A., and Naik, A. (2011). Study on modifications of PLS approach for process monitoring. *IFAC Proceedings Volumes*, 44(1), 12389–12394.

10

Assessment of Analytical Method Robustness: Statistical versus Practical Significance

Binbing Yu, Lingmin Zeng, and Harry Yang

CONTENTS

10.1 Introduction

Analytical methods play a critical role in the drug discovery, biopharmaceutical, and manufacture process development. Results of analytical testing provide a basis for key decision-making. For instance, in early drug discovery, analytical results are used to guide the selection of the lead drug candidates. In both preclinical and clinical development, analytical methods aid optimal dose selection and assess study endpoints. Furthermore, analytical methods are also widely used in formulation and process development and optimization, and in quality control of marketed products. Since the quality of analytical methods have a direct and significant impact on the successful development of a new drug, analytical methods must be developed and validated for their intended use.

One of the assay performance characteristics is robustness. Robustness is a measure of an analytical method. It is defined as "a measure of its capacity to remain unaffected by small, but deliberate variations in method parameters and provide an indication of its reliability during normal usage" (USP 1995; ICH 2005). Another similar but slightly different term is ruggedness. Although ruggedness and robustness are often used interchangeably, there are some distinctions between the two terms. Ruggedness refers to "the degree of reproducibility when the procedure is subjected to changes in external conditions such as different laboratories, analysts, instruments" (USP 1995). Therefore, ruggedness refers to the performance of an analytical method when a noninherent factor, for example, column, instrument, operators, laboratories, is changed while robustness characterizes the behavior of an analytical method when the inherent experimental factors are deliberately modified (Cuadros-Rodriguez et al. 2005).

A robustness test may be viewed as either a part of method validation that is performed at the end of method development or at the beginning of the validation procedure (Dejaegher and Vander Heyden 2007). The robustness assessment procedure includes selecting factors based on the experience of the assay developers, and determining the likely assay variability between analysts and laboratories during repeated runs over time. It also includes choosing appropriate levels or magnitudes that these factors may change, and the assay responses or reportable values to measure these changes.

Since the publication of the guidance for robustness/ruggedness tests in method validation by Vander Heyden et al. (2001), there have been extensive discussions and developments on the design, analysis and evaluation of robustness assessment. In this chapter, we review the common procedure of conducting a robustness study and popular experimental design options. Although innovative statistical methods can provide valuable input in the design and analysis of robustness studies, the decision-making should be based on scientific judgement, taking into consideration the intended use of the assay and regulatory guidance (Cowan 2013).

10.2 Common Steps of a Robustness Assessment

The robustness test used to be considered a part of the method validation related to the precision (reproducibility) determination of the method. However, performing a robustness test late in the validation procedure increases the risk that a method is found not to be robust and has to be redeveloped and optimized. At this stage, much effort and resources have already been spent in the optimization and validation, and therefore the unnecessary redevelopment should be avoided. As such, robustness tests have been shifting to an earlier time in the life cycle of the method (Vander Heyden et al. 2001) and are typically performed at the end of method development prior to method validation.

The robustness studies should tease out which small changes to the assay can be tolerated, and which cannot. If a robustness test is well designed, correctly performed, and appropriately analyzed, the analysis results may provide valuable information on whether the method is in fact sufficiently robust for its intended use, or whether additional modifications to the method are necessary to minimize the impact of these factors on assay performance. Each assay behaves differently, and the impact of these risk factors may be different depending on the parameters and their levels tested (Cowan 2013). The strategy of a robustness study may use either the one-factor-at-a-time approach (OFAT) or the statistical design of experiments (DoE) approaches. For example, a screening design such as the Plackett–Burman design may allow the evaluation of multiple factors in one experiment.

Vander Heyden et al. (2001) presented a comprehensive review on the steps for a robustness assessment. Borman et al. (2011) described a risk-based approach for method ruggedness and robustness studies. A typical robustness study may include the following steps (Nijhuis et al. 1999):

1. Study design
    1.1 Selection of risk factors and their levels
    1.2 Selection of assay responses
    1.3 Statistical experimental design with appropriate sample size
    1.4 Experimental protocol
2. Study execution
3. Analysis and interpretation
    3.1 Statistical analysis and graphical presentation
    3.2 Evaluation and interpretation

To examine potential sources of variability, a number of factors are selected from the operating procedure and examined in an interval that slightly exceeds the variations which can be expected when a method is transferred from one instrument to another or from one laboratory to another. These factors are then examined in an experimental design and the effect of the factors on the response(s) of the method is evaluated. In this way, the factors that may negatively impact the method performance are discovered. The analyst then knows that such factors must be more strictly controlled during the execution.

10.3 Design of Experiments

Both the OFAT approach and the statistical design of experiments (DoE) approach have been used in analytical method robustness studies. Because the OFAT approach usually requires more experiments and is less efficient, especially when the number of risk factors becomes large, the DoE approach is preferred in robustness assessment (Deegher and Heyden 2007). DoE is a systematic method to determine the relationship between factors affecting a process and the output of that process. A strategically planned and executed experiment may provide a great deal of information about the effect on a response variable due to one or more factors.

The popular statistical designs include the Plackett–Burman design, (fractional) factorial designs, super-saturated design, and response surface design (Ragonese et al. 2002; Ferreira et al. 2007). These screening designs allow a fast testing for robustness (Hund et al. 2000). An interaction between two factors may occur when the effect of one factor depends on the level of the other. The evaluation of such interactions is more important in method optimization, where factors are evaluated over much broader interval ranges and thus interactions can be much more important. In a robustness study, the effects of the interactions are often assumed to be negligible, and usually it is the case in practice.

Therefore, the interactions are usually not considered in a screening design, but they may be examined by an appropriate design with higher resolutions.

In practice, there are some other alternative statistical designs. When there are constraints on time and cost, a super-saturated design where the number of experiments is less than or equal to the number of study factors may be used (Dejaegher et al. 2007a, 2007b). Response surface methodology has been used extensively in the optimization and validation of analytical method (Ferreira et al. 2007). Once the optimal conditions are established, the robustness of the analytical method may be determined and confirmed using a second experimental design, for example, a Box–Behnken design (Ragonese et al. 2002).

If one is more concerned about the main effects of factor, and is interested in determining whether a method is robust to possible changes of multiple factors, Plackett–Burman designs are very efficient screening designs in which only main effects are considered. For this reason a two-level Plackett–Burman design is chosen to study the main effects of the variables studied. Taking into account the limited interval range of the variables, we may assume their interactions insignificant, and confounding with the main effects is neglected (Galeano-Diaz et al. 2007).

Two types of risk factors (variables) can be distinguished in the experimental design context: Quantitative and qualitative. The values of quantitative variables are measured in a continuous numeric scale, for example, incubation time and temperature. Qualitative variables are also called categorical variables, which take on values that are names or labels, for example, columns of a chromatographic method. The different levels of the variables are usually expressed as coded values, such as 0, +1, –1, in the design matrix. The nominal level of normal operation is usually 0, whereas the positive (+1) and negative (–1) values are deviations from this nominal level.

The design may be created for $k = 4h - 1$ factors with $h \geq 1$, and thus may be used for 3, 7, 11, 15, or 19 factors, where a greater number may not be practical and necessary. Let N be the number experiments. Up to $N - 1$ factors can be allowed in a Plackett–Burman design with N experiment runs. If $k = N - 1$, it is only possible to estimate the main effects; however, if $k < N - 1$, the effects of some interactions may be estimated including $N - k - 1$ dummy variables. If the effect associated with these variables is significant, they may be confounded with two-factor interaction effects. If the effect is not significant, it is a way to obtain the total error. It is recommended to choose a design that allows at least three dummies. Table 10.1 shows the specifications of factor level for an eight-run Plackett–Burman design.

Factors A–G may be a risk factor with a potential impact on assay responses, for example, column or incubation time, or a dummy factor. A dummy factor is an imaginary factor

TABLE 10.1

The Eight-Run Plackett–Burman Design

Run	Factor A	Factor B	Factor C	Factor D	Factor E	Factor F	Factor G
1	+	+	+	−	+	−	−
2	−	+	+	+	−	+	−
3	−	−	+	+	+	−	+
4	+	−	−	+	+	+	−
5	−	+	−	−	+	+	+
6	+	−	+	−	−	+	+
7	+	+	−	+	−	−	+
8	−	−	−	−	−	−	−

for which the change from one level to the other has no physical meaning. The effect of factor X on the response Y can be calculated as

$$E_X = \frac{\sum Y(+)}{N/2} - \frac{\sum Y(-)}{N/2} \tag{10.1}$$

where X can represent the factors A, B, .., G, and $\Sigma Y(+)$ and $\Sigma Y(-)$ are the sums of the responses where X is at the high and low levels (+) and (−), respectively.

10.4 Evaluation of Assay Robustness

The objective of a robustness test is to evaluate factors potentially causing variability in the assay responses of the method, for example, content determinations. For this purpose, small variations in method parameters are introduced. Therefore, the variance of the assay response measured from the experiments with a statistical design can be used as a potential measure of method robustness (Dejaegher et al. 2005). Both graphical and statistical evaluation methods are described.

Graphical methods are often useful, particularly in presenting the results to others. Rigorous statistical analysis and tests may be performed to validate the conclusion and results. Statistical methods such as regression analysis and ANOVA (analysis of variance) are popular tools for analyzing robustness data.

10.4.1 Graphical Evaluation by Half-Normal Plot

The graphical identification of important effects is usually applied with a half-normal plot. Under the null hypothesis of no significant effects, the nonsignificant effects are normally distributed around zero and the nonsignificant effect values tend to fall on a straight line through zero, while significant effects deviate from the line.

To create the half-normal plot, the k-factor effects are ranked according to increasing absolute value. The rth value of effect sizes is plotted against a scale defined by partitioning the right half of the normal distribution in k parts of equal area and by taking the median of the rth slice. This value is called the Rankit. For an eight-run Plackett–Burman design, the Rankits are 0.09, 0.27, 0.46, 0.66, 0.9, 1.21, and 1.71. The half-normal plot is generated by plots the calculated factor effects E_X against the Rankits.

The graphical evaluation of robustness may not be reliable; it is often used as a screening tool.

10.4.2 Dong's Method

In order to identify the potential impactful factors, Dong (1993) proposed comparing factor effects with margin of error (ME) and simultaneous margin of error (SME) to determine the significance of a factor. An initial estimate of the error on an effect is obtained as

$$s_o = 1.5 \cdot \underset{i}{median} |E_i| \tag{10.2}$$

where E_i is the value of effect i. From s_0, a final estimation of the *standard error* (s_1) is derived as

$$s_1 = \sqrt{m^{-1}\sum E_i^2} \text{ for all } |E_i| \leq 2.5s_0 \tag{10.3}$$

where m is the number of absolute effects smaller than $2.5s_0$. Next, the s_1 value is used to calculate the ME:

$$ME = t_{(1-\alpha/2,df)} \cdot s_1 \tag{10.4}$$

where $1 - \alpha/2 = 0.975$ and $df = m$. The ME is statistically a valid criterion for significance testing when only one effect has to be tested. When multiple effects are tested the chance for nonsignificant effects that exceed the *ME* increases. To compensate for multiplicity of several factors, the significance level has to be adjusted and the SME

$$SME = t_{(1-\alpha^*/2,df)} \cdot s_1 \tag{10.5}$$

where $\alpha^* = 1 - (1 - \alpha)^{(1/m)}$, the adjusted significance level. An effect that exceeds the ME, but is below the SME, is determined to be possibly significant and an effect that is above the SME is determined to be significant.

The standard error estimate S_1 in Dong's method is obtained from the effects of negligible factor effects. The method assumes that the negligible effects are not related to the responses and therefore can be attributed to the experimental error.

10.4.3 Linear Model

When there are independent replicates for each run, the standard error of the responses can be obtained from a generalized linear model. Without loss of generality, we assume that there are J replicates at each run. Let $y_{i1}, ..., y_{ij}$ be the independent replicates and let $A_i, B_i, ..., G_i$ be the factor levels at the ith run. The linear model for the responses can be written as

$$y_{ij} = A_i + B_i + \cdots + G_i + \varepsilon_{ij}, \varepsilon_{ij} \sim N(0,\sigma_\varepsilon^2), \tag{10.6}$$

where $A_i, B_i, ..., G_i = \pm 1$ are categorical variables for the factor values and ε_{ij} represents the random assay variability. The dummy variables may be dropped from Equation 10.6 as they contribute to the random assay variability. The statistical significance of the factor effects can be determined from the linear regression. The estimates and test of significance can be obtained from SAS `proc glm` or R function `lm`.

10.4.4 Statistical vs. Practical Significance

Scientific knowledge should be integrated into the analysis process and result interpretation. Statistical methods alone cannot prove that a factor has a practically meaningful impact. They only provide guidelines for making decisions. Statistical techniques together with good knowledge for the intended use of the analytical method. Common sense will usually lead to sound conclusions. Without common sense, pure statistical models may be misleading.

If the effect of a factor is statistically significant, does that mean that the analytical method is sensitive to the change of the significant factor? That is a legitimate question. A significant factor does indicate the factor has noticeable impact on the response, but is this impact practically meaningful? Probably a more meaningful question might be whether the effect is practically significant.

Practical significance means the actual difference will affect a decision to be made, for example, is the analytical method too variable to be used for release testing? Statistical significance often depends on the sample size. A factor effect of 0.1% may become statistically significant if the sample size is big enough, but it may not be practically significant. In short, statistical significance depends on the sample size and the precision of the method. A very accurate and precise method may be penalized by discerning miniscule differences due to the change of a factor level.

10.5 Case Study

The A280 method is a spectrophotometric method to determine the protein concentration in solution. The absorbance measure at 280 nm (A280) is used to calculate protein concentration by comparison with a standard curve for that protein. In the application, we evaluated the robustness of the A280 method for a monoclonal antibody regarding Factors Lamp Warping (A), Measurement Wavelength (B), Sample Pipetting Volume (C), and Dilution Scheme (D). The target nominal level and the associate low and high levels for each factor are shown in Table 10.2. An eight-run Plackett–Burman design is used. The first four factors A–D are the risk factors of interest and the rest factors E–G are dummy factors. The dummy factors are not confounded with the factors of interest and are used in the analysis to measure random measurement error. Three replicate measurements of total protein concentration are obtained for each run. The data are shown in Table 10.3.

First, Dong's method is applied to evaluate the robustness. The average of the three replicates is used as the response variable for the analysis. The ME is 0.35 mg/ml and the SME is 0.55 mg/ml. Figure 10.1 shows the half-normal plot of the ranked factor effects. We see that the wavelength (Factor B) is outside the simultaneous margin of error (SME) limit, therefore the wavelength has a significant impact on protein concentration measurement.

However, Dong's method only shows the statistical significance of the effects of a risk factor compared to other negligible factors. The statistical significance does not necessarily mean practical significance.

TABLE 10.2

Factors and Factor Levels for the A280 Robustness Study

Factor	Factor Description	Nominal Level	Low (−)	High (+)
A	Lamp Warping	45	30	60
B	Measurement Wavelength (nm)	280	278	282
C	Sample Pipetting Volume (μL)	40	30	50
D	Dilution Scheme (x100)	N/A	5	20

TABLE 10.3

Responses of the A280 Robustness Study with the Plackett–Burman Design

Run	Replicate Responses			Mean Response
	Replicate 1	Replicate 2	Replicate 3	
1	50.9	51.1	51.0	51.1
2	50.8	50.9	51.2	51.0
3	51.6	51.7	51.3	51.5
4	51.8	51.4	51.9	51.7
5	51.3	51.0	51.1	51.1
6	51.8	51.7	52.0	51.8
7	50.7	50.0	51.1	50.6
8	52.0	51.8	51.8	51.9

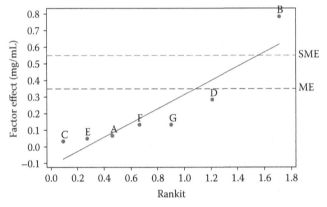

Note: A–D are real factors and E–G are dummy factors.

FIGURE 10.1
Half-normal plot of the ranked factor effects.

When the generalized linear model is applied to the data, the estimates of the factor effects are shown in Table 10.4. We see again Factor B has the strongest effect with a p-value of 0.0006. This shows that Factor B is highly significant, which is consistent with Dong's method. However, the standard deviation of the residual assay variability is $\sigma_\varepsilon = 0.4868$. By comparing the effect of Factor B and $2\sigma_\varepsilon$, we see that the effect of Factor B is within $2\sigma_\varepsilon$. In addition, the mean protein concentration from all eight runs is 51.8 mg/ml. Factor B effect

TABLE 10.4

Factor Effects and p-Value of Four Critical Factors from the Linear Model

Factor	Effect	p-Value
A	−0.0833	0.6797
B	−0.8167	0.0006
C	0.0167	0.9340
D	−0.2667	0.1954

only accounts for 1.6% of the relative change. In addition, the specification of the protein concentration is 48–52 mg/ml. Therefore, Factor B is statistically significant, but may not be practically significant for the A280 method for measuring protein concentration.

10.6 Discussions

Robustness assessment is a critical measure of assay performances. The levels of robustness, reproducibility, and accuracy that are acceptable will depend on the purpose of the assay and must be decided upon by the researcher for his or her intended use. The estimated method variability may also be combined with accumulated knowledge during previous development to set control limits for the continuous verification of the method (Borman et al. 2011).

A successful robustness study requires knowledge of the factors, the operational ranges of these factors, and the appropriate number of levels to use. Generally, this information is not perfectly known before the experiment. Assay development is an iterative process. Therefore, it is suggested to perform experiments iteratively and sequentially. Statistical design and analysis are valuable tools for robustness assessment. However, interpretation of the analysis results requires both statistical and scientific knowledge.

References

Aybar-Muñoz, J., A.M. Garcıá-Campaña, and L. Cuadros-Rodrıǵuez. 2002. Evaluating the significance threshold in robustness testing. A critical discussion on the influence of time in molecular fluorescence spectrometry. *Talanta* 56 (1): 123–36.

Borman, P.J., M.J. Chatfield, I. Damjanov, and P. Jackson. 2011. Method ruggedness studies incorporating a risk based approach: A tutorial. *Analytica Chimica Acta* 703 (2): 101–13.

César, I. de Costa, and G. Antônio Pianetti. 2009. Robustness evaluation of the chromatographic method for the quantitation of lumefantrine using Youden's test. *Brazilian Journal of Pharmaceutical Sciences* 45 (2): 235–40.

Cowan, K.J. 2013. On assay robustness: The importance of early determination and science-driven decision-making. *Bioanalysis*, 5 (11): 1317–1219.

Cowan, K.J., R. Erickson, B. Sue, R. Delarosa, B. Gunter, D.A. Coleman, H. Gilbert, A. Song, and S.K. Fischer. 2012. Utilizing design of experiments to characterize assay robustness. *Bioanalysis*. 4(17): 2127–39.

Cuadros-Rodriguez, L., R. Romero, and J.M. Bosque-Sendra. 2005. The role of the robustness/ruggedness and inertia studies in research and development of analytical processes. *Critical Reviews in Analytical Chemistry* 35 (1): 57–69.

Dejaegher, B., X. Capron, J. Smeyers-Verbeke, and Y. Vander Heyden. 2006. Randomization tests to identify significant effects in experimental designs for robustness testing. *Analytica Chimica Acta* 564 (2): 184–200.

Dejaegher, B., X. Capron, and Y. Vander Heyden. 2007. Fixing effects and adding rows (FEAR) method to estimate factor effects in supersaturated designs constructed from Plackett–Burman designs. *Chemometrics and Intelligent Laboratory Systems* 85 (2): 220–31.

Dejaegher, B., J. Smeyers-Verbeke, and Y. Vander Heyden. 2005. The variance of screening and supersaturated design results as a measure for method robustness. *Analytica Chimica Acta* 544 (1): 268–79.

Dejaegher, B., M. Dumarey, X. Capron, M.S. Bloomfield, and Y. Vander Heyden. 2007. Comparison of Plackett–Burman and supersaturated designs in robustness testing. *Analytica Chimica Acta* 595 (1): 59–71.

Dejaegher, B., and Y. Vander Heyden. 2007. Ruggedness and robustness testing. *Journal of Chromatography A* 1158 (1): 138–57.

Dong, F. 1993. On the identification of active contrasts in unreplicated fractional factorials. *Statistica Sinica* 3 (1): 209–17.

Ferreira, S.L.C., R.E. Bruns, H.S. Ferreira, G.D. Matos, J.M. David, G.C. Brandao, E.G. Paranhos da Silva, L.A. Portugal, P.S. Dos Reis, and A.S. Souza. 2007. Box–Behnken design: An alternative for the optimization of analytical methods. *Analytica Chimica Acta* 597 (2): 179–86.

Freeny, A.E., and V.N. Nair. 1992. Robust parameter design with uncontrolled noise variables. *Statistica Sinica*: 313–34.

Galeano-Díaz, T., M.-I. Acedo-Valenzuela, N. Mora-Díez, and A. Silva-Rodríguez. 2007. Comparative study of different approaches to the determination of robustness for a sensitive-stacking capillary electrophoresis method. Estimation of system suitability test limits from the robustness test. *Analytical and Bioanalytical Chemistry* 389 (2): 541–53.

Goupy, J. 2005. What kind of experimental design for finding and checking robustness of analytical methods? *Analytica Chimica Acta* 544 (1): 184–90.

Hund, E., Y. Vander Heyden, M. Haustein, D.L. Massart, and J. Smeyers-Verbeke. 2000a. Comparison of several criteria to decide on the significance of effects in a robustness test with an asymmetrical factorial design. *Analytica Chimica Acta* 404 (2): 257–71.

———. 2000b. Comparison of several criteria to decide on the significance of effects in a robustness test with an asymmetrical factorial design. *Analytica Chimica Acta* 404 (2): 257–71.

———. 2000c. Robustness testing of a reversed-phase high-performance liquid chromatographic assay: Comparison of fractional and asymmetrical factorial designs. *Journal of Chromatography A* 874 (2): 167–85.

Hund, E., D.L. Massart, and J. Smeyers-Verbeke. 2002. Robust regression and outlier detection in the evaluation of robustness tests with different experimental designs. *Analytica Chimica Acta* 463 (1): 53–73.

ICH Harmonized Tripartite. 2005. Validation of analytical procedures: Text and methodology. *Q2 (R1)*.

Karageorgou, E., and V. Samanidou. 2014. Youden test application in robustness assays during method validation. *Journal of Chromatography A* 1353: 131–9.

Lonardo, A. J., A. Srivastava, S. Singh, and J. Goldstein. 2012. Robustness index score: A new stability parameter for designing robustness into biologic formulations. *Journal of Pharmaceutical Sciences* 101 (2): 485–92.

Nijhuis, A., H.C.M. Van der Knaap, S. De Jong, and B.G.M. Vandeginste. 1999. Strategy for ruggedness tests in chromatographic method validation. *Analytica Chimica Acta* 391 (2): 187–202.

Picardi, A., E. Mazzotti, and P. Pasquini. 2006. Prevalence and correlates of suicidal ideation among patients with skin disease. *Journal of the American Academy of Dermatology* 54 (3): 420–6.

Questier, F., Y. Vander Heyden, and D.L. Massart. 1998. RTS, a computer program for the experimental set-up and interpretation of ruggedness tests. *Journal of Pharmaceutical and Biomedical Analysis* 18 (3): 287–303.

Ragonese, R., M. Macka, J. Hughes, and P. Petocz. 2002. The use of the Box–Behnken experimental design in the optimisation and robustness testing of a capillary electrophoresis method for the analysis of ethambutol hydrochloride in a pharmaceutical formulation. *Journal of Pharmaceutical and Biomedical Analysis* 27 (6): 995–1007.

Rakić, T., B. Jančić-Stojanović, A. Malenović, D. Ivanović, and M. Medenica. 2012. Demasking large dummy effects approach in revealing important interactions in Plackett–Burman experimental design. *Journal of Chemometrics* 26 (10): 518–25.

Rakić, T., A. Malenović, B. Jančić-Stojanović, D. Ivanović, and M. Medenica. 2012. Avoiding the false negative results in LC method robustness testing by modifications of the algorithm of dong and dummy factor effects approach. *Chromatographia* 75 (7–8): 397–401.

Rakić, T., S. Vemić, B. Jančić-Stojanović, and M. Medenica. 2013. Multi-level robustness evaluation approach: From robustness criterion to adapted algorithm of dong. *Chromatographia* 76 (5–6): 267–77.

United States Pharmacopeia. 1995. *Validation of Compendia Method*. United States Pharmacopeia Convention, Rockville.

Vander Heyden, Y., M. Jimidar, E. Hund, N. Niemeijer, R. Peeters, J. Smeyers-Verbeke, D.L. Massart, and J. Hoogmartens. 1999. Determination of system suitability limits with a robustness test. *Journal of Chromatography A* 845 (1): 145–54.

Vander Heyden, Y., A. Nijhuis, J. Smeyers-Verbeke, B.G.M. Vandeginste, and D.L. Massart. 2001. Guidance for robustness/ruggedness tests in method validation. *Journal of Pharmaceutical and Biomedical Analysis* 24 (5): 723–53.

Vander Heyden, Y., F. Questier, and D.L. Massart. 1998. A ruggedness test strategy for procedure related factors: Experimental set-up and interpretation. *Journal of Pharmaceutical and Biomedical Analysis* 17 (1): 153–68.

Vander Heyden, Y., S. Kuttatharmmakul, J. Smeyers-Verbeke, and D.L. Massart. 2000. Supersaturated designs for robustness testing. *Analytical Chemistry* 72 (13): 2869–74.

Zeaiter, M., J.-M. Roger, V. Bellon-Maurel, and D.N. Rutledge. 2004. Robustness of models developed by multivariate calibration. Part I: The assessment of robustness. *TrAC Trends in Analytical Chemistry* 23.

11

cGMP Sampling

Harry Yang

CONTENTS

11.1 Regulatory Guidance

Since biopharmaceutical is a strictly regulated industry, adherence to governmental regulations such as the U.S. current Good Manufacturing Practice (cGMP) is essential in ensuring product safety, efficacy, and quality. The cGMP stipulates that modern standards and technologies be adopted in the design, monitoring, and control of manufacturing processes and facilities (FDA, 1995). To this end, the use of statistically and scientifically sound sampling plans is necessary for inspection of raw materials, release of intermediate and finished products, process validation, justification of process changes postapproval, root cause analysis, assessment of manufacturing process efficiency, and state of control of manufacturing environment. The World Health Organization (WHO) also published a guideline for the sampling of pharmaceutical products and related materials (WHO, 2005). It stresses that "the choice of a sampling plan should always take into consideration the specific objectives of the sampling and the risks and consequences associated with inherent decision errors."

11.2 Risk-Based Sampling Plans

To be strictly compliant with regulatory guidelines, a sampling plan must be prespecified and written. Since a variety of factors may impact a manufacturing process, care should be taken to ensure samples are representative of the population. Of equal importance is to use appropriate statistical methods to select sampling plans so that both consumer's and producer's risks can be protected. It is also advisable to use a risk-based method. For instance, if an attribute is critical to the quality of the product, a heightened inspection might be warranted. Therefore, a risk-based approach should be adopted for the development of sampling plans. It includes assessment of criticality of product quality attributes and understanding of historical performance of vendors or manufacturing processes. A risk-based sampling plan needs to be implemented when there is a change of suppliers of raw materials and devices for the product. Initially a stringent plan may be used. As new vendors demonstrate that they can consistently provide quality raw materials, a less strict sampling plan may be employed. It is important to note that acceptance sampling in itself does little to the quality improvement as this has been inherent to the product. However, it may indirectly improve overall quality of materials and finished products by eliminating or rejecting lots of poor quality vendors or vendors of low quality assurance. Today, acceptance sampling plans are more often used as tactical elements in overall strategies designed to achieve desired quality systems by manufacturers. Such strategies usually encompass continual stabilization and improvement of processes through effective process monitoring and quality control based on computer automation, application of statistical and probabilistic theory, and industrial psychology (Yang and Carlin, 2001).

11.3 Applications

11.3.1 Raw Material, Drug Substance, and Finished Product Release

One of the most common applications of acceptance sampling is to ascertain that material under inspection conform to prespecified quality requirements. To illustrate, consider the influenza vaccine, FluMist® Quadrivalent, which is indicated for active immunization for the prevention of influenza disease caused by influenza A subtype viruses and type B viruses contained in the vaccine (FDA, 2003). The product is delivered intranasally and prefilled in a specially designed sprayer, shown in Figure 11.1.

The sprayers are provided by a vendor. To qualify an incoming batch of sprayers, a battery of tests is conducted on a randomly selected sample. One of these is a visual inspection of sprayer integrity. This includes examination of whether the tip protector and

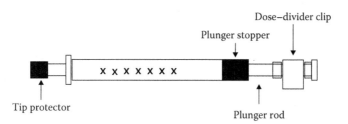

FIGURE 11.1
Diagram of a nasal sprayer.

dose-divider clip are in place. This can be accomplished through inspection of a sample of the batch according to a predetermined sampling plan.

11.3.2 Process Efficiency

Bioburden is a measure of viable microbial containment, which may be introduced at any step of manufacturing processes from nonsterile raw materials, handling of containers and closures, and manufacturing environment. Among many other measures, the risk of bioburden can be mitigated through a sterile filtration process, which utilizes sterilizing-grade filters to remove bioburden. However, a high concentration of bioburden in the prefiltration drug solution may compromise the sterilizing filters, making the filtration process ineffective. The issue can be resolved through an acceptance sampling testing before the final filtration.

11.3.3 Environmental Monitoring

Sampling is also widely utilized to ensure manufacturing processes for sterile drug production are in a state of control. Unlike the acceptance sampling for lot release, samples taken in rooms where the product is manufactured are used to monitor the cleanliness of the rooms. How to collect samples from various locations and in different times is of great interest. It is also important to use historical samples collected when the environment was in the state of control and appropriate statistical methods to establish alert and action limits so that microbial excursions can be effectively detected. A typical control chart for environmental monitoring consists of an alert limit and an action limit as shown in Figure 11.2. An excursion of the alert limit triggers a warning but may not require corrective measures. However, exceeding an action limit is indicative of a probable drift of the environment from its normal state of control and requires immediate root cause analysis and corrections.

11.3.4 Stability Testing

Stability of quality attributes may affect a drug product's safety or efficacy over its labeled use period (shelf life). Effective utilization of stability testing plays a critical role throughout the life cycle of a drug product. During early development, well-designed stability studies can help gain a deep understanding of the product's degradation pathways. In late phase development, stability testing provides information regarding how a variety of environmental factors such as temperature, humidity, and light impact the product quality over time. These data are also used to establish the shelf life and storage conditions of the

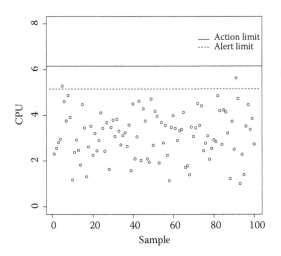

FIGURE 11.2
Control chart of microbial recovery.

product in support of regulatory licensure. For marketed products, stability studies can be used to update shelf life or release limit(s), if needed, to warrant product quality through a specified (shortened or extended) period, and provide assurance of robustness of the manufacturing process after process changes (including site, scale, formulation, storage, shipping conditions, or delivery device). A typical stability study consists of (1) selecting time points at which stability samples are collected and tested; (2) fitting a statistical model to the measured results; (3) estimating or making an inference about the product stability profile. Figure 11.3 shows a plot of potency values from a stability study which was run over a course of 30 weeks. The data were fitted using a linear model. The 95% confidence

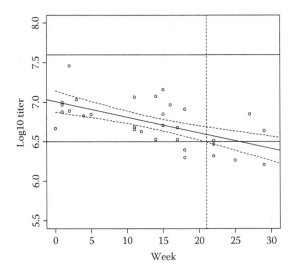

FIGURE 11.3
Stability plot.

interval of the predicted response is plotted along with the stability trend line. Shelf life can be estimated as the point at which the lower 95% confidence limit intersects the lower limit. Since estimation of the stability characteristics such as degradation slope and shelf life depends on the sampling points taken, stability design based on optimal statistical criteria would render more robust estimate of the product stability profile.

11.4 Acceptance Sampling for Lot Inspection

The most common application of acceptance sampling is for lot inspection. This includes acceptance testing of incoming raw materials or devices and disposition of an intermediate and finished product lot. A number of procedures have been developed for said purposes. In the following, we discuss key concepts and elements of these procedures.

11.4.1 Acceptance Sampling Plan

An acceptance sampling plan is a written document detailing a number of samples or volume of samples, method of sampling, tests used to determine conformance to requirement, and a set of rules for disposition of the batch. Since a sample only represents a fraction of the batch, there are two types of errors or risks associated with the acceptance or rejection of the batch. They are described in Table 11.1.

Type I error is a false rejection of a good batch while Type II error is false declaration of a bad batch. Type I and II errors correspond to producer's risk (PR) and consumer's risk (CR), respectively. A large Type I error would financially impact the producer. Such a risk may be potentially mitigated through a retesting process in which the cause of the initially failed test is investigated and additional testing may be conducted to aid disposition of the batch. Type II error is of greater concern due to both the potential for harm and inability to retest the batch after its release (Henson, 2013).

Through proper selection of sample size or volume, a sampling plan can keep both Type I and Type II errors below predetermined levels. As noted by Yang and Carlin (2001), in practice, the costs or consequences of making the two types of errors might be different. For example, if drug A is the only product on the market that treats a life-threatening disease, the cost of rejecting a good batch of product is far greater than accepting a batch which is less potent. As a remedy, a sampling plan can be designed to incorporate the costs of two kinds of errors, thus achieving a more meaningful trade-off between the two risks.

TABLE 11.1

Risks Associated with Acceptance Sampling

Disposition	True State	
	Good Batch	**Bad Batch**
Accept batch	Correct decision	Type II error
Reject batch	Type I error	Correct decision

11.4.2 Quality Level

Design of an acceptance sampling plan requires specification of two levels of quality. The first is the acceptable quality level (CQL), which is quality level desired by the consumer. The second is the lot tolerance percent defective (LTPD). It represents the worst quality level the consumer can tolerate. In literature, LTPD is also referred to as producer quality level (PQL). The producer's and consumer's risks are related to PQL and CQL. The PR is the probability that a sampling plan rejects a lot whose quality is no worse than AQL, and CR is the probability that the sampling plan accepts a lot whose quality is no better than LTPD. An acceptance sampling plan is to ensure neither risk exceeds its prespecified limit.

11.4.3 Operating Characteristic Curve

A sampling plan is usually selected through the operating characteristic (OC) curve. As shown in Figure 11.4, for any sampling plan, this curve displays the probability of accepting a batch per the plan against a range of quality level. When the quality levels PQL and CQL are specified, the risks PR and CR can be directly identified from the curve. The sampling plan is a viable choice if PR and CR are within their prespecified limits. Construction of the OC curve is based on a statistical model of the sampling test outcomes and the acceptance/rejection rules, which is discussed in the next two sections.

11.4.4 Single Attribute Sampling

Attribute sampling is related to situations in which inspection outcomes are dichotomous, for instance, defective or nondefective. It is straightforward to develop a single attribute sampling plan. Typically, a random sample of size n is taken from a batch of size N and the batch is accepted if the number of defective units x is no greater than the acceptance number of failures c. The sample size n and acceptance number c are chosen such that both PR and CR are within prespecified limits. The OC curve can be used to aid the selections of n

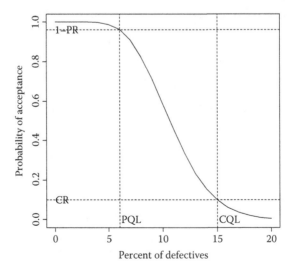

FIGURE 11.4
Operating characteristic curve.

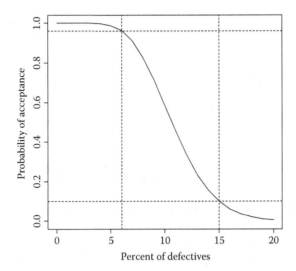

FIGURE 11.5
OC curves of single sampling plan with $n = 100$ and $c = 10$. At defect rates of 6% and 15%, the acceptance probabilities are 96% and 10%, respectively.

and c. The variable x follows a hypergeometric distribution. However, when the batch size N is sufficiently large, the distribution can be approximated by a binomial distribution. Let p be the true percent of defectives in the batch. The probability of acceptance is given by

$$P_a = \sum_{i=0}^{c} \binom{n}{i} p^i (1-p)^{n-i}. \tag{11.1}$$

For example, with a plan of $n = 10$ and $c = 0$, assuming $p = 1\%$, it can be calculated that $P_a = (1 - 0.01)^{10} = 0.904$. That is, there is a little over 90% probability to accept the batch. The OC curve of an acceptance sampling plan with $n = 100$, and $c = 10$ is shown in Figure 11.5.

Assuming that PQL = 6%, CQL = 15%, $\alpha = 5\%$, and $\beta = 10\%$, the above plan is a viable choice.

11.4.5 Variables Sampling

Many quality attributes such as potency and impurity are continuous measures. It is often of interest to understand the percent of the measured quality attribute that is within acceptance limits. Attribute sampling plans can be used in this situation. Alternatively, acceptance sampling plans can be directly constructed based on the continuous measures, resulting in considerable savings in sample size (Schilling and Neubauer, 2009). Such plans involve determining the sample size n, and acceptance limits, and comparing a statistic based on the measured values such as sample mean to the limits. The acceptance limits can be either one-sided (lower or upper limit) or two-sided. Consider an acceptance plan based on an impurity test with a specification limit of U. Let p denote the proportion of the product that exceeds U, thus $U = z_{1-p}$, where z_{1-p} is the $100(1-p)^{th}$ percentile of the standard normal distribution. Let $\bar{X}$ denote the sample mean of a sample $(X_1, \ldots X_n)$ with $X_i \sim N(\mu, \sigma^2)$, $i = 1, \ldots n$. It is further assumed that standard deviation σ

is known and the acceptance limit is A is expressed as $A = U - k\sigma$. The probability of acceptance is given by

$$P_a = \Pr\left[\bar{X} \le U - k\sigma\right]$$
$$= \Pr\left[\frac{\sqrt{n}\left(\bar{X} - \mu\right)}{\sigma} \le \sqrt{n}\left(\frac{\left(z_{1-p} - \mu\right)}{\sigma} - k\right)\right] \tag{11.2}$$

which can be easily calculated from the standard normal distribution.

The OC curve corresponding to the plan (n, k) can be obtained by plotting the above probability of acceptance against a range of p-values. The OC curve of a variable sampling plan $(n, k) = (8, 1.44)$ is plotted in Figure 11.6 along with that of an attribute sampling plan $(n, c) = (22, 1)$.

From the plot, it is evident that both plans have about the same performance characteristics, providing nearly the same protection to consumer's and producer's risks. From the economical perspective, the variables plan is more preferable as it uses much smaller sample size as the attribute plan.

Key to the development of variables plans is the selection of sample size n and factor k in the acceptance limits. Shilling and Neubauer (2009) derived a formula that can be readily used to calculation (n, k). For illustration, suppose that a plan is to be developed with a producer's quality level LTPD = p_1 and the consumer's quality level CQL = p_2. It is also assumed that the measured attribute is deemed to be acceptable if it does not exceed an upper limit U. Furthermore, the Type I and II errors are required to be bound by α and β, respectively. Under the above conditions and normality assumption of the measurements, a plan can be developed by randomly selecting a random sample of size n and comparing the sample mean $\bar{X}$ to the quantity $U - k\sigma$ when the standard deviation of the measurements σ is known or to $U - kS$ with S being the sample standard deviation when σ is unknown. Formula for calculating the sample size n and factor k are given in Table 11.2.

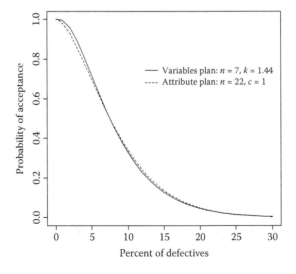

FIGURE 11.6
OC curves of a variable and an attribute acceptance sampling plans.

TABLE 11.2

Calculation of Factor k and Sample Size n for One-Sided Acceptance Limit

Sampling Plan	Standard Deviation	
	Known	Unknown
Factor k	$\dfrac{Z_{LTPD}Z_\alpha + Z_{CQL}Z_\beta}{Z_\alpha + Z_\beta}$	$\dfrac{Z_{LTPD}Z_\alpha + Z_{CQL}Z_\beta}{Z_\alpha + Z_\beta}$
Sample Size n	$\left(\dfrac{Z_\alpha + Z_\beta}{Z_{CQL} + Z_{LTPD}}\right)^2$	$\left(\dfrac{Z_\alpha + Z_\beta}{Z_{CQL} + Z_{LTPD}}\right)^2\left(1 + \dfrac{k^2}{2}\right)$

As an illustration, suppose that LTPD = 0.01 and CQL = 0.1. For $\alpha = 0.05$ and $\beta = 0.1$, it can be determined that

$$k = \frac{2.33 \times 1.65 + 1.65 \times 1.28}{1.65 + 1.28} = 1.87$$

$$n = \left(\frac{1.65 + 1.28}{2.33 - 1.28}\right)^2 = 7.85 \approx 8$$

$$n = \left(\frac{1.65 + 1.28}{2.33 - 1.28}\right)^2\left(1 + \frac{1.87^2}{2}\right) = 21.54 \approx 22.$$

The OC curve corresponding to the above plan $(n, k) = (22, 1.87)$ is shown in Figure 11.7.

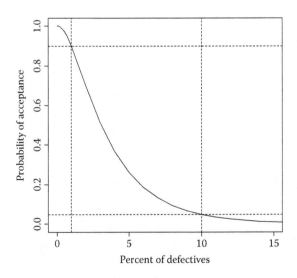

FIGURE 11.7
OC curve of a variable sampling plan with LTPD = 0.01 and CQL = 0.1; $\alpha = 0.05$ and $\beta = 0.1$.

11.4.6 Selection of Sampling Plan

After the quality levels CQL and QPL are specified, selection of a sampling plan is to determine the sample size and batch disposition rules. Therefore it is important to understand the impact of sample size and decision rules on both the consumer's and producer's risks. Figure 11.8 shows three sampling plans with sample size $n = 50$, 100, and 150, and a decision rule that rejects a batch when five or more defective units are identified. In general, the larger the sample size n is, the lower the acceptance probability is. This implies a large sample size renders more protection for the consumer's risk.

Consider a situation in which PQL and CQL are 1% and 7%, respectively, and acceptable consumer's and producer's risks are both 5%. Thus a viable sampling plan should accept a batch with probabilities over 95% and no more than 5% at PQL and CQL, respectively. From the plot in Figure 11.8, the acceptance probabilities are obtained and presented in Table 11.3.

It is clear that the sampling plan with a sample size of 150 is the only plan out of the three that warrants consumer's and producer's risks to be within the prespecified limit of 5%. Therefore, it can be used for lot disposition.

The impact of decision rules can be similarly evaluated. Figure 11.9 displays three OC curves for sampling plans with $n = 100$ and cutoff point in the decision rule $c = 3$, 5, and 7.

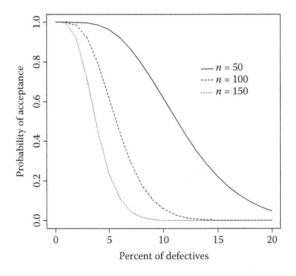

FIGURE 11.8
Operating characteristic curves of single sampling plans with $c = 5$ and $n = 50$, 100, and 150.

TABLE 11.3

Acceptance Probabilities of Three Sampling Plans

Quality Level	Sample Size (n)		
	50	100	150
1%	100%	100%	100%
5%	86%	29%	4.5%

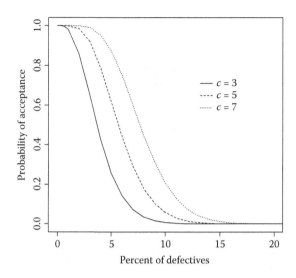

FIGURE 11.9
Operating characteristic curves of single sampling plans with $n = 100$ and $c = 3, 5,$ and 7.

It can be seen the acceptance probability decreases as c decreases, thus rendering more protection to the consumer's risk.

Designing an acceptance sampling plan is an iterative process involving trials and errors. A clear understanding on how the sample size and acceptance criterion impacts the acceptance probability provides guidance on the selection of the final sampling plan. For this purpose, the OC curve is a useful tool.

11.4.7 Double Sampling Plan

A double sampling plan is an extension of a single sampling plan. It allows disposition of a batch to be based on one or two samples. One advantage of such a plan is that a batch can be accepted or rejected with a small initial sample. This occurs more often when the batch is either extremely good or bad. Theoretically it can be shown that on the average a double sampling plan requires a smaller sample size while providing the same level of protection for the consumer's and producer's risks. It is particularly useful for raw materials and components of a product acceptance testing when the suppliers are known to have provided quality supplies. For example, some products are provided in prefilled syringe. Usually the syringes are sourced from other vendors. If the vendors historically provided high-quality syringes, use of double sampling plans could help the drug maker reduce overall inspection costs.

To demonstrate, consider the case where the quality attribute is an attribute variable. Figure 11.10 presents a flow chart for a double sampling plan for the attribute. Let Ac_i and Re_i be the batch acceptance and rejection thresholds for the ith stage of sampling ($i = 1$ and 2). The double sampling plan Ac_2 is chosen to be equal to Re_2 so that the decision concerning acceptance or rejection of the batch can be definitively made at the conclusion of the second acceptance testing. Let d_i denote the number of defectives in the ith sample ($i = 1$ and 2). According to the flow chart, an initial sample of size n_1 is taken and the batch is accepted (rejected) if $d_1 \le Ac_1$ ($d_1 \ge Re_1$). When $Ac_1 < d_1 < Re_1$, a second sample of size n_2 is taken. If the total number of defectives satisfies $d_1 + d_2 \le Ac_2$, the batch is accepted; otherwise, it is rejected.

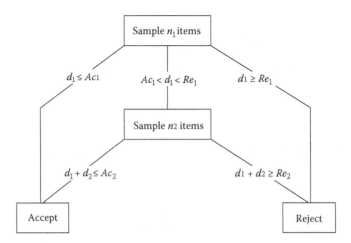

FIGURE 11.10
Procedure for double sampling.

Assuming the sample follows a binomial distribution B(p, N), where N and p are the batch size and the percent of defectives in the batch, respectively, it can be shown that the probability of acceptance is

$$P_a = P(x_1 \le Ac_1) + P(x_1 = Ac_1 + 1)P(x_2 = Ac_2 - x_1) + \ldots$$
$$+ P(x_1 = Re_1)P(x_2 \le Ac_2 - x_1)]$$
$$= \sum_{i=0}^{Ac_1} \binom{n_1}{i} p^i (1-p)^{n_1-i} + \sum_{j=Ac_1+1}^{Re_1} \binom{n_1}{j} p^j (1-p)^{n_1-j} \qquad (11.3)$$
$$\sum_{k=0}^{Ac_2-j} \binom{n_2}{k} p^k (1-p)^{n_2-k}$$

As an illustration, suppose an incoming batch of vials has size N = 200 and percent of defective p = 0.1. Suppose the decision rules of the double sampling plan consist of $n_1 = n_2 = 10$, $Ac_1 = 0$, $Ac_2 = 1$, $Re_1 = Re_2 = 2$. The probability of acceptance is

$$P_a = \binom{10}{0} 0.1^0 0.9^{10} + \binom{10}{1} 0.1^1 0.9^9 \times \binom{10}{0} 0.1^0 0.9^{10} = 0.48.$$

Double sampling plans also can be constructed when the acceptance/rejection decisions are made based on continuous variables. Several procedures have been developed. For detail, please refer to Schilling and Neubauder (2009) and Burdick and Ye (2017). Like single sampling, the OC of the sampling plan can be constructed using the above acceptance probability.

An important application of double sampling concerns out-of-specification (OOS) results, which may be observed during the production of the drug substance and drug product. They may also occur when conducting stability testing. Since OOS results may have a significant impact on data interpretation and product lot disposition, the FDA guidance recommends a step-wise approach to OOS investigation (FDA, 2006). It starts with an assessment of potential laboratory errors. A full-scale investigation is conducted if the initial laboratory assessment does not yield a root cause. As stated in the FDA guidance, "Part of the investigation may involve *retesting* a portion of the original sample. The sample used for the retesting should be taken from the same homogenous material that was originally collected from the lot, tested, and yielded the OOS results." Furthermore, additional tests based on resampling may be warranted. In this context, a double-sampling plan may be prespecified for OOS investigation.

11.5 Acceptance Sampling of Liquid Product

11.5.1 Prefiltration Bioburden Control

Sterile biological drug products (finished dosage forms) are usually manufactured by sterile filtration followed by aseptic processing. Critical for ensuring product quality and safety is the control of the microbial load, which is often referred to as prefiltration bioburden level, at the sterile filtration step. A high prefiltration bioburden level would have the potential to compromise the sterilizing filters, thus causing safety concerns. Both FDA (FDA, 1993, 1997, 2004) and EMA (EMA, 1996, 1997, 2001, 2006, 2012) regulatory guidelines require that a maximum acceptable bioburden level be specified at the point immediately prior to the sterile filtration step. The EMA guideline further states that a bioburden limit of no more than ten colony-forming units (CFU) per 100 mL will be considered acceptable in most situations while sample volume of less than 100 mL may be tested if justified. The primary purpose of the prefiltration bioburden test is to reject drug solution with undesirably high bioburden before the final sterilizing filtration.

Ideally, multiple samples may be taken from a batch of solution and tested according to prespecified acceptance sampling plan. However, for biological products, particularly a for clinical products and products produced in small lot sizes, a sample volume of 100 mL can represent a significant proportion of the batch and a high cost. In general, a single with lower sample volume (~10 mL) would be preferable. However, it is understood that this single sample testing plan is not adequate to provide safety assurance. The residual uncertainty of a solution that passes the prefiltration sampling test is removed through the sterilizing filtration step. A risk-based approach was suggested by Yang, Li, and Chang (2013), based on understanding the factors that impact both prefiltration risk, which is defined as the probability of accepting a batch of drug substance for the final filtration when it has an undesirable level of bioburden, and postfiltration risk, which is the probability of having bioburden break through the sterilizing filter.

Let X be the viral count in a test sample drawn from drug solution under evaluation, AL the bioburden acceptance limit, and D the bioburden concentration of the drug substance. The prefiltration can be quantified as

$$R_{Pre} = \Pr\left[X \leq AL | D\right] \tag{11.4}$$

while the postfiltration risk can be readily calculated by

$$R_{Post} = \Pr\left[Y \geq 1 | X \leq AL\right]. \tag{11.5}$$

where Y is the number of CFUs in the final filtrated solution.

11.5.2 Performance of Prefiltration Test Procedures

Typically bioburden is described through a Poisson distribution. However, this model requires that the bacteria are distributed uniformly throughout the bulk volume, which in reality is seldom true. The phenomenon that variability in the observed number of bacteria from a given sample is larger than that under the Poisson assumption is called *overdispersion* and can be modeled using a negative binomial distribution. For the purpose of illustration, we assume that the bioburden concentration in the drug solution follows a negative binomial distribution with a variance twice as large as its mean. The acceptance probability based on testing a single sample is given by

$$P_a = \sum_{xi=0}^{AL} g\left(x|\lambda, 1/\lambda\right) \tag{11.6}$$

where $g\left(x|\lambda, 1/\lambda\right) = \dfrac{\Gamma(\lambda+x)}{x!\Gamma(\lambda)2^{\lambda+x}}$ is the density function of the negative binomial distribution with its mean twice as large as the variance, where λ is the unknown mean bioburden concentration in the drug solution. A plot of the acceptance probability against various values of λ is given in Figure 11.11, based on the acceptance limit of AL = 10 CFU/100 mL.

From the OC curve, the acceptance probabilities when the true bioburden concentration is at 10 CFU/100 mL and 24 CFU/100 mL are 58.8% and 1%, respectively. An acceptance sampling plan can be developed. For example, the following procedure may be used: (1) Take a sample of volume 100 mL, (2) determine the bioburden concentration, and (3) accept the batch if the bioburden concentration in the sample is no more than 10 CFU. According to the OC curve, if there CFU concentration of the drug solution is more than 24 CFU/100 mL, there is more than 99% probability that the batch would be rejected.

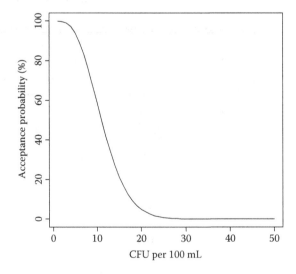

FIGURE 11.11
OC curve of single testing of a prefiltration sample based on a negative binomial distribution with overdispersion parameter = 2 and an acceptance limit of AL = 10 CFU/100 mL.

11.5.3 Risk Mitigation through Sterile Filtration

After a batch of drug solution passes the acceptance testing described previously, there is high confidence that the bioburden concentration is no more than the acceptance level, say, 24 CFU/100 mL. Since the product needs to be sterile, a filtration step which utilizes sterilizing filters to remove the bioburden in the drug solution is employed. As required by regulatory guidance, these filters should be demonstrated to reproducibly remove microorganisms from a carrier solution containing a high concentration of at least 10^7 CFU per cm². The validation is carried out under the worst-case production conditions and should result in no passage of the microorganisms used in the studies. Based on the above observations, the postfiltration risk probability of having one CFU in the final filtered solution can be calculated (Yang et al., 2013) as

$$R_{post} = \Pr\left[Y \geq 1 | X \leq AL\right]$$
$$= 1 - (1 - p_0)^{(S-V) \times D}$$

(11.7)

where Y is the total number of CFUs in the drug solution after the final filtration, which is assumed to follow a binomial distribution $b[(S - V) \times D, p_0]$, with S, V, D, and $(S - V) \times D$ being the batch size of the unfiltered drug solution, volume of the sample for the prefiltration bioburden testing, CFU concentration of the number of CFUs in the drug solution that passes the filtration test, and the total number of CFUs in the unfiltered drug solution. The parameter p_0 is the probability for a CFU to penetrate the sterilizing filter.

Although the parameter is p_0 unknown, an upper $100 \times (1 - \alpha)\%$ confidence limit for p_0 was derived by Yang, Li, and Chang (2013). Let N be the total number of CFUs used in the filter validation study, and n_1 be the number of CFUs that penetrate the filter. Because the FDA guidance requires that a challenge concentration of at least 10^7 CFU/cm² be used, resulting in no passage of the challenge microorganism, we have

$$N \geq A \times 10^7 \text{ and } 100 \times (1 - \alpha)\%$$

(11.8)

where A is the area of the filter (cm²). As a result, a one-sided upper $100 \times (1 - \alpha)\%$ exact confidence limit for p_0 can be constructed, using the Clopper–Pearson method (1934):

$$p_0 \leq 1 - \left[1 - \frac{N - n_1}{(n_1 + 1)F\left[\alpha, 2(,(n_1 + 1), 2(N - n_1)\right]}\right]^{-1} = \frac{F(\alpha, 2, N)}{N + F(\alpha, 2, N)}$$

(11.9)

where $F(\alpha, 2, N)$ is the $100 \times (1 - \alpha)^{th}$ percentile of an F distribution with degrees of freedom of 2 and N.

Since the FDA guidance requires that a challenge concentration of at least 10^7 CFU/cm² be used, $N = A \times RC \geq A \times 10^7$ with RC and A being the retention capability and the effective filter area of the sterilizing filter, respectively. Combining Equations 11.7 and 11.9, a one-sided $100 \times (1 - \alpha)\%$ upper limit on the probability of post-filtration bioburden risk is

$$R_{post} \leq 1 - \left[1 - \frac{F(\alpha, 2, N)}{N + F(\alpha, 2, N)}\right]^{(S-V) \times D}$$

(11.10)

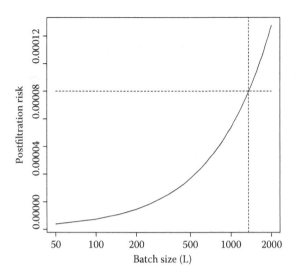

FIGURE 11.12
Plot of upper bound of postfiltration risk again batch size. The dashed line corresponds to risk of 10^{-4} with the corresponding batch size being 1336 L.

It is apparent that postfiltration bioburden risk is dependent on both the sterilizing filter efficiency and the unfiltered drug solution batch size. A plot of the upper bound of postfiltration risk is presented in Figure 11.12. The plot is constructed based on the filter retention efficiency of 10^7 CUF/cm^2 and filter size of 1000 cm^2. As the batch size increases, the risk also increases. If the tolerance of the postfiltration risk is 10^{-4}, from the plot it can be determined that the maximum batch size is 1336 L. Therefore, controlling batch size can help mitigate postfiltration.

11.6 Sampling for Stability Testing

Stability studies play a critical role at every stage of a drug product life cycle. Data from stability studies can be used for (1) development of drug formulation; (2) establishment of the shelf life, storage conditions, and release limit of the product; (3) demonstration of comparability after a manufacturing process. An important aspect of stability study design is to select sampling time points. Since stability studies are costly and time-consuming, appropriate selection of the sampling points can greatly help save resources. Consider an example that assumes a linear model between the potency of a vaccine product and time:

$$y_i = \beta_0 + \beta_1 x_i + \varepsilon_i \tag{11.11}$$

where y_i are potency values measured at times x_i, $i = 1,\ldots, n$, β_0 and $\beta_1(<0)$ are the intercept and degradation slope parameters, and ε_i are measurement errors which are assumed to be independently and identically distributed (*iid*) according to a normal distribution $N(0, \sigma^2)$. The slope estimate $\hat{\beta}_1$ follows a normal distribution with mean β and standard deviation

$$\sigma / S_{xx} \tag{11.12}$$

with $S_{xx} = \sum_{i=1}^{n}(x_i - \bar{x})^2$ and $\bar{x} = \dfrac{1}{n}\sum_{i=1}^{n}x_i$. One criterion that can be used to select design is to collect samples at $X_0 = (x_1,\ldots,x_n)^T$ such that the precision of the degradation slope estimate given in (11.11) is minimized. This is equivalent to maximize the quantity $S_{xx} = \sum_{i=1}^{n}(x_i - \bar{x})^2$.

Since either per regulatory requirements or out of logistic concerns, all sampling points are chosen as whole numbers, the optimization can be achieved through enumeration of S_{xx} over a discrete grid of values of x_i values. To demonstrate, assume that the study is an accelerated stability study with testing done at times, 0, x_2, x_3, and 6 months with x_2 and x_3 being integers satisfying $0 < x_2 \le x_3 < 6$. There are 20 pairs of (x_2, x_3), which satisfy the above constraints. Through enumeration, it can be shown that S_{xx} achieves its maximum 70.65 when $x_2 = 1$ and $x_3 = 5$.

When the stability study involves multiple batches, Murphy (1996) suggested a moment measure:

$$M = \sum_{i,j}(x_{ij} - \bar{x})^2 \tag{11.13}$$

where x_{ij} is the jth time point of the ith batch.

In addition, several other matrices, including D-efficiency, uncertainty, G-efficiency (Murphy, 1996), and statistical power (Nordbrock, 1992) were also proposed. The method based on statistical power calculation is particularly useful for selecting an optimal stability design for a comparability study. For example, assume that stability data are collected at the same time points $X_0 = (x_1,\ldots,x_n)^T$ before and after a process change. The statistical power for detecting a significant difference δ between the degradation slopes before and after the change is given by

$$\text{Power} = 1 - \Phi\left(z_{1-\alpha/2} - \frac{\delta}{\sqrt{2}\sigma}\sqrt{S_{xx}} \right) + \Phi\left(-z_{1-\alpha/2} - \frac{\delta}{\sqrt{2}\sigma}\sqrt{S_{xx}} \right) \tag{11.14}$$

where Φ and $z_{1-\alpha/2}$ are the cumulative probability function and $100 \times (1 - \alpha)^{th}$ percentile of the standard normal distribution.

The optimal design is the one that maximizes the above power. Using the above example, and assuming $\alpha = 0.05$, $\delta = 0.25$ and $\sigma = 1$, it can be shown that the maximum power is obtained when the sampling time points $X_0 = (0, x_2, x_3, 6)^T = (0, 1, 5, 6)^T$, which is the same as the previous example.

11.7 Sampling and Environmental Monitoring

Production of sterile products requires strict controls for the manufacturing environment to ensure sterility. Regulatory guidance (FDA, 2004) stipulates that all unit operations of aseptic processing mush be designed, monitored, and controlled for bioburden. These may include sterile filtration as discussed in Section 11.6, rigorous control of air flow and direction, surface areas that the product contacts, sterilization of equipment and containers, and training of manufacturing personnel to follow standard operating procedure (Henson, 2013). However, despite these efforts, opportunistic contaminations are unavoidable. Therefore it is necessary to establish an environmental monitoring (EM) program. Several sampling concerns exist for EM program, including sampling locations, timing, and frequency testing. The primary objective of collecting EM data is to set up alert and action limits. For this purpose, it is important to apply appropriate statistical methods that account for the non-normal nature of the data and heterogeneity.

11.7.1 Sampling Site, Timing, and Frequency

International Organization for Standardization (ISO) 14644-1 (ISO, 2015) recommends a method to determine the number of sampling sites for clean room qualification study. Specifically the number of sites is determined as

$$n = \sqrt{A} \tag{11.15}$$

where A is the area of the room in square meters when the sterile product is produced.

The clean room is validated if there are no negative findings from testing samples from the n selected sites. Figure 11.13 depicts the acceptance probability of this sampling plan based on a clean room of a total area of 1200 m^2.

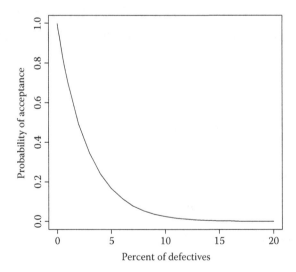

FIGURE 11.13
OC curve of acceptance sampling plan with a sample size equal to the square root of the room area, 1200 m^2.

From the plot, the percent of defectives or average quality level corresponding to $P_a = 95\%$ is 0.8%. Therefore the plan appears reasonable. The plan also makes intuitive sense if one likens the validation of the clean room to performing an acceptance testing of a batch of size A, accepting the batch if there is no defectives identified after testing $n = \sqrt{A}$ items. After the number of sites is determined, there is a need to identify sampling sites. Several general recommendations are provided in various regulatory guidelines. For example, FDA guidance on aseptic processing states that

> It is important that locations posing the most microbiological risk to the product be a key part of the program. It is especially important to monitor the microbiological quality of the critical area to determine whether or not aseptic conditions are maintained during filling and closing activities. Air and surface samples should be taken at the locations where significant activity or product exposure occurs during production. Critical surfaces that come in contact with the sterile product should remain sterile throughout an operation. When identifying critical sites to be sampled, consideration should be given to the points of contamination risk in a process, including factors such as difficulty of setup, length of processing time, and impact of interventions.

Considerations should be also given to timing of sampling, which specifies when the sample is taken—during or at the end of manufacturing operation. At minimum, duplicate samples need to be taken at each site. This allows for use of statistical models that account for intrasample variability when setting up alert and action limits.

11.7.2 Alert and Action Limits

A key component of an EM program is to set the alert and action limits based on facility quantification data. Alert limit is a microbial level, and when exceeded, is indicative of a possible drift of a process or system from its normal operation condition; whereas an action limit is a threshold that when exceeded indicates a process or system has drifted from its normal operation range. Setting robust alert and action limits depends not only on data that reflect the state of the manufacturing environment but also statistical methods that take into account the distribution of the data, and various sources of variations that affect the distribution of the data. Common statistical models for setting alert and action limit include: (1) Normal distribution, (2) Poisson, (3) negative binomial, (4) hierarchical model, (5) zero-inflated Poisson or binomial model, and (6) nonparametric methods. When data are normally distributed, the alert and action limits can be estimated as $\bar{X} \pm 2\hat{\sigma}$ and $\bar{X} \pm 3\hat{\sigma}$, respectively, where $\bar{X}$ and $\hat{\sigma}$ are sample mean and standard deviation. When the normality assumption does not hold, serval parametric and nonparametric methods can be explored and used. For instance, the negative binomial and hierarchical models are particularly useful to account for variations both within and between sampling location. For clean room monitoring, as microbial excursions are rare, data often contain excess of zeros. Under such circumstances, a zero-inflated negative binomial model may be more appropriate to use.

Yang (2017) provides a systematic review of current statistical methods and suggests a procedure that can be used for determining data distribution and an appropriate model for estimating alert and action limits. Through a simulation study, Yang, Zhao et al. (2013) demonstrated the zero-inflated negative binomial model shows a superior performance in setting alert and action limits when compared to other methods.

11.8 Concluding Remarks

Sampling plays an important role in ensuring product quality and quality system effectiveness. An effective sampling plan is developed based on many considerations, including the consumer's and producer's risk, quality systems of vendors, and manufacturing history. Although traditionally acceptance sampling is in general used for disposing a batch of raw materials, intermediate, or finished product, it has been increasingly utilized for selection of optimal stability study design, establishment of an effective and comprehensive environmental monitoring program, and assessment of quality systems of aseptic product manufacturing. Perhaps more importantly, sampling needs to be coupled with other quality strategies to achieve cGMP compliance.

References

Burdick, R.K. and Ye, F. (2017). Acceptance sampling, in *Nonclinical Statistics for Pharmaceutical and Biotechnology Industries*, ed. L. Zhang. Springer.

Clopper, C.J. and Pearson, E.S. (1934). The use of confidence or fiducial limits illustrated in the case of the binomial. *Biometrika*, 26(4), 404–413.

EMA. (1996). CPMP note for guidance on manufacture of finished dosage form.

EMA. (1997). ICH Topic Q5A (R1) Quality of biotechnological products: Viral safety evaluation of biotechnology products derived from cell lines of human or animal origin. *CPMP/ICH/295/95*. Canary Wharf, London. Accessed April 17, 2016, from http://www.ema.europa.eu/docs/en _GB/document_library/Scientific_guideline/2009/09/WC500002801.pdf.

EMA. (2001). Note for guidance on plasma-derived medicinal products.

EMA. (2006). Guideline on virus safety evaluation of biotechnological investigational medicinal products.

EMA. (2012). Guideline on the requirements for quality documentation concerning biological investigational medicinal products in clinical trials.

FDA. (1993). Points to consider in the characterization of cell lines used to produce biologicals. Bethesda, MD.

FDA. (1995). Current good manufacturing practice in manufacturing, processing, packing, or holding of drug: Amendment of certain requirements for finished pharmaceuticals. *Federal Registry*, 60 (13), 4087–4091.

FDA. (1997). Points to consider in the manufacture and testing of monocloncal antibody products for human use.

FDA. (2003). Prescribing information for FluMist® Quadrivalent. Accessed August 18, 2017, from https://www.fda.gov/downloads/BiologicsBloodVaccines/Vaccines/ApprovedProducts /ucm294307.pdf.

FDA. (2004). FDA guidance for industry: Sterile drug products produced by aseptic processing— Current good manufacturing practice. Accessed from https://www.fda.gov/ohrms/dockets /dockets/05d0047/05d-0047-bkg0001-Tab-09-GDL-vol2.pdf.

FDA. (2006). Guidance for industry investigating out-of-specification (OOS) test results for pharmaceutical production. Accessed August 18, 2017 from https://www.fda.gov/downloads/drugs /guidances/ucm070287.pdf.

Henson, E. (2013). A pocket guide to cGMP sampling: The basics. Accessed August 18, 2017, from http://www.ivtnetwork.com/article/pocket-guide-cgmp-sampling.

International Organization for Standardization. (2015). Cleanrooms and associated controlled environments—Part 1: Classification of air cleanliness by particle concentration. Accessed July 15, 2017 from https://www.iso.org/standard/53394.html.

Murphy, J.R. (1996). Uniform matrix stability study designs. *Journal of Biopharmaceutical Statistics*, 6, 477–494.

Nordbrock, E. (1992). Statistical comparison of stability designs. *Journal of Biopharmaceutical Statistics*, 2, 91–113.

Schilling, E.G. and Neubauer, D.V. (2009). *Acceptance Sampling in Quality Control.* 2nd ed. CRC Press.

World Health Organization (2005). WHO guidelines for sampling of pharmaceutical products and related materials. WHO Technical Report Series, No. 929. Accessed August 18, 2017, from http://www.who.int/medicines/areas/quality_safety/quality_assurance/GuidelinesSamplingPharmProductsTRS929Annex4.pdf?ua=1.

Yang, H. (2017). *Emerging Non-Clinical Biostatistics for Biopharmaceutical Development and Manufacturing.* Chapman & Hall/CRC Press.

Yang, H. and Carlin, D. (2001). *Acceptance Sampling Plan by Attributes in Applied Statistics in the Pharmaceutical Industry*, ed. S. Millard and A. Krause, pp. 475–502. Springer-Verlag.

Yang, H., Li, N., and Chang, S. (2013). A risk-based approach to setting sterile filtration bioburden limits. *PDA Journal of Pharm. Science and Technology*, 67, 601–609.

Yang, H., Zhao, W., O'Day, T., and Fleming, W. (2013). Environmental monitoring: setting alert and action limits based on a zero-inflated model. *PDA Journal of Pharm. Science and Technology*, 67(1), 1–9.

Index

Page numbers followed by f and t indicate figures and tables, respectively.

Printed in the United States
by Baker & Taylor Publisher Services